Human Health: Nutrition and Pharmacology

Human Health: Nutrition and Pharmacology

Editor: Christopher Herald

AMERICAN
MEDICAL PUBLISHERS
www.americanmedicalpublishers.com

AMERICAN
MEDICAL PUBLISHERS
www.americanmedicalpublishers.com

Cataloging-in-publication Data

Human health : nutrition and pharmacology / edited by Christopher Herald.
p. cm.
Includes bibliographical references and index.
ISBN 979-8-88740-191-1
1. Clinical pharmacology. 2. Health. 3. Nutrition. 4. Clinical medicine. I. Herald, Christopher.
RM301.28 .H86 2023
615.1--dc23

American Medical Publishers,
41 Flatbush Avenue,
1st Floor, New York,
NY 11217, USA

ISBN 979-8-88740-191-1 (Hardback)

Contents

Preface

The main aim of this book is to educate learners and enhance their research focus by presenting diverse topics covering this vast field. This is an advanced book which compiles significant studies by distinguished experts in the area of analysis. This book addresses successive solutions to the challenges arising in the area of application, along with it; the book provides scope for future developments.

Human health refers to the total state of social, physical as well as mental well-being rather than just the absence of illness, infirmity or disease. Nutrients are components found in food that drive biological activity and are therefore necessary for human health. Good nutrition is required for a person to develop physically and maintain proper health. Nutrients can be classified as carbohydrates, proteins, minerals, lipids as well as vitamins, which are helpful in performing essential functions of the body. They are helpful in growth and maintenance of body parts like teeth, bone and muscle, as well as the generation of energy. Eating a range of foods including grains, fruits, vegetables and wild foods like berries and fish are essential for maintaining good health. This book explores all the important aspects of pharmacology and nutrition in the modern day. It aims to shed light on the role of nutrition and pharmacology in human health. Researchers and students in this field will be assisted by this book.

It was a great honour to edit this book, though there were challenges, as it involved a lot of communication and networking between me and the editorial team. However, the end result was this all-inclusive book covering diverse themes in the field.

Finally, it is important to acknowledge the efforts of the contributors for their excellent chapters, through which a wide variety of issues have been addressed. I would also like to thank my colleagues for their valuable feedback during the making of this book.

Editor

1

Metabolism Changes as Indicated by the Erythrocytes of Patients with Alzheimer's Disease

Erland Johansson, Tuomas Westermarck,
Paul Ek and Faik Atroshi

1. Introduction

The aging processes proceed in small steps making it difficult to separate aging symptoms from early pathological processes. Cell metabolism involves metal ions and trace elements together with compounds necessary for optimal function. In case of imbalance in cells both compounds and distribution of metal ions may be changed but the change of metal ions and trace elements may probably be easier to identify than the large quantity of metabolized compounds. In cells there are distributions of elements, an elemental profile, indicating normal metabolism. Brain has a high demand of oxygen supply and need optimal supply of protection of reactive products. The erythrocytes pass brain many times and other organs accumulating information of elements during their way. We have chosen erythrocytes because oxygen dependent cells need regular supply of oxygen for a stable metabolism. Erythrocytes collect information for about 120 days and then will be replaced by new cells. Elemental profiles of erythrocytes reflect information in their own metabolism (limited metabolism) but may also give important information from other cells by deviations in the homeostasis, the element profile. For monitoring elemental profiles of the erythrocytes we have used inductively coupled plasma mass spectrometry (ICP-MS) which is selective, sensitive and allow analysis of elements in low concentration in a short time.

2. Material and methods

2.1. Patients

Thirteen diagnosed Alzheimer patients, 9 men and 4 women (mean age 61 y) and age matched controls (mean age 58 y) were selected for the study living in the same area. All patients participated voluntarily according to Helsinki declaration.

2.2. Samples

Whole blood (2x7 ml) was drawn into Vacutainer tubes for trace element analysis (BDH, with sodium heparin as anticoagulant). Centrifugation was started half an hour after venopuncture. The erythrocytes were separated by centrifugation at 120xg at 4 C for 15 minutes. After removing the buffy coat the erythrocytes were washed twice with 0.9 % NaCl at 1000xg for 5 minutes. The erythrocytes were transferred to cryo vials (Nunc) weighed and freezed at-18 C. The samples (0.6-0.8g, wet weight) were digested with nitric acid and hydrogen peroxide (both ultra pure) in microwave oven. The samples were diluted with Milli-Q water in 25 ml polypropylene bottles.

2.3. ICP-MS instrumentation

For the elemental analysis of the erythrocytes ICP-MS, Elan 6100 DRC was used in peak hopping mode. The isotopes monitored: ^{107}Ag, ^{114}Cd, ^{208}Pb and ^{238}U. Integration time: 5 sweep, 100 msek. Internal standard 10 ppb Rh was supplied by externally feeding. ^{114}Cd was corrected for ^{114}Sn. The analytical technique used is described in more details [1, 2, 3].

2.4. Reagents and standards

Ultra pure nitric acid and hydrogen peroxide was obtained from Merck. ICP-MS standards were obtained from Johnson & Matthey, SRM 1566a and 1577a from NIST. The different isotopes were validated against Oyster tissue 1566a, Bovine liver 1577a.

The estimated accumulated mean error in the analysis of samples was ± 10 % or less generated in the sampling procedure, preparation, digestion, volumetric and weighing errors and error in the ICP-MS analysis. For statistical calculations of ICP-MS results Wilcoxon's nonparametric test was used.

3. Results

3.1. Elemental profiles of erythrocytes

The main transport of erythrocytes is oxygen from the lungs to cells and carbon dioxide back to lungs serving different organs including brain. The elemental profile of the erythrocytes reflect metabolism of oxygen supplied cells but also the metabolism of the erythrocyte itself.

As erythrocytes carry ferro ions in hemoglobin and other divalent elements e.g. zinc, magnesium, calcium they will also reflect external influence of metabolism. The elemental profile of erythrocytes will be a status report of cell metabolism translated in terms of metal ions and trace elements. In this study we report accumulated ions: silver, cadmium, lead and uranium in the erythrocytes of patients with Alzheimer's disease. The concentration of lead (wet weight) in the erythrocytes of patients with Alzheimer's disease is demonstrated in Figure 1. The result of cadmium analysis (wet weight) of the erythrocytes is shown in Figure 2. The concentration of silver in the erythrocytes is indicated in Figure 3. The concentration of uranium in the erythrocytes was significant higher that of controls Figure 4. In summary the concentrations of Pb, Cd, Ag and U were significant higher than those of controls.

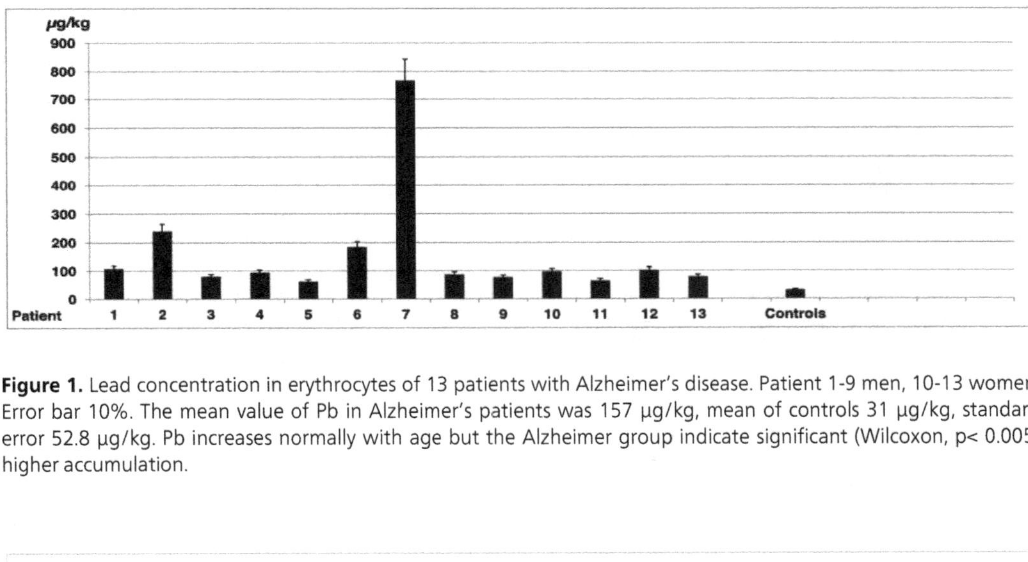

Figure 1. Lead concentration in erythrocytes of 13 patients with Alzheimer's disease. Patient 1-9 men, 10-13 women. Error bar 10%. The mean value of Pb in Alzheimer's patients was 157 μg/kg, mean of controls 31 μg/kg, standard error 52.8 μg/kg. Pb increases normally with age but the Alzheimer group indicate significant (Wilcoxon, $p < 0.005$) higher accumulation.

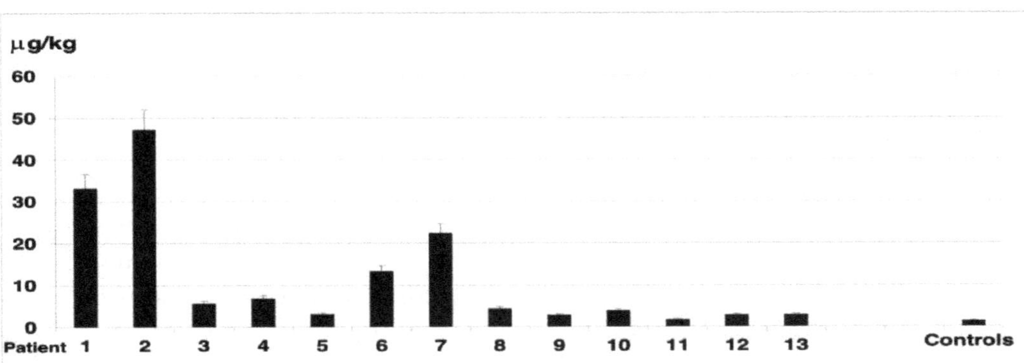

Figure 2. Distribution of cadmium in erythrocytes of 13 patients with Alzheimer's disease. Patient 1-9 men, 10-13 women. Error bar 10%. The mean value of Cd in Alzheimer's patients was 11.5 μg/kg, standard error 3.9 μg/kg, mean of controls 1.3 μg/kg, The concentration of Cd in the erythrocytes of patients with Alzheimer's disease was significant higher (Wilcoxon, $p < 0.05$) than that of controls.

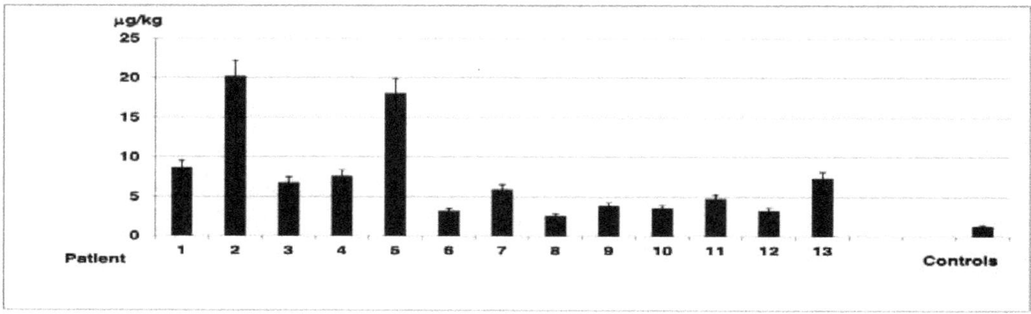

Figure 3. Distribution of silver in erythrocytes of 13 patients with Alzheimer's disease. Patient 1-9 men, 10-13 women. Error bar 10%. The mean value of Ag in Alzheimer's patients was 7.4 µg/kg, standard error 1.5 µg/kg, mean of controls 1.3 µg/kg, The concentration of silver in the erythrocytes of patients was significant higher (Wilcoxon, $p< 0.005$) than that of controls.

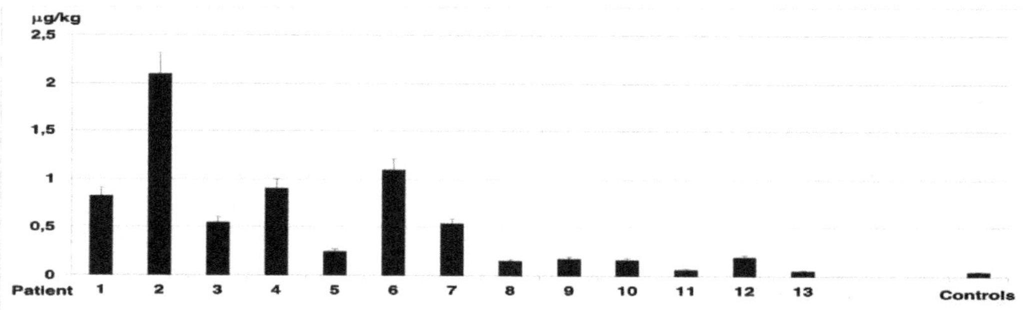

Figure 4. Concentration of uranium in erythrocytes of 13 patients with Alzheimers disease. Patient 1-9 men, 10-13 women. Error bar 10 %. The mean value of U in Alzheimer's patients was 0.55 µg/kg, standard error 0.16 µg/kg, mean of controls 0.11 µg/kg, The concentration of uranium in the erythrocytes of patients with Alzheimer's disease was significant higher (Wilcoxon, $p<0.01$) than that of controls

4. Discussion

Brain has low storing capacity of oxygen though it is a demanding consumer: brain uses about 20 % of oxygen total supply. In degenerative diseases like Alzheimer's, Parkinson's disease the etiology often are not fully known. In Alzheimer's disease pathophysiological theories have been proposed e.g. heat shock protein interactions [4], Tau-protein abnormality [5] neuroinflamation and neuronal loss [6, 7], β-amyloid interactions [8], mitochondrial misfunction [9]. An overlooked possibility may be using ICP-MS for analysis of elemental profiles of erythrocytes as biomarker for Alzheimer 's disease. Small changes in metabolism of oxygen dependent cells may give symptoms difficult to identify due to lack of suitable biomarkers [10, 11, 12. 13, 14]. Erythrocytes carrying excess lead, cadmium, silver and uranium ions may induce damages in cells including brain cells. Accumulation of elements in the human erythrocytes are a result of low exposure and not of a sudden insult which calls for sensitive biomarkers.

4.1. Effects of accumulated lead, cadmium, silver and uranium in the erythrocytes

At present there is lack of methods to describe the accumulated effects of metal ions in erythrocytes in terms of stability constants or conditional constants. There is lacking information of e.g. solvent properties, pH, temperature, redox properties, lack of knowledge of interacting compounds. Elemental profiles of erythrocytes may be an alternative to estimate changes of trace elements and metal ions at the cellular level. The discussion below will be focused on some effects on membrane integrity by lead, cadmium, silver and uranium because it is not fully known how these ions are associated to other compounds.

4.2. Initiation of eryptosis by accumulated lead, cadmium silver and uranium in erythrocytes

It has been suggested that mature erythrocytes may enter programmed death without the aid of caspase systems [15,16]. Heavy metal ions and organic compounds may be involved in early senescence [17, 18, 19]. When erythrocytes are growing old they will change gradually, fragments will be cleaned up [20, 21], mainly in spleen, liver, bone marrow by the macrophages. Most material of captured senescent erythrocytes e.g. iron and metabolized organic material will be reused [22, 23].

Silver, cadmium ions induce suicidal erythrocyte death [24, 25] and it is likely that erythrocytes and cells dependent on erythrocytes of patients with Alzheimer's disease with accumulated silver and also lead, cadmium and uranium may show early eryptosis. Eryptosis may also be initiated via formation of phosphatidylserine by lead, cadmium, hemin as stimulator [26, 27, 28].

4.3. Erythrocyte channels exposed to accumulated ions of lead, cadmium, silver and uranium

The accumulated lead, cadmium, silver and uranium may interfere the activity in the erythrocyte channels for cations, anions and water. Cadmium, lead, silver may interfere with potassium, calcium [29, 30] and other ions in erythrocyte membranes [31, 32]. Binding in vitro of cadmium to β-amyloid channels was reported by [33]. Exposure to accumulated lead, cadmium, silver, uranium ions to β-amyloid or other compounds is likely to support the pathophysiological process by association to available binding sites.

Anions e.g. chlorides, carbonates ions are transported in anion channels [34, 35, 36] may react with silver, lead, cadmium and uranium disturbing channel transport and oxygen handling.

Aquaporin channels in the erythrocyte membrane are important for flow of water and shape [37, 38, 39]. Accumulated cadmium, lead, silver, uranium ions associated to erythrocyte aquaporin channels may decrease the capacity to shrink and expand. Water exchange may also be important for osmotic regulation when the erythrocytes enter capillaries. It cannot be excluded that lead, cadmium, silver, uranium may release important elements. e.g. calcium from their association sites. Released calcium may form non-selective channels in membranes [40].

4.4. Accumulated cadmium, lead, silver and uranium ions may compete with essential elements in carrier systems

Cadmium is known to compete with zinc in e.g. metallothionein (MT), carrier of zinc. Metal ions having higher affinity than zinc may interact with the binding sites in MT or other carrier. Lead and uranium ions is known to compete with calcium metabolism. Magnesium and calcium ions in calmodulin (calcium carrier) may be displaced by accumulated lead, cadmium, silver, uranium ions and release essential elements e.g. Mg, Ca, Zn. Release of secondary messenger e.g. Mg may disturb ATP metabolism, Ca may activate translocases flippases, floppases, scramblases and start apoptosis signals. Ca may also activate platelets and make them sticky, ready for clot. Sticky platelets may associate to proteins and form placks.

4.5. Sources of cadmium, lead, silver and uranium — Food and implants

The food intake is not known for individual patients. In Finland cadmium uptake from food is about 5-10 μg/day, lead 20-66 μg /day, uranium and, silver was not mentioned [41]. In Sweden is reported cadmium uptake from wheat, rice, potatoes, root-crops 10-20 μg /day, lead 15-30 μg /day, uranium 1-4 μg /day, silver not indicated [42]. Cd uptake from nutrition may disturb the heme synthesis. Cadmium rich diet in Nigeria decreased Hb and erythrocyte counts in mice [43]. It cannot be excluded that cadmium, lead, silver, uranium contaminated food may accumulate in human erythrocytes and in similar manner decrease erythrocyte counts and hemoglobin synthesis. Smoker may have higher cadmium values in blood but there was no information about smoking habits. Elevated uranium in drinking water may damage the kidneys and increase protein loss in urine [44, 45].

In Finland some districts have drinking water with high uranium concentrations (> 100 μg/L) which together with cadmium, lead and silver may increase kidney damage and disturb erythrocyte metabolism. Uranium in the drinking water may explain the significant elevated uranium concentrations of erythrocytes of Alzheimer patients.

Implants may be a source of metal ion supply. Amalgam is an alloy which is not stable [2, 3, 46, 47, 48] (release mercury, silver). Guttapercha may sometime contain cadmium [2] but the released amount is not known for the examined patients. Mercury was not analyzed as mercury will associate strong to liver, kidney also to pituary, low mercury will be found in blood. Mercury has also capacity to displace secondary messenger e.g. Mg, Ca, Zn, Fe when not properly associated.

4.6. Elemental profiles of erythrocytes as biomarkers of Alzheimer's disease by ICP-MS

The early diagnosis of a neurological disease like Alzheimer's and Parkinson's disease is difficult. In Parkinson's disease about 25 % of the patients may get wrong diagnosis [49]. The present study indicate that the elemental profile of erythrocytes may be used as a support in the diagnosis and pathophysiology of Alzheimer's disease. Changes in the elemental profile should be possible to identify earlier due to high sensitivity of ICP-MS. Monitoring elements in the erythrocytes may also be used to observe effects of applied pharmacy and effects on secondary messengers. More research is needed to interpret early symptoms of Alzheimer disease and pathophysiological processes.

5. Conclusions

Monitoring changes of elements in the erythrocytes by ICP-MS may be used as an early biomarker of Alzheimer's disease and may support the pharmaceutical treatment. The accumulated lead, cadmium, silver and uranium may interfere with channel activities, have effects on apoptosis, react with secondary messenger and support pathophysiological processes.

Acknowledgements

We thank Crafoord foundation for economic support and Åbo Academy for putting instrumental facilities to our disposal. We also thank dr Sture Brishammar, Evert Karlsson for discussions.

Author details

Erland Johansson[1*], Tuomas Westermarck[2], Paul Ek[3] and Faik Atroshi[4]

*Address all correspondence to: erland.johansson@uppsala.mail.telia.com

1 EJSelenium Consultant Ltd, Uppsala, Sweden

2 Rinnekoti Research Center, Helsinki, Finland

3 Laboratory of Analytical Chemistry, Åbo Academy, Finland

4 Department of Pharmacology and Toxicology, University of Helsinki, Finland

References

[1] Johansson E, Westermarck T, Hasan MY, Nilsson B et.al. Alterations in nickel and cadmium concentrations in erythrocytes and plasma of patients with Parkinson's disease. Trends in Biomedicine in Finland 2007; XXI 2(4),17-32.

[2] Johansson E and Liljefors T. Heavy elements in root tips from teeth with amalgam fillings: in TEMA 7 (ed. Momcilovic B), pp 11-18-11-20. Zagreb 1991.

[3] Johansson E, Liljefors T, Plantin L-O. Comparative ICP-MS estimation of elements using quantitative and conditional Saha factors: in Trace Element Analytical Chemistry in Medicine and Biology, vol.7. (eds. Brätter P, Ribas B, Schramel P) pp 141-146. Madrid 1995.

[4] Ji-Sook H. The Hsp90 chaperone machinery from structure to drug development BMB reports 2009;342(10), 623-630.

[5] Lee VM, Goedert M and Trojanowski JQ Neurodegenerative Taupathies Annu Rev Neurosci 2001; 24,1121-1159.

[6] Eikelenboom P, Verhuis R, Scheper W, Roozemuller AJ, van Gool WA et.al. The significance of neuroinflammation in understanding Alzheimer's disease J Neurol Transm 2006; 113(11), 1685-1695.

[7] Eikelenboom PR, van Exel E, Hoozemans JJM, Verhuis R, Roozemuller AJM et.al. Neuroinflammation, an early event in both the history and pathogenesis of Alzheimer's disease. Neurodegenerative disease 2010; 7(1-3), 38-41.

[8] Gharibyan A. Amyloids here, amyloids there.....whats wrong with them? PhD thesis. University of Umeå, Sweden, 2012.

[9] Hedskog L. Mitochondria in Alzheimer disease:regulatory mechanisms and cell-death. PhD thesis, Karolinska Institute, Stockholm, Sweden, 2012.

[10] Bosman GJ, Van der Linden PA, Bartholomeus IG. De Man A.J, De Grip WJ, Van Kalmthout PJ. Erythrocyte aging in the demented elderly: a fluctuating process? Mech Ageing Dev 1998;100(1), 53-58.

[11] Franco RS. The measurement and importance of red cell survival. Am J Haematol 2009;84, 109-114.

[12] Bosman GJ, Willekens FL, Werre JM. Erythrocyte aging: a more than superficial resemblance to apoptosis? Cell Physiol Biochem 2005; 16(1-3), 1-8.

[13] Huang Y-X, Wu Z-J, Marishi J, Huang B-T, Chen X-Y et.al. Human red blood cell aging: correlative changes in surface charge and cell properties J Cell Mol Med 2010; 15(12), 2634-2642.

[14] Daniels G. Structure and function of red cell surface antigens Science Series 2006;1, 3-8.

[15] Bratosin D, Estaquier J, Petit F, Arnoult D, Quatannens B et.al. Programmed cell death in mature erythrocytes: a model for investigating death effector pathways operating in the absence of mitochondria Cell Death Differ 2001; 8(12), 1143-1156.

[16] Lang F, Lang KS, Lang PA, Huber SM, Wieder T. Mechanisms and significance of eryptosis Antioxid Redox Signal 2006; 8(7-8), 1183-1192.

[17] Lang F, Gulbins E, Lang FA, Zappulla D, Föller M. Ceramide in suicidal death of erythrocytes Cell Physiol Biochem 2010;26(1), 21-28.

[18] Föller F, Bobbala D, Koka S, Huber SM, Lang F. Suicide for survival-death of infected erythrocytes as a host mechanisms to survive malaria Cell Physiol Biochem 2009; 24,133-140.

[19] Gatidis S, Fšller M, Lang F. Hemin-induced suicidal erythrocyte death Ann Hematol 2009; 88, 721-725.

[20] Ryter ST, Alami J, Choi AMK. Heme oxygenase-1/Carbon monoxide: from basic science to therapeutic applications Physiol Rev 2006; 86, 583-656.

[21] Koizumi S, Gong P, Suzuki K, Murata M. Cadmium responsive element of the human heme oxygenase-1 mediates heat shock dependent transcriptional activation J Biol Chem 2007:282(12), 8715-8723.

[22] Kay MMB. Mechanism of removal senescent cells by human macrophages in situ Proc Natl Acad Sci USA 1973;72(9), 3521-3525.

[23] Tenhunen R, Marver HS, Schmidt R The enzymatic conversion of heme to bilirubin by microsomal heme oxygenase Proc Natl Acad Sci USA 1968; 61(2), 748-755.

[24] Sopjani M, Föller M, Haendeler J, Gštz F, Lang F. Silver ion-induced suicidal erythrocyte death J Appl Toxicol 2009;29(6), 531-536.

[25] Sopjani M, Fšller M, Dreischer P, Lang F. Stimulation of eryptosis by cadmium ions Cell Physiol Biochem 2008; 22(1-4), 245-252.

[26] Kempe SD, Lang PA, Eisele K., Klart BA., Wieder T., Huber SM. Stimulation of erythrocyte phosphatidylserine exposure by lead ions. Am.J.Physiol Cell Physiol 2005;288(2), C396-C402.

[27] Nguyen DB. Phosphatidylserine exposure in red cells: a suggestion for the active role of red blood cells in blood clot formation PhD thesis. University of Saarland, Saarbrücken, Germany. 2010.

[28] Boas FL, Forman L, Beutler E. Phosphatidylserine exposure and red cell viability in red cell aging and in hemolytic anemia ProcNatl Acad Sci USA. 1998; 95, 3077-3081.

[29] Gardos G. The function of calcium in the permeability of human erythrocytes Biochem Biophys Acta 1958; 30, 653-654.

[30] Lijnen P, Staessen J, Fagard R. Amery A. Effect of cadmium on transmembrane Na+ and K+-transport systems in human erythrocytes Br J Ind Med 1991; 48, 392-398.

[31] Leinders T., van Kleef RGDM,Vijberberg HPM. Distinct metal ion binding sites on Ca2+activated K+channels in inside-out patches of human erythrocytes Biochem BiophysActa 1992; 11-12,75-82.

[32] Lang PA, Kaiser S, Mysaina S, Wieder T, Lang F, Huber SM. Ca2+ -activated K+-channels in human erythrocyte apoptosis. Am J Physiol.Cell Physiol 2003;285(6), C1553-C1560.

[33] Gabriella N, Enrico G, Silvia M, Daniela M. Effect of cadmium ions on amyloid beta peptide 1-42 channels activity J Environ Chem Ecotoxicol. 2011;. 3(12), 309-319.

[34] Akkaya C, Shumulina E, Bobballa D, Brand VB, Mahmud H et.al. The Plasmodium falciparum-induced anion channel of human erythrocytes is an ATP-release pathway Eur J Physiol 2009; 457,1035-1047.

[35] Yamaguchi T, Ikeda Y, Abe Y, Kuma H, Kang DM, Hamasaki N, Hirai T. Structure of the membrane domain of human erythrocyte anion exchanger-1 revealed by electron crystallography J Mol Biol 2010; 397(1), 179-189.

[36] Obaid AL and Crandall ED. HCO_3^- and Cl^-. Exchange across the human erythrocyte membrane: effects of pH and temperature J Membrane Biol 1979; 50, 23-41.

[37] Roudier N, Verhavatz J-M, Maurel C, Ripoche P, Tacnet F. Evidence for the presence of Aquaporin-3 in human red cells J Biol Chem 1998;273, 8407-8412.

[38] Murata K, Mitsuoka K, Walz T, Agre P, Heymann JB, Engel A, Fujiyoshi Y. Structural determinants of water permeation through aquaporin-1 Nature 2000; 407, 599-605.

[39] Bietz S, Montila I, Przyborski JM, Lingelbach K. Recruitment of human aquaporin 3 to internal membranes in the Plasmodium falciparum infectant erythrocyte Mol Biochem Parasitol 2009;167(19), 48-53.

[40] Mironova GD, Gateau-Rosch O, Levrat C, Gritsenko E, Pavlov E, Lazareva AV, Linarenko E, Rey C, Louisot P, Saris N-E. Palmitic and stearic acids bind Ca^{2+} with high affinity and form nonspecific channels in black-lipid membranes, possible relation to Ca^{2+} -activated mitochondrial pores. J Bioenergetics and Biomembranes; 2000; 33(4), 319-330.

[41] Varo P and Koivistonen P Mineral element composition of Finnish Foods in Acta Agr Scand. Suppl.22 (ed. Koivistonen P) pp165-171, Stockholm 1980.

[42] Bielak AT, Holmes J, SavgŒrd J, Schaefer KA Comparison of European and North American approaches to the management and communication of environmental research. Swedish Environmental Protection Agency Report 2009; 5958.

[43] Asagba SO and Eriyamremu GE. Oral cadmium exposure alters haematological and liver function parameters of rats fed a Nigerian-like diet J Nutr Environ Med 2007;16(3-4), 267-274.

[44] Kurttio P, Auvinen A, Salonen L, Saha H, Pekkanen J et.al. Renal effects of uranium in drinking water Environ Health Perspective 2002;110(4), 337-342.

[45] Karpas Z, Paz-Tao O, Lorber A, Komulainen H, Auvinen A. et.al. Urine, hair, and nails as indicators for ingestion of uranium in drinking water Health Phys 2005;88(3), 229-242.

[46] Johansson E. Selenium and its protection against the effects of mercury and silver J Trace Elem Electrolytes Health Dis 1991;5(4): 273-274.

[47] Johansson E. The biochemistry of selenium in humans. In: Palmieri Y(ed) Selenium-Tellurium Development Association, Brussels, pp 359-365, 1994.

[48] Johansson E. and Lindh U. Mercury in blood cells-altered elemental profiles Biol-Trace Elem Res 1987;12, 309-321.

[49] Holmberg B. The diagnostic challenge of Parkinsonian syndrome PhD thesis. University of Gothenborg, Sweden, 2000.

2

The Pharmacology and Biochemistry of Selenium in Cancer

T. Westermarck, Arno Latvus and Faik Atroshi

1. Introduction

Cancer is the leading cause of death in economically developed countries and the second leading cause of death in developing countries (WHO)[1]. It is extraordinarily complex with novel mutations and phenotypes that are often unique to an individual. It is a disease of the chromosomes and the problem is, in almost all cancers, it isn't just one mutation but may be much more. Cancer may be regarded as a complex metabolic deficiency disease [9, 10, 11, 12, 13, 14]

Cancer diet is also used as a complementary approach to cancer that involves the use of special nutritional supplements. Selenium (Se) and cancer is a term that can be referred to the approach or associations between cancer and nutrition that is to lower an individual's risk of cancer. Selenium was first recognized as having some nutritional importance almost six decades ago [15]. Selenium is found in food as selenoamino acids or selenoproteins, and as selenide, selenite, or selenate [16]. Selenium is a critical cofactor in the activity of gluthathione peroxidase and is also important in the management of peroxynitrite. The selenium content of food depends upon soil content and varies regionally and nationally, with soil levels relatively low in most European countries [17, 18, 19]. Soil conditions have been associated with clinical selenium toxicity in animals (selenosis) in some areas with very high selenium content, and with selenium deficiency syndromes in animals and humans in areas of low soil selenium [17].

Selenium is essential nutrient that act as cofactor in enzyme oxidation–reduction reactions (e.g. iodothyronine deiodinase and glutathione peroxidases) [20]. It maintains the specific configuration of proteins, is incorporated into the structure of hormones, and plays a structural and catalytic role in gene expression and transcriptional regulation. The trace element selenium is contained in soil and drinking water varies from area to area, which determines the variation in intake seen in different communities and the amount and chemistry of dietary constituents eaten with the this element affect the absorption efficiency of the selenium is said be 'the only trace element to be specified in the genetic code' [21].

Selenocysteine is a vital component of 35 or more selenoproteins, some of which are important enzymes [22]. Selenium functions as a redox centre, an example of which is the reduction of hydrogen peroxide and lipid and phospholipid hydroperoxides to nondamaging water and alcohols by the glutathione peroxidases [23]. Functions of this kind help maintain membrane integrity, and protect prostacyclin production. Prevention of the oxidative chain reactions in this way prevents further damage to lipids, lipoproteins, and DNA; hence its antioxidant function helps prevent atheroma and cancer, among other things [24, 25, 26].

2. Clinical applications

Selenium deficiency results in impaired immunity [27], and supplementation is immune stimulant. Deficiency increases the virulence of some viruses such as in Keshan disease [28, 29] by altering their genome to a more virulent one. Deficiency may also be associated with low mood [30], increased cognitive decline in older people, and susceptibility to epilepsy [31], exacerbates hypothyroidism in iodine deficiency [32], protective against cardiovascular disease and cancer [33, 34], beneficial in a variety of inflammatory conditions by reducing oxidative stress, and in male fertility [35] through testosterone synthesis and spermatozoa function.

The conventional cancer therapies currently available are surgery, radiotherapy, and chemotherapy. Chemotherapy is typically the main regimen for most cancers. However, many tumours develop resistance to these harsh drugs, known as chemo resistance, which can lead to other complications [36]. A number of natural products and compounds have been shown to act as effective chemo sensitizers. However, taking antioxidants during cancer treatment could interfere with the way chemotherapy work and diminish their benefits to the patient [37]. It was conclude that the use of supplemental antioxidants during chemotherapy and radiation therapy should be discouraged because of the possibility of tumour protection and reduced survival [37].This is because radiation and some chemotherapy agents work by generating free radicals, which then kill rapidly dividing cancer cells. Since antioxidants scavenge free radicals, they might interfere with the therapeutic effects of these treatments. However, oxidation supports the proliferation of malignant cells and may itself interfere with treatment [38]. People who hold this view maintain that antioxidants may counter the harmful effects of oxidation in the malignant process and thereby increase the effects of drugs or radiation therapy to the benefit of the patient. Moreover, they note that some evidence suggests that antioxidant supplements offer patients protection from the toxic effects of therapy [39].

The balance between oxidants and antioxidants can be a key issue in the development of cancer [40] and reactive oxygen species (ROS) are involved in aging, chronic illness, and cancer. Oxidants also cause free radical damage, thus the body generates large amounts of antioxidants to prevent harm and maintain health. However, Watson [41] reported that antioxidants can promote cancer growth of late stage metastatic cancers. The process is explained in terms of redox signalling, redox being a term used for reduction and oxidation. Healthy cells and also malignant ones benefit from intact Keapl/Nrf2 signalling, making a dysregulated hydroperoxide signaling a plausible explanation for the increased cancer risk in selenium deficiency [42]. Therefore, a research agenda to investigate the synergistic operation of such substances in cancer treatment is required.

3. Cancer and oxidation

Cancer is a generic term for a large group of diseases that can affect any part of the body and it can exist in many different forms and types, some of which are brought on by the destructive choices people make while others are less predictable and are not the result of destructive decisions. It can be broadly grouped into different types (Carcinomas, Sarcomas, Lymphomas and Leukaemia's), depending on which tissues they come from [43, 44]. Cancer develops when cells multiply in the presence of oxidation and other damage. According to micro-evolutionary models, cells become damaged and change their behaviour, growing uncontrollably, and act like the single-celled organisms from which they originally evolved. The cancer cells' individualism overwhelms the cooperative control processes that are essential to a complex multicellular organism [45, 46]. As cancers become malignant, they exhibit incredible genetic diversity. Whereas a benign tumour is like a colony of similar abnormal cells, a malignant tumour is a whole ecosystem. At this late stage, some (but not all) antioxidants can indeed promote cancer cell growth. Thousands of different cell types coexist: cooperating, competing, and struggling to survive. A consequence of the anaerobic conditions that prevail during the early development of a malignancy is that cancer cells differ from healthy cells, in that they have been selected for the way they generate energy (i.e. anaerobically, using glucose) [47, 48].

The sulfhydryl group is the most sensitive to the oxidizing effects of ROS among the amino acid side chains in protein; it is often involved in the intracellular transduction machinery of redox signals in response to physiological and oxidative stimuli. In fact, a variety of biological functions, not directly related to peroxidase activity, have also been reported for the Prx family [49]. Oxidative damage in DNA can cause cancer. Several antioxidant enzymes such as superoxide dismutase, catalase, glutathione peroxidase, glutathione reductase, glutathione S-transferase etc. protect DNA from oxidative stress. It has been proposed that polymorphisms in these enzymes are associated with DNA damage and subsequently the individual's risk of cancer susceptibility [50].

Nutrition and physical activity and major lifestyle changes can reduce the risk of cancer [51, 52]. Antioxidants are becoming an increasingly common choice as a hopeful cancer prevention agent. Importantly, antioxidants limit oxidative damage and thus inhibit early benign cancer growth, preventing cancer from developing. Selenium has received publicity over the past decades based on some confusing and contradictory research about whether low-selenium diets are implicated in cancer risk. To date, this is still a question without a clear answer. However, selenium is required for the proper activity of a group of enzymes collectively called glutathione peroxidase. Each of these enzymes helps to turn toxic hydrogen peroxide into harmless water. Of the eight known glutathione peroxidase enzymes, five of them require selenium. It is a necessary component for appropriate function of the immune system, muscle function, successful reproduction, and peak brain function. Also, selenium produces valuable antioxidant enzymes. Deficiencies in selenium have been linked to decreased thyroid function, cardiovascular disease, and cancers [24]. Research shows selenium, especially when used in conjunction with vitamin C, vitamin E and beta-carotene, works to block chemical reactions that create free radicals in the body (which can damage DNA and cause degenerative change in cells, leading to cancer). Also research has demonstrated that selenium is also linked to reduction in risk to some carcinomas [6, 7].

4. Pathophysiology of cancer and causes

Cancer is a disease of regulation of tissue growth. In this disease, the cells of the body display uncontrolled growth, invasion that intrudes and destroys adjacent tissues and spreads to other body locations. In order for a normal cell to transform into a cancer cell, genes which regulate cell growth and differentiation must be altered and DNA repair genes are altered and turned off [53, 54]. The pathophysiology of cancer is a complicated issue. Genes that are influenced in the pathogenesis of cancer are proteins that are involved in a variety of processes including cell growth and differentiation, cell cycle processes, and angiogenesis, which is the formation of new blood vessels [55]. These proteins also play a role in tumour progression, immune regulation, and apoptosis. Since the cells involved are complex and have such a broad range of functions, the pathophysiology of cancer has been hard to determine precisely.

Understanding what causes cancer is a complex process. Cancer has been linked to many factors, such as environmental exposures, lifestyle practices, medical interventions, genetic traits, viruses, familial susceptibility, and aging. Cancer is most probably the result of interactions between repeated carcinogenic exposures and an individual's susceptibility status [56]. Environmental exposures and lifestyle practices have been determined to be the major risk factors in the development of cancer [57, 58]. The major lifestyle factors that contribute to cancer include smoking, alcohol, diet, medical practices, and ultraviolet exposures.

Genes that are influenced in the pathogenesis of lung cancer are proteins that are involved in a variety of processes including cell growth and differentiation, cell cycle processes, and angiogenesis, which is the formation of new blood vessels. The proteins also play a role in tumour progression, immune regulation, and apoptosis [59, 60]. Since the cells involved are complex and have such a broad range of functions, the pathophysiology of lung cancer has been hard to determine precisely. A healthy cell becomes a cancer cell by undergoing the following processes in which proto-oncogenes are changed to oncogenes. Proto-oncogenes are genes that are coded to maintain normal cell growth. In cases of a developing cancer, oncogene takes its place. Oncogene is a gene that makes cells grow and divide rapidly [61]. Pharmaceutical companies are continuing to develop approaches for targeting oncogene activity in the ongoing war on cancer [61]. Pathology of cancers and other complex disorders have undergone a big change after development of technologies like immunohistochemistry, flow cytometry, and molecular biologic approaches to cancer diagnosis. Cancer is not a singular, specific disease but a group of variable tissue responses that result in uncontrolled cell growth [56].

5. Selenium mechanism

The biochemistry of selenium differs from other dietary minerals and trace elements. Selenium is not a structural component nor a metal coordination complex and the biosynthesis of selenocysteine is regulated by four genes and begins with the aminoacylation of the amino acid serine by the enzyme serine synthetase to produce Ser-tRNASec [62, 63]. However, selenocysteine is the active site in which, at physiological pH, selenium is fully ionized and is a very efficient redox catalyst [64]. Selenium exists in elemental, organic, and inorganic forms, with four important oxidation states: selenide (Se 2−), elemental (Se0) selenite (Se+4), and selenate (Se+6) [62, 65]. Selenium compounds inhibit signaling enzymes such as protein kinase C (PKC) [66] that play crucial roles in tumor promotion. The selenium-containing nutrient, selenomethionine has been shown to regulate the tumor suppresser p53 by the redox factor refl-dependent redox mechanism. Studies continue to support evidence that one important pathway is that many selenium-containing nutrients can be converted in the body to methylselenol. Methylselenol has been shown to block expansion of pre-malignant cells forming into fully developed cancers [67]. Several pathways have been proposed that could explain how selenium-containing compounds could block mutated cells from progressing to cancer. Methylseleninic acid has been shown to inhibit NF-kappa B and regulate I kappa B in prostate cancer cells [68]. Selenium compounds inhibit signaling enzymes such as protein kinase C (PKC) [66] that play crucial roles in tumor promotion. A representative of the hydrogen selenide metabolic pool has been found to protect liver cells against damage to DNA. The cellular redox-milieu involves several metabolic, antioxidative and regulatory aspects that are maintained and regulated largely by two enzyme-based systems: the glutathione and thioredoxin systems [69] The thioredoxin and glutathione systems constitute a balanced redox network. The thioredoxin system may influence virtually all phases of tumorgenesis via its involvement in transcription and translation [69].

There are several possible mechanisms for the protective effect of selenium. Selenium activates an enzyme in the body called glutathione peroxidase that protects against the formation of free radicals—those loose molecular cannons that can damage DNA. There appear to be at least two distinct families of selenium-containing enzymes [70, 71]. The first includes glutathione peroxidases Bermano et al [72] and thioredoxin reductase [73], which are involved in controlling tissue concentrations of highly reactive oxygen-containing metabolites. These metabolites are essential at low concentrations for maintaining cell-mediated immunity against infections but highly toxic if produced in excess.

The role of selenium in the cytosolic enzyme glutathione peroxidase (GPx) was first illustrated [74, 75]. During stress, infection, or tissue injury, selenoenzymes may protect against the damaging effects of hydrogen peroxide or oxygen-rich free radicals. This family of enzymes catalyses the destruction of hydrogen peroxide or lipid hydroperoxides according to the following general reactions:

Selenium-containing glutathione peroxidases (GPx) constitute a family of anti-oxidative enzymes that are capable of reducing organic and inorganic hydroperoxides to the corresponding hydroxy compounds utilizing glutathione or other hydrogen donors as reducing equivalents

$$\begin{array}{l} H_2O_2 + 2GSH \cdots\cdots\cdots\cdots 2H_2O + GSSG \\ ROOH + 2GSH \cdots\cdots\cdots\cdots ROH + H_2O + GSSG \end{array} \quad (1)$$

Where GSH is glutathione and GSSG is its oxidized form. At least four forms of GPx exist; they differ both in their tissue distribution and in their sensitivity to selenium depletion [72]. The GPx enzymes of liver and blood plasma fall in activity rapidly at early stages of selenium deficiency. In contrast, a form of GPx associated specifically with phospholipid-rich tissue membranes is preserved against selenium deficiency and is believed to have broader metabolic roles (e.g., in prostaglandin synthesis) [76]. In concert with vitamin E, selenium is also involved in the protection of cell membranes against oxidative damage. The selenoenzyme thioredoxin reductase is involved in disposal of the products of oxidative metabolism [77]. It contains two selenocysteine groups per molecule and is a major component of a redox system with a multiplicity of functions, among which is the capacity to degrade locally excessive and potentially toxic concentrations of peroxide and hydroperoxides likely to induce cell death and tissue atrophy [76].

There is strong evidence that oxidative free radicals have a role in the development of degenerative diseases including CHD [78]. Oxidative free radicals increase the peroxidation of low density lipoprotein thereby increasing its uptake by macrophages with increased foam cell formation and atherosclerosis [79], though other mechanisms may exist. Anti-oxidants in the diet include vitamin A (carotenoids, which are metabolised to retinol), vitamin C (ascorbate), vitamin E (tocopherol), and selenium, which is an integral part of the antioxidant enzyme glutathione peroxidase:

6. Selenium function

Despite an evident progress in cancer diagnosis and treatment, there is a constant need of a drug which could arrest the premalignant process, thus reducing the risk of cancer. However, the role of selenium (Se) as an antioxidant and anticancer agent is well documented [80]. In addition, it has been proven that an adequate concentration of selenium can restore the sensitivity to chemotherapeutic agents of cytostatic-resistant malignant cells [81]. Selenium can exist with oxidation state-2,+2,+4,+6, and Se (II) is the dominant form in organoselenium chemistry [82]. The highest activity as a free radical scavenger and anticancer agent is assigned to selenium compounds containing selenium at the+4 oxidation level [83]. Other essential role of selenium in human and animal nutrition is well established. In humans, it has been demonstrated that an endemic cardiomyopathy (Keshan disease) prevalent in certain areas of China is correlated with selenium deficiency [84, 85]. Selenium is often thought to be a dietary antioxidant, but the antioxidant effects of selenium are most likely due to the antioxidant activity of proteins that have this element as an essential component (i.e., selenium-containing proteins), and not to selenium itself [86]. The damage to cells caused by free radicals, especially the damage to DNA, may play a role in the development of cancer and other health conditions [40]. Many observational studies, including case–control studies and cohort studies, have been conducted to investigate whether the use of dietary antioxidant supplements is associated with reduced risks of cancer in humans. Overall, these studies have yielded mixed results [87]. Healthy Chinese men and women at increased risk of developing esophageal cancer and gastric cancer were randomly assigned to take a combination of 15 milligrams (mg) beta-carotene, 30 mg α-tocopherol, and 50 micrograms (μg) selenium daily for 5 years or to take no antioxidant supplements. The initial results of the trial showed that people who took antioxidant supplements had a lower risk of death from gastric cancer but not from oesophageal cancer. However, their risks of developing gastric cancer and/or esophageal cancer were not affected by antioxidant supplementation [88].

As an essential trace element in humans [89], it's only established function is its presence in the enzyme glutathione peroxidase [90]. Using GSH2 as the reducing equivalent, this enzyme plays a significant role in detoxification of peroxides induced by oxygen radicals. As such it may be important in the toxicity of anticancer treatments that generate such reactive molecules [91]. In addition, epidemiological and experimental data suggest an anti-carcinogenic activity by selenium [92]. Considerable epidemiological data suggests that cancer mortality is inversely correlated with selenium consumption. Chemoprotective effect of diphenylmethyl selenocyanate against cyclophosphamide (CP) induced cellular toxicity and antitumor efficacy was evaluated in mice bearing Ehrlich ascites carcinoma [93], their results indicate that diphenylmethyl selenocyanate has the potential to reduce the cellular toxicity of CP at the same time improving its antitumor efficacy. Supplementation of a torula yeast-based diet with 2.5 or 5.0 ppm Selenium as Na_2SeO_3 also significantly increased the survival time of EAT-bearing mice [94]. Their data show that the form and mode of administration of selenium influence the antitumorigenic properties of this trace element. In addition, they suggested that some intermediate in the normal pathway for selenium detoxification is probably responsible for this trace element's antitumorigenic properties [94]. The ability of selenium to inhibit or prevent the growth of Ehrlich as cites tumour cells was highly dependent upon the form and quantity of selenium administered [95]. The only significant alteration that has been observed in mice treated with quantities of selenium at dosages of 4μg 3 times weekly was a slight reduction in intestinal weights. The reduction in intestinal weights was not attributable to a reduction in the intestinal macro constituents, suggesting that selenium may have altered rapidly dividing cells [95]. In fact selenocystine was used in the treatment of human leukaemia in 1956 with some short term success [96, 97]. The mechanism of its effect was thought to be competitive deprivation of cystine, but this was not proven. Others have shown that selenium compounds can cause chromosome breaks and inhibit critical DNA synthetic enzymes [98]. Specific incorporation of selenium into RNA molecules has been observed in several bacterial species. Since in a number of instances modified bases in RNAs have been shown to be involved in regulatory functions of the RNAs, the selenium-modified bases may have similar roles.

Furthermore, some RNA viruses, as well as leader mRNAs contain RNA-like segments that may interact with specific enzymes and, thus, play regulatory roles [99]· Hence, it is reasonable to assume that detailed information concerning selenium-modified RNAs may contribute to the understanding of the biological roles of selenium [100]. Near toxic levels of selenium have been reported to produce tumours in rats but other studies indicated that these concentrations of selenium created chronic toxic hepatitis that resembled hyperplasia.

In mammals glutathione peroxidase is the only selenium-dependent enzyme so far identified, but it seems unlikely that the complicated biological effects of selenium in man and animals are attributable solely to variations in the level of this enzyme. In fact, at least two other seleno proteins of unknown catalytic activity have been detected in animals. Investigations in a variety of animal systems have suggested that there is a significant interaction of selenium with glutathione independent of the enzyme glutathione peroxidase [101]. White muscle disease (WMD), a degenerative muscle disease, found in domestic animals [102, 103]. It is caused by a deficiency of selenium and/or vitamin E. Selenium and vitamin E deficiencies can produce symptoms of ill thrift and reproductive losses: lower conception rates, fetal reabsorption, dystocia, retained placenta, reduced milk production, and reduced semen quality, poor rate of growth or ill thrift in young lambs, low wool yields and have increased incidence of periodontal disease [102, 103]. Selenium appears to be a key nutrient in counteracting the development of virulence and inhibition of HIV progression to AIDS. It is required for sperm motility and may reduce the risk of miscarriage. Selenium deficiency has been linked to adverse mood states and some findings suggest that selenium deficiency may be a risk factor in cardiovascular diseases [104]. Studies continue to confirm that people with higher levels of selenium in their blood have lower rates of prostate and lung cancers [105].

Selenium is synergistic with vitamin E; they serve related metabolic functions and share in common the role of endogenous antioxidants [106]. Vitamin E has a free radical Scavenger, and Se as a component of the peroxide reducing enzyme, glutathione peroxidase. Vitamin E restricts the formation of peroxides by neutralizing free radicals, an integral component of glutathione peroxidase, an enzyme responsible for the removal of hydrogen peroxide and organic hydroperoxides [107].

Selenium and vitamin C; CH_3SeH is thought to be a critical metabolite in Se chemoprevention [108, 109]. The family of selenoenzymes called thioredoxin reductases catalyze the NADPH-dependent reduction of oxidized thioredoxin, hyperoxides, dehydroascorbate, ubiquinol and other substrates [110].The action of thioredoxin reductases in recycling dehydroascorbate to ascorbate (vitamin C) now explain the synergistic action of selenium and vitamin C [111]. The thioredoxin system is also capable of regenerating proteins inactivated by ROS. Daily supplementation with vitamin C (120 mg), vitamin E (30 mg), beta-carotene (6 mg), and the minerals selenium (100 μg) and zinc (20 mg) for a median of 7.5 years had no effect on the incidence of cancer or cardiovascular disease or on all-cause mortality [112]. Antioxidant and mineral supplementation was associated with lower total cancer incidence and all-cause mortality among men but not among women, and with an increase in skin cancer incidence, including melanoma, among women but not among men [113].

Selenium and Silver; Selenium serves as a major protective factor in precipitating the silver in a highly insoluble and hence inert form of silver selenide. Although some of this may be taken up in lysosomes in macrophages, the deposits are essentially long lived or permanent [114]. A lack of positive effect of Se supplementation on the prostate cancer incidence was observed in this study.

7. Conclusion

Selenium as non-metals is an essential nutrient that acts as cofactor in enzyme oxidation–reduction reactions. It maintains the specific configurations of proteins, is incorporated into the structure of hormones, and plays a structural and catalytic role in gene expression and transcriptional regulation. In the physiological dosage range, Se appears to function as an antimutagenic agent, preventing the malignant transformation of normal cells and the activation of oncogenes. These protective effects of Se seem to be primarily associated with its presence in the glutathione peroxidases, which are known to protect DNA and other cellular components from damage by oxygen radicals. Selenoenzymes are also known to play roles in carcinogen metabolism, in the control of cell division, oxygen metabolism, detoxification processes, apoptosis induction and the functioning of the immune system. Other modes of action, either direct or indirect, may also be operative, such as the partial retransformation of tumor cells and the inactivation of oncogenes.

Author details

T. Westermarck[1*], Arno Latvus[2] and Faik Atroshi[3]

*Address all correspondence to: tuomas.westermarck@ppa.inet.fi

1 Rinnekoti Research Center, Espoo, Finland

2 Hankintatukku Oy, Museokatu, Helsinki, Finland

3 Pharmacology & Toxicology, University of Helsinki, Finland

References

[1] WHO, World Health Organization. The Global Burden of Disease: 2004 Update. Geneva: World Health Organization; 2008.

[2] Meyskens, F. L., Jr., & Szabo, E. Diet and cancer: the disconnect between epidemiology and randomized clinical trials. Cancer Epidemiol Biomarkers Prev, 2005, 14(6), 1366-1369.

[3] Bjelakovic, G; Nikolova, D; Gluud, LL; Simonetti, RG; Gluud, C (2012). "Antioxidant supplements for prevention of mortality in healthy participants and patients with various diseases". In Bjelakovic, Goran. Cochrane database of systematic reviews (Online) 3: CD007176.

[4] Imlay JA. Pathways of oxidative damage. Annu Rev Microbiol. 2003;57:395-418.

[5] Rayman MP. Food-chain selenium and human health. Br J Nutr. 2008;100:254-268.

[6] Clark LC, Combs GF Jr, Turnbull BW, Slate EH, Chalker DK, Chow J, Davis LS, Glover RA, Graham GF, Gross EG, Krongrad A, Lesher JL Jr, Park HK, Sanders BB Jr, Smith CL, Taylor JR. Effects of selenium supplementation for cancer prevention in patients with carcinoma of the skin. A randomized controlled trial. Nutritional Prevention of Cancer Study Group. JAMA. 1996 Dec 25;276(24):1957-63.

[7] Clark LC, Jacobs ET. Environmental selenium and cancer: risk or protection? Cancer Epidemiol Biomarkers Prev. 1998 Oct;7(10):847-8.

[8] Combs G.F. Selenium in global food systems. Br. J. Nutr. 2001;85:517–547.

[9] Tallberg T, Westermarck T, Atroshi F. Cancer Treatment, Based on Active Nutritional Bio-Modulation, Hormonal Therapy and Specific Autologous Immunotherapy.In: Heavy Metals in the Environment (editors: Zueng-Sang Chen, Dar-Yuan Lee, Tser-Sheng Lin). Publisher, National Taiwan UniversityTaipei, Taiwan.

[10] DeBerardinis RJ. Is cancer a disease of abnormal cellular metabolism? New angles on an old idea. Genet Med. 2008 Nov;10(11):767-77.

[11] Anand P, Kunnumakkara AB, Kunnumakara AB, Sundaram C, Harikumar KB, Tharakan ST, Lai OS, Sung B, Aggarwal BB (September 2008). "Cancer is a preventable disease that requires major lifestyle changes". Pharm. Res. 25 (9): 2097–116.

[12] Seyfried TN, Shelton LM. Cancer as a metabolic disease. Nutr Metab (Lond). 2010 Jan 27;7:7. doi: 10.1186/1743-7075-7-7.

[13] Tallberg, T and Atroshi F. Prostate Cancer, the Long Search for Etiologic and Therapeutic Factors: Dietary Supplementation Avoiding Invasive Treatment. In: Prostate Cancer – From Bench to Bedside, 33-52, 2011.

[14] Crohns M, Westermarck T and Atroshi F. Prostate Cancer, Inflammation and Antioxidants. In :Advances in Prostate Cancer. (Gerhard Hamilton, ed.), 2013, INTECH Publisher, Croatia. 978-953-51-0932-7.

[15] Schwarz, K., and C. M. Foltz. 1957. Se as an integral part of factor against dietary liver degeneration. J. Am. Chem. Society 79:3292-3296.

[16] Sunde RA. Regulation of glutathione peroxidase-1 expression. In: Hatfield DL, Berry MJ, Gladyshev VN, editors. Selenium: its molecular biology and role in human health. 2nd ed. New York: Springer Science Media; 2006. p. 149–60.

[17] Kabata-Pendias A. Geochemistry of selenium. J Environ Pathol Toxicol Oncol. 1998;17(3-4):173-7.

[18] Haug A, Graham RD, Christophersen OA, Lyons GH. How to use the world's scarce selenium resources efficiently to increase the selenium concentration in food. Microb Ecol Health Dis. 2007 Dec;19(4):209-228.

[19] Sioen, I., Boon, P.E., Huybrechts, I. et al. (2010) Long-term dietary exposure to selenium in young children living in different European countries. Scientific Report submitted to EFSA.

[20] Kraus RJ, Prohaska JR, Ganther HE. Oxidized forms of ovine erythrocyte glutathione peroxidase. Cyanide inhibition of a 4-glutathione:4-selenoenzyme. Biochim Biophys Acta. 1980 Sep 9;615(1):19-26.

[21] Hatfield DL, Gladyshev VN. How selenium has altered our understanding of the genetic code. Mol Cell Biol. 2002 Jun;22(11):3565-76.

[22] Johansson L, Gafvelin G, Arnér ES. Selenocysteine in proteins-properties and biotechnological use. Biochim Biophys Acta. 2005 Oct 30;1726(1):1-13.

[23] Stadtman TC. Discoveries of vitamin B12 and selenium enzymes. Annu Rev Biochem. 2002;71:1-16.

[24] Rayman MP. The importance of selenium to human health.Lancet. 2000 Jul 15;356(9225):233-41.

[25] Donovan J, Copeland PR. The efficiency of selenocysteine incorporation is regulated by translation initiation factors. J Mol Biol. 2010 Jul 23;400(4):659-64.

[26] Bjelakovic G, Nikolova D, Gluud LL, Simonetti RG, Gluud C. Antioxidant supplements for prevention of mortality in healthy participants and patients with various diseases. Cochrane Database Syst Rev. 2012 Mar 14;3:CD007176. doi: 10.1002/14651858.CD007176.pub2.

[27] Arthur JR, McKenzie RC, Beckett GJ. Selenium in the immune system. J Nutr. 2003 May;133(5 Suppl 1):1457S-9S.

[28] Diplock AT. Metabolic and functional defects in selenium deficiency. Philos Trans R Soc Lond B Biol Sci. 1981 Aug 14;294(1071):105-17.

[29] Chen X. Selenium and cardiomyopathy (Keshan disease). Acta Pharmacol Toxicol (Copenh). 1986;59 Suppl 7:325-30.

[30] Hawkes WC, Hornbostel L. Effects of dietary selenium on mood in healthy men living in a metabolic research unit. Biol Psychiatry. 1996 Jan 15;39(2):121-8.

[31] Majkowski J, Atroshi F, Westermarck T. Effects of Epileptic Seizures and Antiepileptic Drugs on Oxygen Stress. Factors Attenuating the Effects of Oxygen Stress. EPILEPTOLOGY 2011, 19:143-157.

[32] Zimmermann MB, Köhrle J. The impact of iron and selenium deficiencies on iodine and thyroid metabolism: biochemistry and relevance to public health. Thyroid. 2002 Oct;12(10):867-78.

[33] Whanger PD. Selenium and its relationship to cancer: an update.Br J Nutr. 2004 Jan; 91(1):11-28.

[34] Aboul-Fadl T. Selenium derivatives as cancer preventive agents. Curr Med Chem Anticancer Agents. 2005 Nov;5(6):637-52.

[35] Hansen JC, Deguchi Y. Selenium and fertility in animals and man--a review. Acta Vet Scand. 1996;37(1):19-30.

[36] Gupta D, Raina V, Rath GK, Shukla NK, Mohanti BK, Sharma DN. Clinical and pathological response rates of docetaxel-based neoadjuvant chemotherapy in locally advanced breast cancer and comparison with anthracycline-based chemotherapies: eight-year experience from single centre. Indian J Cancer. 2011 Oct-Dec;48(4):410-4.

[37] Lawenda BD, Kelly KM, Ladas EJ, Sagar SM, Vickers A, Blumberg JB. Should supplemental antioxidant administration be avoided during chemotherapy and radiation therapy? J Natl Cancer Inst. 2008 Jun 4;100(11):773-83. doi: 10.1093/jnci/djn148. Epub 2008 May 27.

[38] Borek C, Ong A, Mason H. In vitro transformation of human cells by radiation. Toxicol Ind Health. 1987 Sep;3(3):397-404.

[39] Casciari JJ, Riordan NH, Schmidt TL, Meng XL, Jackson JA, Riordan HD. Cytotoxicity of ascorbate, lipoic acid, and other antioxidants in hollow fibre in vitro tumours. Br J Cancer. 2001 Jun 1;84(11):1544-50.

[40] Valko M, Rhodes CJ, Moncol J, Izakovic M, Mazur M. Free radicals, metals and antioxidants in oxidative stress-induced cancer. Chem Biol Interact. 2006;160:1–40.

[41] Watson J. Oxidants, antioxidants and the current incurability of metastatic cancers. Open Biol. 2013 Jan 8;3(1):120144.

[42] Brigelius-Flohé R, Kipp AP. Selenium in the redox regulation of the Nrf2 and the Wnt pathway. Methods Enzymol. 2013;527:65-86.

[43] Cancer Research UK "How many different types of cancer are there? CancerHelp UK". Retrieved 11 May 2012.

[44] Lebeau A, Kriegsmann M, Burandt E, Sinn HP. [Invasive breast cancer: the current WHO classification]. Pathologe. 2014 Feb;35(1):7-17. doi: 10.1007/s00292-013-1841-7.

[45] Hanahan, D ; Weinberg, R A. (2011). "Hallmarks of Cancer: The Next Generation". Cell 144 (5): 646–74.

[46] Danaei G, Vander Hoorn S, Lopez AD, Murray CJ, Ezzati M (2005). "Causes of cancer in the world: comparative risk assessment of nine behavioural and environmental risk factors". Lancet 366 (9499): 1784–93

[47] Warburg O. On the origin of cancer cells. Science. 1956 Feb 24;123(3191):309-14.

[48] Villalba M, Rathore MG, Lopez-Royuela N, Krzywinska E, Garaude J, Allende-Vega N. From tumor cell metabolism to tumor immune escape. Int J Biochem Cell Biol. 2013 Jan;45(1):106-13.

[49] Butterfield LH, Merino A, Golub SH, Shau H. From cytoprotection to tumor suppression: the multifactorial role of peroxiredoxins. Antioxid Redox Signal. 1999 Winter; 1(4):385-402.

[50] Asim M, Khan LA, Husain SA, Husain S, Sarma MP, Ahmad I, Sharma JK, Sharma A, Sharma S, Thayumanavan L, Kar P. Genetic polymorphism of glutathione S transferases M1 and T1 in Indian patients with hepatocellular carcinoma.Dis Markers. 2010;28(6):369-76.

[51] Doyle C, Kushi LH, Byers T, Courneya KS, Demark-Wahnefried W, Grant B, McTiernan A, Rock CL, Thompson C, Gansler T, Andrews KS. Nutrition and physical activity during and after cancer treatment: an American Cancer Society guide for informed choices. CA Cancer J Clin. 2006 Nov-Dec;56(6):323-53.

[52] Anand P, Kunnumakkara AB, Sundaram C, Harikumar KB, Tharakan ST, Lai OS, Sung B, Aggarwal BB. Cancer is a preventable disease that requires major lifestyle changes. Pharm Res. 2008 Sep;25(9):2097-116.

[53] Braig M, Schmitt CA. Oncogene-induced senescence: putting the brakes on tumor development. Cancer Res. 2006 Mar 15;66(6):2881-4.

[54] Baylin SB, Ohm JE. Epigenetic gene silencing in cancer-a mechanism for early oncogenic pathway addiction? Nat Rev Cancer. 2006 Feb;6(2):107-16.

[55] Suzuki H, Asakawa A, Amitani H, Fujitsuka N, Nakamura N, Inui A. Cancer cachexia pathophysiology and translational aspect of herbal medicine. Jpn J Clin Oncol. 2013 Jul;43(7):695-705. doi: 10.1093/jjco/hyt075. Epub 2013 Jun 4.

[56] Fraumeni JF Jr. Epidemiologic approaches to cancer etiology. Annu Rev Public Health. 1982;3:85-100.

[57] Chlebowski RT. Reducing the risk of breast cancer. N Engl J Med. 2000 Jul 20;343(3): 191-8.

[58] Lichtenstein GR. Reduction of colorectal cancer risk in patients with Crohn's disease. Rev Gastroenterol Disord. 2002;2 Suppl 2:S16-24.

[59] Wick, M., Dubey, P., Koeppen, H., Siegel, C. T., Fields, P. E., Chen, L., Bluestone, J. A., Schreiber, H. Antigenic cancer cells grow progressively in immune hosts without evidence for T cell exhaustion or systemic anergy J. Exp. Med. 1997,186,229-238.

[60] Rosenberg, S. A. Progress in human tumour immunology and immunotherapy Nature, 2001, 411,380-384.

[61] Chin L, Gray JW. Translating insights from the cancer genome into clinical practice. Nature. 2008 Apr 3;452(7187):553-63. doi: 10.1038/nature06914.

[62] Rotruck JT, Pope AL, Ganther HE, Swanson AB, Hafeman DG and Hoekstra WG. Selenium: biochemical role as a component of glutathione peroxidase. Science 1973 Feb 9;179(73):588-90.

[63] Leinfelder, W., Forchhammer, K., Veprek, B., et al., In vitro synthesis of selenocysteinyl-tRNA (UCA) from seryl-tRNA (UCA): involvement and characterization of the selD gene product. Proc. Natl. Acad. Sci. USA 1990:87;543-547.

[64] Reddy CC, Massaro EJ. Biochemistry of selenium: a brief overview. Fundam Appl Toxicol. 1983 Sep-Oct;3(5):431-6.

[65] Stadtman TC. SELENIUM BIOCHEMISTRY. Annu. Rev. Biochem. 1990. 59:111-127.

[66] Gopalakrishna R, Gundimeda U. Antioxidant regulation of protein kinase C in cancer prevention. J Nutr. 2002 Dec;132(12):3819S-3823S.

[67] Zeng H, Cheng WH, Johnson LK. Methylselenol, a selenium metabolite, modulates p53 pathway and inhibits the growth of colon cancer xenografts in Balb/c mice. J Nutr Biochem. 2013 May;24(5):776-80.

[68] Pillai SS, Sugathan JK, Indira M. Selenium downregulates RAGE and NFκB expression in diabetic rats. Biol Trace Elem Res. 2012 Oct;149(1):71-7.

[69] Gromer S., Arscott L.D., Williams C.H., Jr, Schirmer R.H., Becker K. Human placenta thioredoxin reductase. Isolation of the selenoenzyme, steady state kinetics, and inhibition by therapeutic gold compounds. J. Biol. Chem. 1998, 273:20096–20101.

[70] Chu FF. "The human glutathione peroxidase genes GPX2, GPX3, and GPX4 map to chromosomes 14, 5, and 19, respectively". Cytogenet Cell Genet, 1994, 66 (2): 96–8.

[71] Müller C, Wingler K, Brigelius-Flohé R. "3'UTRs of glutathione peroxidases differentially affect selenium-dependent mRNA stability and selenocysteine incorporation efficiency". Biol. Chem, 2003,384 (1): 11–8.

[72] Bermano G, Arthur JR, Hesketh JE. Role of the 3' untranslated region in the regulation of cytosolic glutathione peroxidase and phospholipid-hydroperoxide glutathione peroxidase gene expression by selenium supply. Biochem J. 1996 Dec 15;320 (Pt 3):891-5.

[73] Lacey BM, Eckenroth BE, Flemer S, Hondal RJ. Selenium in thioredoxin reductase: a mechanistic perspective. Biochemistry. 2008 Dec 2;47(48):12810-21.

[74] Mills GC. Hemoglobin catabolism. I. Glutathione peroxidase, an erythrocyte enzyme which protects hemoglobin from oxidative breakdown. J Biol Chem. 1957 Nov; 229(1):189–197.

[75] Ganther HE, Kraus RJ. Oxidation states of glutathione peroxidase. Methods Enzymol. 1984;107:593-602.

[76] Maiorino M, Chu FF, Ursini F, Davies KJ, Doroshow JH, Esworthy RS. Phospholipid hydroperoxide glutathione peroxidase is the 18-kDa selenoprotein expressed in human tumor cell lines. J Biol Chem. 1991 Apr 25;266(12):7728-32.

[77] Arteel GE, Sies H. The biochemistry of selenium and the glutathione system. Environ Toxicol Pharmacol. 2001 Sep;10(4):153-8.

[78] Ames. B N, Shigenaga MK, and Hagen TM. Oxidants, antioxidants, and the degenerative diseases of aging. Proc. Natl. Acad. Sci. USA,1993, 90:7915-7922.

[79] Aviram, M. (1995) Oxidative modification of low density lipoprotein and its relation to atherosclerosis. Isr. J. Med. Sci. 31:241-249.

[80] Tapiero H, Townsend DM, Tew KD. The antioxidant role of selenium and seleno-compounds. Biomed Pharmacother. 2003 May-Jun;57(3-4):134-44.

[81] Jönsson-Videsäter K, Björkhem-Bergman L, Hossain A, Söderberg A, Eriksson LC, Paul C, Rosén A, Björnstedt M. Selenite-induced apoptosis in doxorubicin-resistant cells and effects on the thioredoxin system. Biochem Pharmacol. 2004 Feb 1;67(3): 513-22.

[82] Wallschläger D, Feldmann J. Formation, occurrence, significance, and analysis of organoselenium and organotellurium compounds in the environment. Met Ions Life Sci. 2010;7:319-64. doi: 10.1039/BK9781847551771-00319. Epub 2010 Jan 30.

[83] Suchocki P, Misiewicz I, Skupinska K, Waclawek K, Fijalek Z, Kasprzycka-Guttman T. The activity of Selol in multidrug-resistant and sensitive human leukemia cells. Oncol Rep. 2007 Oct;18(4):893-9.

[84] Beck MA, Levander OA, Handy J (May 2003). "Selenium deficiency and viral infection". J. Nutr. 133 (5 Suppl 1): 1463S–7S. PMID 12730444.

[85] Ren LQ, Li XJ, Li GS, Zhao ZT, Sun B, Sun F (November 2004). "Coxsackievirus B3 infection and its mutation in Keshan disease". World J. Gastroenterol. 10 (22): 3299–302.

[86] Davis CD, Tsuji PA, Milner JA. Selenoproteins and cancer prevention. Annu Rev Nutr. 2012 Aug 21;32:73-95.

[87] Patterson BH, Levander OA. Naturally occurring selenium compounds in cancer chemoprevention trials: a workshop summary. Cancer Epidemiol Biomarkers Prev. 1997 Jan;6(1):63-9.

[88] Blot WJ, Li JY, Taylor PR, Guo W, Dawsey S, Wang GQ, Yang CS, Zheng SF, Gail M, Li GY, et al. Nutrition intervention trials in Linxian, China: supplementation with specific vitamin/mineral combinations, cancer incidence, and disease-specific mortality in the general population. J Natl Cancer Inst. 1993 Sep 15;85(18):1483-92.

[89] Young VR. Selenium: a case for its essentiality in man. N Engl J Med. 1981 May 14;304(20):1228-30.

[90] Hafeman DG, Sunde RA, Hoekstra WG. Effect of dietary selenium on erythrocyte and liver glutathione peroxidase in the rat. J Nutr. 1974 May;104(5):580-7.

[91] Batist G, Norton J, Katki AG, Wagman L, Ferrans VJ, Maher M, Myers CE. Cardiac and red blood cell glutathione peroxidase: results of a prospective randomized trial in patients on total parenteral nutrition. Cancer Res. 1985 Nov;45(11 Pt 2):5900-3.

[92] Schrauzer GN. Selenium and cancer: a review. Bioinorg Chem. 1976;5(3):275-81.

[93] Chakraborty P, Sk UH, Bhattacharya S. Chemoprotection and enhancement of cancer chemotherapeutic efficacy of cyclophosphamide in mice bearing Ehrlich ascites carcinoma by diphenylmethyl selenocyanate. Cancer Chemother Pharmacol. 2009 Oct; 64(5):971-80. doi: 10.1007/s00280-009-0950-8. Epub 2009 Feb 17.

[94] Poirier KA, Milner JA. Factors influencing the antitumorigenic properties of selenium in mice. J Nutr. 1983 Nov;113(11):2147-54.

[95] Greeder GA, Milner JA. Factors influencing the inhibitory effect of selenium on mice inoculated with Ehrlich ascites tumor cells. Science. 1980 Aug 15;209(4458):825-7.

[96] Weisberger, A. S.. and Suhrland, L. G. Studies on analogues of L-cysteine and L-cystine. The effect of selenium cystine on leukemia. Blood, / /: 19-30, 1956.

[97] Batist G, Katki AG, Klecker RW Jr, Myers CE. Selenium-induced cytotoxicity of human leukemia cells: interaction with reduced glutathione. Cancer Res. 1986 Nov; 46(11):5482-5.

[98] Weitberg AB, Weitzman SA, Clark EP, Stossel TP. Effects of antioxidants on oxidant-induced sister chromatid exchange formation. J Clin Invest. 1985 Jun;75(6):1835-41.

[99] Hendrickson W.A., Horton,J.R. and LeMaster,D.M. (1990) Selenomethionyl proteins produced for analysis by multiwavelength anomalous diffraction (MAD): a vehicle for direct determination of three-dimensional structure. EMBO J., 9, 1665–1672.

[100] Ching WM. Characterization of selenium-containing tRNAGlu from Clostridium sticklandii. Arch Biochem Biophys. 1986 Jan;244(1):137-46.

[101] Chung AS, Maines MD. Effect of selenium on glutathione metabolism. Induction of gamma-glutamylcysteine synthetase and glutathione reductase in the rat liver. Biochem Pharmacol. 1981 Dec 1;30(23):3217-23.

[102] Lagace A. Effect of selenium on white muscle disease in lambs.J Am Vet Med Assoc. 1961 Feb 15;138:188-90

[103] Schwarz S. Essentiality and metabolic functions of selenium. Med Clin North Am. 1976 Jul;60(4):745-58.

[104] Ferencík M, Ebringer L. Modulatory effects of selenium and zinc on the immune system. Folia Microbiol (Praha). 2003;48(3):417-26.

[105] Vogt TM, Ziegler RG, Graubard BI, Swanson CA, Greenberg RS, Schoenberg JB, Swanson GM, Hayes RB, Mayne ST. Serum selenium and risk of prostate cancer in U.S. blacks and whites. Int J Cancer. 2003 Feb 20;103(5):664-70.

[106] Hoekstra, W. G. Biochemicalfunction of seleniumand its relation to vitamin E. Fed. Proc., 34: 2083-2089,1975.

[107] Tappel AL. Biological antioxidant protection against lipid peroxidation damage. Am J Clin Nutr. 1970 Aug;23(8):1137-9.

[108] Ip C. Interaction of Vitamin C and Selenium Supplementation in the Modification of Mammary Carcinogenesis in Rats. JNCI J Natl Cancer Inst (1986) 77 (1): 299-303.

[109] Spallholz JE, Palace VP, Reid TW (2004) Methioninase and selenomethionine but not Se-ethylselenocysteine generate methylselenol and superoxide in an in vitro chemiluminescent assay: implications for the nutritional carcinostatic activity of selenoamino acids. Biochem Pharmacol 67:547–554.

[110] Stadtman TC. Selenium biochemistry. Mammalian selenoenzymes. Ann N Y Acad Sci. 2000;899:399–402.

[111] Badmaev V, Majeed M, Passwater RA. Selenium: a quest for better understanding. Altern Ther Health Med. 1996 Jul;2(4):59-62, 65-7.

[112] Hercberg S, Galan P, Preziosi P, Bertrais S, Mennen L, Malvy D, Roussel AM, Favier A, Briançon S. The SU.VI.MAX Study: a randomized, placebo-controlled trial of the health effects of antioxidant vitamins and minerals. Arch Intern Med. 2004 Nov 22;164(21):2335-42.

[113] Hercberg S, Kesse-Guyot E, Druesne-Pecollo N, Touvier M, Favier A, Latino-Martel P, Briançon S, Galan P. Incidence of cancers, ischemic cardiovascular diseases and mortality during 5-year follow-up after stopping antioxidant vitamins and minerals supplements: a postintervention follow-up in the SU.VI.MAX Study. Int J Cancer. 2010 Oct 15;127(8):1875-81.

[114] Sato S, Sueki H, and Nishijima A. "Two unusual cases of argyria: the application of an improved tissue processing method for X-ray microanalysis of selenium and sulphur in silver-laden granules," British Journal of Dermatology, vol. 140, no. 1, pp. 158–163, 1999.

3

Anti Oxidative, Anti Peroxidative and Hepatoprotective Potential of *Phyllanthus amarus* Against Anti Tb Drugs

Sangeeta Shukla, Neelu Sinha and Amita Jaswal

1. Introduction

The liver plays an astonishing array of vital functions in the maintenance and performance of the body. Additionally, it is also handling the metabolism and excretion of drugs and other xenobiotics from the body thereby providing protection against foreign substances by detoxifying and eliminating them (saleem et al., 2010). Large numbers of xenobiotics are reported to be potentially hepatotoxic. Free radicals generated from the xenobiotic metabolism can induce lesions of the liver and react with the basic cellular constituents such as proteins, lipids, RNA and DNA (Ajith *et al.,* 2007). A growing international health concern is Tuberculosis caused by *Mycobacterium tuberculosis* (Abdelaal *et al.,* 2009).India is the highest TB burden country accounting for one fifth (21%) of the global incidence (WHO, 2010). The first line anti-tuberculosis drugs isoniazid (INH), rifampicin (RIF), pyrazinamide (PZA) and Ethambutol(ETH)continues to be the effective drugs in the treatment of tuberculosis, however, the use of these drugs is associated with toxic reactions in tissues, particularly in the liver, leading to hepatitis (Eminzade *et al.,* 2008). This is one of the most serious adverse effects of anti-tuberculosis drugs (ATD). Liver injury or liver dysfunction is a major health problem that challenges not only health care professionals but also the pharmaceutical industry and drug regulatory agencies (saleem *et al.,* 2010). It has great capacity to detoxify and synthesize useful substances, and therefore damage to the liver has grave consequences (Devaraj *et al.,* 2011). Currently, there is no effective treatment against ATD induced hepatic damage. Plants are an important component of the health care system in India and have been found to be effective in the treatment of different diseases and are the beacon of the therapeutic sources for curing diseases from times immemorial (Merina *et al.,* 2012). *Phyllanthus amarus* Linn. is commonly known as *bhumi amla* (Joshi&Parle2007). It is reported to possess antiviral (Lee *et al.,* 1996), anticancer (Rajeshkumar *et al.,* 2002). But there is no scientific evidence for its hepatoprotective activity against ATD induced liver injury. Hence the present study was undertaken to explore the key behind the use of *P.amarus* as a hepatoprotective formulation against xenobiotics induced hepatic adverse effect.

2. Materials and methods

2.1. Chemicals

Anti TB drug *i.e,* Rifampicin, Isoniazid, Pyrazinamide as anti TB kit was generously obtained from Government TB hospital, Gwalior (M.P.). All the other chemicals used in this study were of analytical grade and were procured from Sigma–Aldrich (USA), E Merck (Germany), Ranbaxy Pvt. Ltd. and BDH Company (India).

2.2. Preparation of plant extract

Whole plant of *Phyllanthus amarus* was obtained from the authenticated ayurvedic dealer and was identified by the experts of Botany Department, Jiwaji University Gwalior, India. The shade dried plant was pulverized and extracted with 75% alcohol for 10 days with concomitant shaking and then filtered. The filtrate was evaporated in vacuum to yield a brownish powder (P. amarus) powder it was stored in refrigerator at 4°C and administered orally according to body weight of animals at different concentration.

2.3. Animal maintenance and feeding

Female albino rats of *Sprague Dawley* strain (160±10 g, b.w.) were used for the present investigation. Animals were housed in polypropylene cages under standard conditions (25±2°C temperature, 60%-70% relative humidity and 14 h light and 10 h dark) and were fed on standard pellet diet (Pranav Agro Industries Ltd., New Delhi, India) and drinking water *ad libitum.* Animals used in this study were treated and cared for in accordance with the guidelines recommended by the Committee for the Purpose of Control and Supervision of Experiments on Animals (CPCSEA), Government of India, Ministry of Culture, Chennai.

2.4. Experimental design

Animals were divided into various groups of six animals each. *P.amarus* and anti TB drugs were given alternatively for 8 weeks (3 days/week). The groups were treated as follows:

Group I: Control (normal saline, 0.9%).

Group II: *Per se* - 400mg/kg, b.w., *P.amarus* (p.o.), daily.

Group III: Experimental control-RIF+INH+PZA+ETH at 52, 70,175,140 mg/kg, b.w., (p.o.), 3days/week.

Group VI- VII: INH+RIF+PZA (as in group III) + *P.amarus* at 100, 200, 300 and 400 mg/kg, b.w., (p.o) 3days/week.

Group VIII: Positive control-Silymerin -50mg/kg b.w. (p.o.), daily.

All the animals were euthanized 24hours after the last treatment to perform various biochemical and histological analysis.

2.4.1. Blood biochemical investigations

Blood was drawn from retro-orbital venous sinus and serum was isolated. Serum Urea, Uric acid and Creatinine determined by commercially prepared kit method (E-Merck, Germany). Serum AST and ALT activity were determined with Reitman and Frankel, 1957.

2.4.2. Tissue biochemical investigations

The tissues viz., liver and kidney were quickly excised, washed in ice cold, normal saline and blotted individually freed from extraneous material on ash-free filter paper. The tissues were then homogenized separately in hypotonic buffer (0.008% NaHCO3), pH 7.4, using a Potter-Elvejham homogenizer at 600-1000 rpm in ice cold conditions.

The crude tissue homogenate was centrifuged at 2000 rpm for 15 min (0-4°C). The supernatant was collected and stored at- 20°C until used for estimating tissue biochemical parameters. Lipid Peroxidation (LPO) was determined by measuring thiobarbituric acid reactive substances (TBARS) in tissues according to Sharma and Krishnamurthy, 1968.SOD and Catalase activity were determined according to Misra and Fridovich, 1972 and Aebi, 1974 respectively.

2.4.3. Histopathological investigations

Tissues were fixed with Bouin's solution. They were later sectioned using a microtome, dehydrated in graded alcohol, embedded in paraffin section, and stained with hemotoxylin and Eosin (H & E).

2.5. Statistical analysis

Results are presented as mean ± S.E. of six animals used in each group. Data were subjected to statistical analysis through one-way analysis of variance (ANOVA) at 5% significance level followed by Student's t-test at $p \leq 0.05$(Snedecor and Cochran,1989).

3. Results — Table 1-6 and histopathology

Treatment	AST (IU/L)	ALT (IU/L)
Group I	69 ± 3.81	52 ± 2.87
Group II	74 ± 4.09	53.6±2.96
Group III	345±19.07#	188 ± 10.39#
Group IV	120.22 ± 6.65* (81.44%)	81 ± 4.48* (78.67%)
Group V	112.34 ± 6.21* (84.29%)	71 ± 3.92* (86.02%)
Group VI	100.7 ± 5.57* (88.51%)	63 ± 3.48* (91.91%)
Group VII	94.4± 5.22* (90.79%)	60 ± 3.32* (94.11%)
Group VIII	83 ± 4.59* (94.92%)	59 ± 3.26* (94.85%)
ANOVA F Value	**141.88@**	**90.172@**

Data are mean ± S.E., n=6.ANOVA (F Values at 5% level). # P≤0.05 vs. Control,*P ≤0.05 vs. ATD, @ Significant

Table 1. Therapeutic effect of *P.amarus* against ATD induced blood biochemical alterations

Treatment	SALP (U/L)	Albumin (g/dl)	Bilirubin(mg/dl)
Group I	193.3±10.68	4.1 ± 0.23	0.19 ± 0.010
Group II	220±12.16	4.0 ± 0.22	0.2±0.011
Group III	462±25.54#	3.0±0.17#	0.8± 0.044#
Group IV	381.3±21.08* (30.03%)	3.5 ± 0.19 (45.45%)	0.65± 0.036* (24.59%)
Group V	305.25±16.87* (58.33%)	3.6 ± 0.199 (54.54%)	0.58 ± 0.032* (36.06%)
Group VI	257±14.21* (76.29%)	3.7 ± 0.20* (63.63%)	0.34± 0.018* (75.4%)
Group VII	236±13.05* (84.10%)	3.8± 0.21* (72.72%)	0.32 ± 0.017* (78.68%)
Group VIII	216±11.94* (91.55%)	4.0± 0.22* (90.9%)	0.3 ± 0.016* (81.96%)
ANOVA F Value	**39.135@**	**3.631@**	**89.61@**

Table 2. Curative effect of *P.amarus* against ATD on selected serological parameters serum

Treatment	Urea (mg/dl)	Uric acid (mg/dl)	Creatinine (mg/dl)
Group I	19.5±1.08	5.3± 0.292	0.4± 0.022
Group II	24±1.33	5.6± 0.309	0.5±0.027
Group III	52.6±2.91#	10±0.552#	0.8± 0.044#
Group IV	47±2.59 (16.91%)	7.6± 0.420* (51.06%)	0.7± 0.038* (25%)
Group V	44.1±2.44* (25.67%)	6.22± 0.343* (80.42%)	0.66± 0.036* (35%)
Group VI	35.7±1.97* (51.05%)	6.1± 0.337* (82.97%)	0.6± 0.033* (66%)
Group VII	30.7±1.70* (66.16%)	6± 0.331* (88.90%)	0.575± 0.032* (75%)
Group VIII	27.8±1.544* (74.92%)	5.8± 0.320* (89.36%)	0.55± 0.030* (83%)
ANOVA F Value	**32.005@**	**20.642@**	**16.887@**

Data are mean ± S.E., n=6.ANOVA (F Values at 5% level).# P≤0.05 vs. Control,*P ≤0.05 vs. ATD,@ Significant

Table 3. *P.amarus* efficiency in reducing Anti TB drugs induced renal alterations.

Treatment	Lipid Peroxidation (n mole of TBARS/mg protein)		Reduced glutathione (µ mole / g)	
	Liver	Kidney	Liver	Kidney
Group I	0.31±0.017	0.3± 0.016	7.97± 0.441	7.5± 0.441
Group II	0.341±0.018	0.33± 0.018	8.136±0.449	7.78± 0.449
Group III	1.94±0.107#	1.28±0.071#	6.8± 0.376#	6.17± 0.376#
Group IV	0.69±0.038* (76.68%)	1.096± 0.061* (18.77%)	7.08± 0.391 (23.93%)	6.69± 0.391 (39.09%)
Group V	0.57±0.034* (84.04%)	1.096± 0.061* (18.77%)	7.18± 0.396 (32.47%)	7.0± 0.397 (62.40%)
Group VI	0.44±0.0243* (92.02%)	0.737± 0.041* (55.47%)	7.4± 0.409 (51.28%)	7.25± 0.409 (81.20%)
Group VII	0.431±0.0238* (92.57%)	0.721± 0.039* (57.04%)	7.75± 0.428 (81.19%)	7.33± 0.428 (87.21%)
Group VIII	0.335±0.018* (98.46%)	0.665± 0.037* (62.75%)	7.85± 0.434 (89.74%)	7.34± 0.434 (87.96%)
ANOVA F Value	**174.79@**	**70.42@**	**1.566**	**1.971**

Data are mean ± S.E., n=6.ANOVA (F Values at 5% level).# P≤0.05 vs. Control,*P ≤0.05 vs. ATD,@ Significant

Table 4. Effect of *P.amarus* against AT drugs treated animals in tissue biochemical estimations.

Treatment	SOD (U/min./mg protein)		Catalase (μ mole of H_2O_2 oxidised/min/mg protein)	
	Liver	Kidney	Liver	Kidney
Group I	70.7±3.908	48.78± 2.696	50.7± 2.802	70.1± 3.875
Group II	76±4.201	51.2± 2.830	51.8±2.863	62.14± 3.435
Group III	37.52±2.074#	24.39±1.348#	38.1± 2.106#	50.8± 2.808#
Group IV	44±2.432 (19.52%)	33.3± 1.840* (36.53%)	42.02± 2.322 (31.11%)	59.67± 3.298 (45.95%)
Group V	45.6±2.520 (24.35%)	35.9± 1.984* (47.19%)	42.5± 2.349 (34.92%)	59.97± 3.315 (47.51%)
Group VI	55±3.040* (52.68%)	41.15± 2.274* (68.71%)	44.05± 2.435 (47.22%)	61.96± 3.425* (57.82%)
Group VII	60.9±3.366* (70.46%)	43.13± 2.384* (76.83%)	45.2± 2.498 (56.34%)	62.1± 3.432* (58.54%)
Group VIII	68±3.759* (91.86%)	41.83± 2.312* (71.50%)	50.6± 2.775* (96.03%)	62.57± 3.458* (58.54%)
ANOVA F Value	**22.664@**	**12.569@**	**4.464@**	**2.911@**

Data are mean ± S.E., n=6.ANOVA (F Values at 5% level).# P≤0.05 vs. Control,*P ≤0.05 vs. ATD,@ Significant

Table 5. Effect of *P.amarus* on SOD, Catalase activity in liver and kidney against anti TB drugs.

Treatment	ATPase Liver	ATPase Kidney
	(mgPi/100gm/min)	
Group I	1971±108.95	2449.99±135.44
Group II	2114±116.86	2257.14±124.77
Group III	1335.71±73.84#	1785.7±98.72#
Group IV	1721.4± 95.16* (60.71%)	1814.28±100.29 (4.30%)
Group V	1864.28±103.06* (83.02%)	1907.14±105.43 (18.28%)
Group VI	1889±104.43* (87.09%)	2042.85±112.93 (38.71%)
Group VII	1966.06±108.69* (99.22%)	2149.99±118.85* (54.83%)
Group VIII	1969±108.85* (99.68%)	2107.14 ±116.48 (48.38%)
ANOVA F Value	**6.350@**	**4.696@**

Data are mean ± S.E., n=6.ANOVA (F Values at 5% level). # P≤0.05 vs. Control,*P ≤0.05 vs. ATD, @ Significant.

Table 6. Therapeutic Effect of *P.amarus* on ATPase against ATD

4. Discussion

The liver diseases remain one of the serious health problems as variedly exposed to xenobiotics. Modern medicines have little to offer for alleviation of hepatic diseases. Although *P. amarus is* reported to possess varied medicinal properties such as antiviral, anticancer, antioxidant, anti-inflammatory, hepatoprotective (Joshi and Parle, 2007), there is no previous report about the hepatoprotective activity of this plant against anti TB drugs. The present investigation reports the hepatoprotective effect of *P.amarus*. In the present study, hepatotoxicity model in albino rats was successfully produced by administering RIF, INH and PZA.

Effects of administration of Anti TB Drugs and *Phyllanthus amarus* orally on selected biochemical parameters in rat tissue and blood serum is presented in Table 1-6.

Significant rise above the normal upper limits in the measured serum transaminases in toxicant group on day 60 of the experiment was a biochemical indication of liver injury. Elevated levels of serum enzymes, AST and ALT are indicative of cellular leakage, and loss of functional integrity of cell membrane in liver (Ranawat *et al.,* 2010). Oral administration of *P. amarus* extract at doses (100, 200, 300 and 400 mg/kg) showed significant recoupment in a dose dependent manner ($P \leq 0.05$) (Table1).

The increased level of serum alkaline phosphatase is reliable marker of liver damage, which occurs due to the *de novo* synthesis by the liver cells (Muriel and Escobar, 2003). Serum albumin concentration is affected by hepatic protein and its synthesis is a typical function of normal liver cells (Thirunavukkarasu and Skthisenkaran, 2003). Bilirubin is one of the most frequent clinical test to evaluate the extent of chemically induced hepatotoxicity (Zimmerman, 1973). Toxicants administration caused significant increase in the serum alkaline phosphatase activity. Stabilization of SALP and bilirubin levels by the treatment of *P.amarus* is clear indication of improvement in functional status of liver cells. Results suggested that *P.amarus* at a dose of 400mg/kg, b.w., have protective effect on plasma membrane of hepatocytes. (Table2)

As a measure of renal function status, serum urea, uric acid and creatinine are often regarded as reliable markers (Adebisi *et al.,* 2000). Serum creatinine has been used to estimate glomerular filtration rate. Thus, elevations in the serum concentrations of these markers are indicative of renal injury (Adebisi *et al.,* 2000; Adewole *et al.,* 2007).The same was observed after toxicant administration. It may be due to dysfunctional and dystrophic changes in the liver and kidney. Experiment has shown that *P.amarus* at different doses, showed significant protective but the highest protection was obsereved at 300 and 400 mg/kg with mere difference indicating normal glomerular filtration rate thereby improved functional status of kidney. (Table 3)

Various biochemical parameters were measured in liver and kidney tissues. The levels of TBARS in liver and kidney tissues of ATD intoxicated rats were significantly elevated when compared to the level of TBARS in control animals. The increased lipid peroxidation results in changes in cellular metabolism of the hepatic and extra hepatic tissues, which ultimately leads to the whole cell deformity and cell death (Arun and Balasubramanian, 2011). The administration of herbal drug *P. amarus* at the different therapeutic doses showed reduction in TBARS level. The standard hepatoprotective drug Silymarin maintained the decreased lipid peroxidation level to the normal limits in the liver.

Concomitant cellular oxidative stress was manifested by reduced GSH levels and increased lipid peroxidation. The inverse linear relationship between the ROS level and the GSH level indicated that free radical species were generated by exposure to anti TB drugs which reduced intracellular antioxidant levels. The results indicate that, the herbal drug *Phyllanthus amarus* has very good hepatoprotective effect in liver damage. The results were presented in the Table 4.

Superoxide dismutase and Catalase mutually function as important enzymes in elimination of Reactive oxygen species (ROS). SOD is the major attractive metalloprotein in the antioxidant family. The defensive antioxidant enzyme next to SOD is CAT. CAT is an enzymatic antioxidant widely distributed in all animal tissues, and the highest activity is found in the red cells and liver. Both are the key component of the antioxidant defense system. In the present study, the observed decrease in SOD and CAT activities were presumably associated with the increased oxidative stress caused by these toxicants that might be due to low level of zinc (a metal constituent of the enzyme SOD) in liver tissue (Arun and Balasubramanian, 2011) Therapy at 200-400 mg/kg b.w. reversed the SOD and CAT activity in the liver tissues and protected from free radical induced oxidative stress. These observations are substantiated by author (Gnanadesigan *et al.,* 2011).(Table 5)

ATPase is a membrane bound enzyme. Since, phosphatase is a constituent of all the body tissues; it plays an important role in inorganic pyrophosphates activity. ATPase activity may be considered as a marker for assessing hepatocellular damage induced by hepatotoxic agents. (Table 6)

In our experiment, a concurrent fall was found in ATPase in liver after toxicants exposure. It might be due to dysfunctional and dystrophic changes in the mitochondria and cell membrane permeability. This damage was also very clearly visible in histopathological studies after toxicant administration. These observations are substantiated by other authors (Gao and Zhou, 2005; Krithika and Verma, 2009).The effect of the extracts on ATPase was as pronounced with 100mg/kg as with 200-400mg/kg b.w.

Liver damage induced by toxicant was associated with a variety of biochemical abnormalities following loss of integrity of the cell membrane or interference with normal hepatocytes metabolism and function.

The reason for hepatoprotective effect of the extracts may be due to presence of lignans and flavonoids which might have scavenged the free radical offering hepato protection.

5. Conclusion

The results of this study showed that common medicinal plant, *P. amarus* even at minimal dose 300mg/kg was found to have beneficial hepatoprotective properties in albino rats as all the major parameters showed percent protection level above 50% at dose levels 300 and 400mg/kg. All these properties make *P. amarus*, a novel herb for treating oxidative stress and anti Tb drug associated hepatic toxicity. There is, however, the need of further experiments for chronic study to exercise on excessive and prolonged use of this plant.

6. Histopathological studies

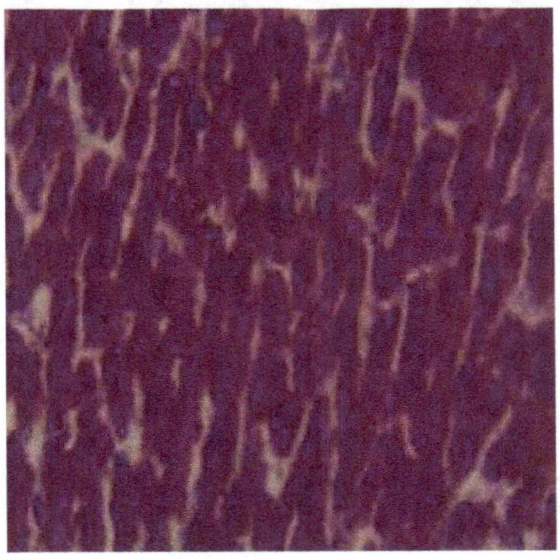

Figure 1. Hepatocytes of the normal control group showed a normal lobular architecture of the liver (400 x).

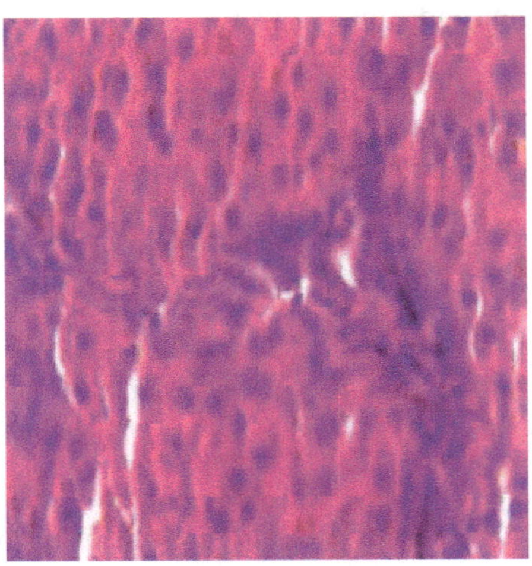

Figure 2. Hepatocytes of the INH + RIF+ PZA treated group showed liver cell necrosis and inflammation also observed in the centrilobular region with portal triaditis (400 x).

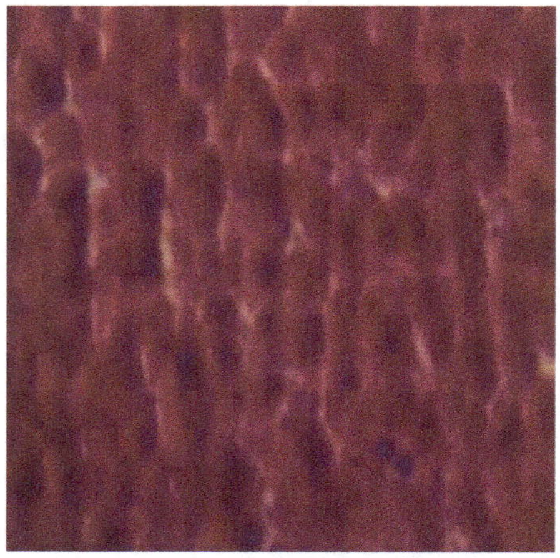

Figure 3. Hepatocytes of the *P.amarus* treated group showed cuboidal hepatocytes with moderate portal triaditis and their lobular architecture was normal (400 x).

Acknowledgements

Authors are grateful to Jiwaji University for providing lab facility and UGC for financial assistance.

Author details

Sangeeta Shukla*, Neelu Sinha and Amita Jaswal

*Address all correspondence to: profsshukla@gmail.com

School of Studies in Zoology, Jiwaji University, Gwalior, India

References

[1] Saleem TSM, Chetty CM, Ramkanth S, Rajan VST, Kumar KM, Gauthaman K (2010).Hepatoprotective Herbs – A Review. Int. J. Res. Pharm. Sci.1:1, 1-5.

[2] Ajith TA, Hema U and Aswathy MS (2007). Zingiber officinale Roscoe prevents acetaminophen-induced acute hepatotoxicity by enhancing hepatic antioxidant status. Food Chem. Toxicol.; 45(11): 2267-72.

[3] Abdelaal A, El-Ghaffar HA, Hosam M, Zaghloul E, El mashad N, Badran E and Fathy A (2009).Genotypic detection of rifampicin and isoniazid resistant Mycobacteri-

um tuberculosis strains by DNA sequencing: a randomized trial. Annals of Clinical Microbiology and Antimicrobials, 8:4.

[4] Eminzade S, Uras F and Izzettin FV. (2008). Silymarin protects liver against toxic effects of anti-tuberculosis drugs in experimental animals. Nutrition & Metabolism, 5:18.

[5] Devaraj VC, Gopala KB, Viswanatha GL, Kamath JV, Kumar S (2011). Hepatoprotective activity of Hepax-A polyherbal formulation. Asian Pacific Journal of Tropical Biomedicine. 142-146.

[6] Joshi H, Parle M (2007). Pharmacological evidences for antiamnesic potentials of *Phyllanthus amarus* in mice. African Journal of Biomedical Research, Vol. 10; 165 – 173.

[7] Lee S B, Bablanian R and Esteban M. (1996). Regulated expression of the interferon-induced protein kinase p68 (PKR) by vaccinia virus recombinants inhibits the replication of vesicular stomatitis virus but not that of poliovirus. Journal of Interferon and Cytokine Research 16, 1073-1078.

[8] Reitman and Frankel. (1957). A colorimetric method for the determination of serum glutamic oxalacetic and glutamic pyruvic transaminases. Amer. J. Clin. Pathol. 28: 56-63.

[9] Sharma SK and Krishnamurthy CR (1968). Production of lipidperoxides of brain. J Neurochem; 15: 147-9.

[10] Misra HP and Fridovich I (1972). The role of superoxide anion in the autoxidation of epinephrine and a simple assay for superoxide dismutase. J Biol Chem. 247: 3170–3175.

[11] Aebi H (1984). Catalase in vitro; Methods Enzymol. 105. 121–126

[12] Ranawat L, Bhatt J and Patel J. (2010). Hepatoprotective activity of ethanolic extracts of bark of Zanthoxylum armatum DC in CCl4 induced hepatic damage in rats. J. Ethnopharmacol. 127(3):777-780.

[13] Muriel P, EscobarY (2003). Kupffer cells are responsible for liver cirrhosis induced by carbon tetrachloride. J. App. Toxicol., 23(2):103-108.

[14] Thirunavukkarasu C, Sakthisekaran D (2003).Influence of sodium selenite on glycoprotein contents in normal and N-nitrosodiethylamine initiated and Phenobarbital promoted rat liver tumors. Pharmacol Res 48(2):167-73.

[15] Zimmerman L (1973).Podiatry and the law.J Am Podiatry Assoc, 63; 691-3.

[16] Adebisi SA, Oluboyo PO, Okesina AB (2000).Effect of drug-induced hyperuricaemia on renal function in Nigerians with pulmonary tuberculosis. Afr J Med Med Sci. 3-4:297-300.

[17] Adewole SO, Salako AA, Doherty OW, Naicker T (2007). Effect of melatonin on carbon tetrachloride-induced kidney injury in Wistar rats. Afr. *J. Biomed. Res.,* 10: 153-164.

[18] Arun K and Balasubramanian U (2011).Comapartive study on hepatoprotective activity of *phyllanthus amarus* and *eclipta prostrata* against alcohol induced in albino rats. International journal of environmental sciences volume 2:1.

[19] Gnanadesigan M, Ananad M, Ravikumar S, Maruthupandy M, Syed Ali M, Vijayakumar V, Kumaraguru AK (2011).Antibacterial potential of biosynthesized silver nanoparticles using *Avicennia marina* mangrove plant, Applied Nanoscience.

[20] Gao H, Zhou YW (2005).World. J. Gastroenterol.11, 3671.

[21] Krithika R and VERMA R J (2009). Ameliorative potential of phyllanthus amarus against carbon tetrachloride-induced hepatotoxicity. Acta Poloniae Pharmaceutica ñ Drug Research, 66(5)-579-583.

[22] Snedecor GW, Cochran, WG (1989).Statistical method.8th edition Ames,IA:Affiliated east-West Press;217-36.

[23] Rajeshkumar NV, Joy KL, Kuttan G, Ramsewak RS, Nair MG, Kuttan R (2002). Antitumour and anticarcinogenic activity of Phyllanthus amarus extract. J Ethnopharmacol.81(1):17-22.

[24] Narah M, Kalita JC, Kotoky J (2012). Medicinal plants with potential anticancer activities: a review. International Research Journal of Pharmacy.3 (6)

4

Copper Deficiency a New Reason of Androgenetic Alopecia?

Margarita G. Skalnaya

1. Introduction

Androgenetic alopecia is the common type of hair loss in men and women since puberty. Typically, AA is the complex result of an androgen-dependent process and this process is located to androgen receptor (AR) areas (frontal and vertex zone). Number of androgen receptors is genetic transmission. The polymorphism involving the CAG triple repeat expansion of the AR protein has been revealed in men with AA. This male pattern hair loss may represents from influence of minimal androgen excess basing on genetically sensitive hair papilla.

Dihydrotestosterone (DHT) is derived from circulating testosterone (T) inhibits cell proliferation in the dermal papilla and local production of vascular endothelial growth factor [1]. As a result, the DHT-dependent process leads to the miniaturization of sensitive hair follicles and progressive thinning the scalp hair. It is known that the follicular dermal papilla controls hair growth. Steroid hormones, including androgens, estrogens and glucocorticoids may influence on timing of hair cycle [2].

More recent studies have focused on androgen-regulated hair growth. But, studies of action of other steroids in the hair follicle have been relatively limited. There are two estrogen receptors (ERα and ERβ) which bind to 17β-estradiol. The effects of estrogens seem complex whereby estrogen prolongs the anagen phase of the hair follicle and stimulates hair shaft elongation [2]. ERβ expression was found in outer root shaft and epithelial matrix. In contrast, ERα and AR were expressed in dermal papilla [3].Therefore, the ratio of ERα to ERβ in dermal papilla cells is extremely important. Estrogen also modifies androgen metabolism. The local production of estrogens from androgen precursors has been converted by the aromatase cytochrome P 450 enzyme complex. It is now clear there is aromatase expression in the dermal papilla and the outer root sheath. The activity of aromatase is higher in women in occipital

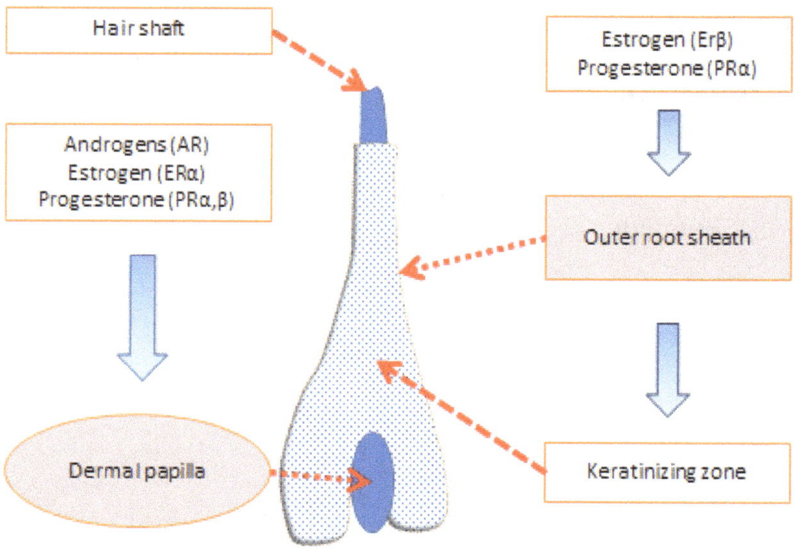

Figure 1. The hair shaft

scalp area compared to the frontal scalp and it has been diminished in AA [4]. Some researchers found that estradiol inhibited 5 alpha-reductase activities [5]. The effects on estrogens might be explained by an increased conversion of T to the weaker androgens such as androstendione and androstendiol. Progesterone is able to modulate activity of DHT in dermal papilla by 75% [4, 6]. Also, progesterone is widely recognized as a marker of estrogen action and has anti-inflammatory properties. Progesterone regulates the expression of matrix metalloproteinases (MMPs) by transforming growth factor-β [7].

However, in women hair loss is not limited to only this location and combined with diffuse alopecia. Except in some cases, treatment of 5 alpha reductase inhibitors is ineffective in women. The origin and mechanisms of AA in women are different and more complicated than in men and remain a challenge.

The aim of the work was to estimate a possible role of trace elements (TE) changes in AA in man and women.

2. Materials and methods

In this study, 97 women and 40 men, ages 20-55 y., with AA were selected for the determination of TE content and CP in serum, hormonal status. Diagnosis of AA was based on clinical findings, pattern of increased hair thinning on frontal/vertex scalp with greater hair density on occipital scalp zone; retention of frontal hairline; and the presence of miniaturized hairs (vellus hair, diameter less 30 μkm). Detailed study of the consumption of drugs, iron intake and thyroid metabolism ruled out other types of alopecia. The degree of AA was determined

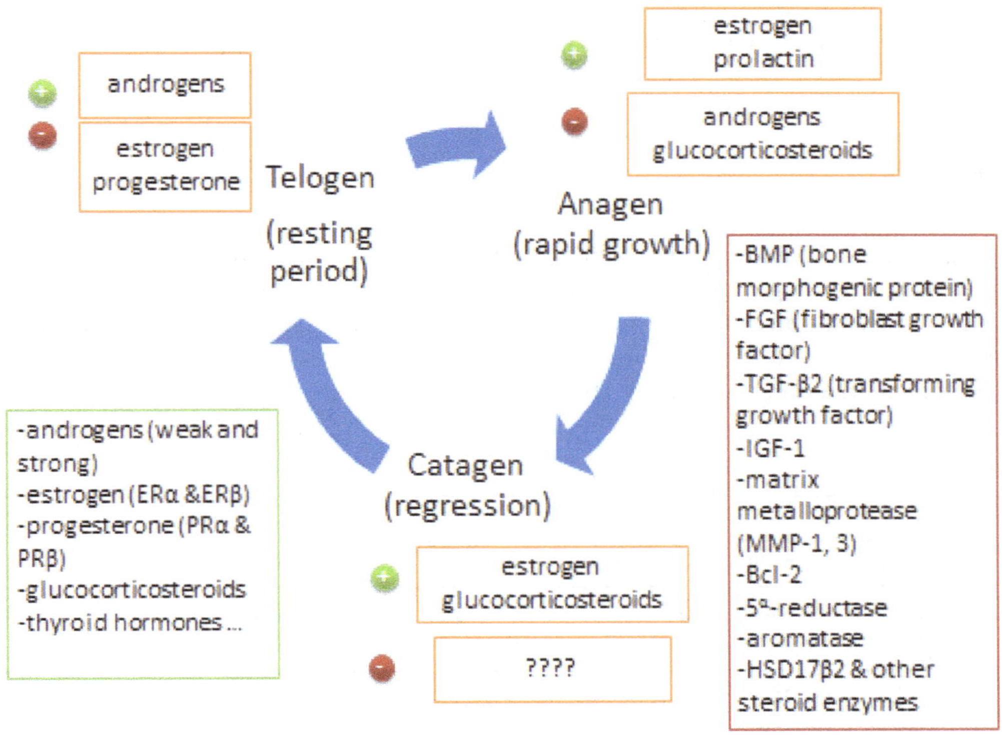

Figure 2. The timing of the hair cycle

by application of Ludwig scales (II–III). Exclusion criteria were: replacement hormone therapy (RHT) with estrogens, progesterone, testosterone, L-thyroxin or corticoids during last 6 months. Women's group was divided by 5 subgroups: women with excess of androgens, ages before 40 and after 40 y.o. (22 and 19 correspondently), women with excess of estrogens before and after 40 y.o. (24 and 17) and women with obesity at age of 20-40 year (16 patients). Women had both AA and the other sings of elevated androgens level (hirsutism and acne) were included in group with excess of androgens (HA 1 and 2). Women in group with excess of estrogens had endometriosis, uterine leiomyoma or combining both of these (HE 1 and 2). Childbearing aged women with abdominal obesity (waist >88 cm.) and excess of ALT concentration in blood were enrolled in group with obesity (O1). Control group included in age-matched men and women (76 and 32 patients correspondently) who presented no diseases at the time of examine. The concentration of TE has been analyzed by ICP mass-spectrometer Nexion-300D and Elan-9000 (Perkin Elmer Corp., USA). Reference materials of serum and hair samples were used. The level of FSH (follicle-stimulated hormone), LT (leuteotpophic), 17β-estradiol (E2), progesterone (PR), prolactin, androstendione (A), dihydrotestosterone (DHT) and sex hormone bound globulin (SHPG) was tested by routine laboratory methods.

Statistical analyses were performed with the ANOVA software (Statistics version 7). We applied non parametrical statistics: median, 25 and 75 percentiles. Student's t-test was used to compare the values of quantitative variables. Correlations among variables were studied using the Pearson's coefficient. $P \leq 0.05$ was considered significant in all analyses.

3. Results

No significant differences of TE serum content in men and women were found between AA patients and control group. The exception was the concentration of copper (Cu) which was statistically significant differences between men and women suffering from AA and matched control (Table 1). In present work in women with hyperandrogenism there are the some trends in TE content in serum than in men. The key disorder was decreased Cu level in frontal zones of scalp hair and serum.

Element	Men				Women			
	AA group, n=40		Control, n=32		AA group, n=97		Control, n=76	
	Median	Persencile (25-75)	Median	Persencile (25-75)	Median	Persencile (25-75)	Median	Persencile (25-75)
As	0,019	0,015-0,025	0,015	0,008-0,028	0,018	0,007-0,028	0,02	0,01-0,032
Ca	92,3	88,2- 98,5	96,1	91,0-101,0	95,8	90,6-102,4	95,3	89,6-103,3
Co	0,0005	0,0004-0,0006	0,0006	0,0004-0,0007	0,006	0,0005-0,0008	0,0006	0,0005-0,0008
Cu	***0,80***	***0,70-0,85***	***0,88****	***0,75-1,06***	***0,85***	***0,77-0,94***	***0,99****	***0,90-1,11***
Fe	1,3	1,0-1,5	1,4	1,3-1,5	1,3	1,0-1,6	1,2	0,78-1,46
K	183	169-196	187	178-199	170	158-193	178	157-204
Mg	20,7	19,9-21,2	20,7	19,3-22,4	20,3	19,1-21,5	20,8	19,4-22,4
Mn	0,0034	0,0030-0,0038	0,0037	0,0031-0,0048	0,0032	0,0027-0,0039	0,0032	0,0026-0,0043
Mo	0,0008	0,0007-0,0012	0,0009	0,0007-0,0012	0,0009	0,0007-0,0012	0,001	0,0008-0,0014
Ni	0,006	0,005-0,007	0,006	0,005-0,008	0,006	0,005-0,007	0,006	0,005-0,008
Se	0,14	0,13-0,16	0,16	0,13-0,17	0,14	0,13-0,17	0,14	0,13-0,16
Zn	0,89	0,83-1,04	0,91	0,82-1,10	0,81	0,72-0,95	0,83	0,69-1,06

*-P<0, 01 (differences between control group and AA's group)

Table 1. Trace elements content (mkg/ml) in serum in men and women with AA

In spite of sex decreased Cu concentration in serum were obtained in patients with AA. However, Cu level in women was higher in comparison to men.

Median, 25-th and 75-th percentiles values in women with AA and accompanying other diseases are summarized in Table 2.

Element	HA1 n=22	HA2 n=19	O1 n=24	HE1 n=17	HE2 n=16	Control n=76
As	0,017 (0,007-0,031)	0,020 (0,008-0,031)	0,016 (0,006-0,038)	0,014 (0,006-0,023)	0,012 (0,007-0,031)	0,020 (0,010-0,032)
Ca	95,8 (91,5-98,0)	101,1 (89,3-104,0)	91,3 (87,2-97,5)	97,8 (87,1-100,5)	93,5 (91,7-97,1)	95,3 (89,6-103,3)
Co	0,0006 (0,0005-0,0007)	0,0005 (0,0004-0,0007)	0,0006 (0,0004-0,0008)	0,0007 (0,0005-0,0008)	0,0007 (0,0005-0,0010)	0,0006 (0,0005-0,0008)
Cu	0,81* (0,72-0,89)	0,85* (0,80-0,91)	0,94 (0,81-1,08)	0,97** (0,86-1,19)	0,99** (0,89-1,21)	0,99 (0,90-1,11)
Fe	1,3 (1,1-1,7)	1,2 (1,1-1,4)	1,2 (0,8-1,6)	1,3 (0,4-1,5)	1,1 (0,6-1,4)	1,2 (0,8-1,5)
K	183 (164-204)	193 (169-291)	183 (165-194)	195 (175-234)	170 (153-190)	178 (157-204)
Mg	20,4 (19,1-21,8)	20,9 (20,1-22,1)	19,6 (18,4-21,4)	20,5 (18,7-22,3)	19,6 (18,1-20,5)	20,8 (19,4-22,4)
Mn	0,0033 (0,0027-0,0040)	0,0035 (0,0030-0,0039)	0,0031 (0,0026-0,0034)	0,0030 (0,0027-0,0035)	0,0033 (0,0027-0,0036)	0,0032 (0,0026-0,0043)
Mo	0,0009 (0,0007-0,0013)	0,0007 (0,0005-0,0010)	0,0009 (0,0006-0,0011)	0,0008 (0,0006-0,0009)	0,0007 (0,0007-0,0008)	0,0010 (0,0008-0,0014)
Ni	0,006 (0,005-0,007)	0,006 (0,005-0,007)	0,006 (0,004-0,007)	0,005 (0,005-0,006)	0,005 (0,004-0,006)	0,006 (0,005-0,008)
Se	0,15 (0,13-0,16)	0,14 (0,14-0,16)	0,15 (0,13-0,16)	0,14 (0,12-0,16)	0,14 (0,13-0,15)	0,14 (0,13-0,16)
Zn	0,93 (0,82-1,05)	0,85 (0,75-1,07)	0,70* (0,66-0,76)	0,89 (0,80-0,95)	0,79 (0,69-1,19)	0,83 (0,69-1,06)
Cu/Mn	239 (187-306)	245 (213-277)	319 (278-369)	336** (300-438)	349** (282-420)	288 (253-370)
Cu/Zn	0,82* (0,73-1,06)	1,01 (0,76-1,14)	1,31* (1,22-1,40)	1,12 (1,04-1,25)	1,12 (0,82-1,50)	1,22 (0,94-1,42)

*-P<0,005 (differences between control group and others)

**-P<0, 05 (differences between groups with excess of androgens (HA1) and estrogens (HE 1 or 2)).

Table 2. TE content and ratio Cu/Mn and Cu/Zn (Median, 25-75th percentiles) in women with AA and associated with different diseases.

When we separated women with AA into subgroups there have obtained differences between control and investigated groups. No significant differences were found between AA patients and control in the majority of TE content in serum. Although the lowest Cu content was observed in group combining AA with other sing of excess of androgens such as hirsutism and acne.

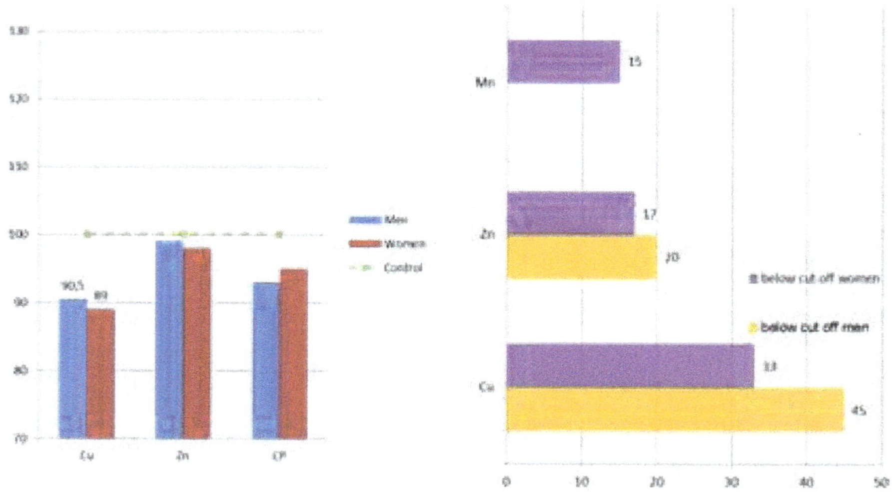

Figure 3. Content of Cu, Zn and ceruloplasmin (CP) in men and women with AA

Cu concentration in groups with elevated androgens level and with appearance of several marks of androgens abundance was lower than in the whole women group with AA. There were statistically significant differences between Cu level in groups with plenty of androgens and estrogen. In case of being endometriosis or uterine leiomyoma (HE1 and 2) in women Cu concentration in serum have maintained the same than in control, although not decreased in patients with AA. The overflowed androgens in women were conducted the reduction Cu content in serum considerably. The zinc (Zn) level was the lowest in women who combined AA and abdominal obesity. There was variety Zn content in serum in women at ages. In women under 40 year of age either elevated androgens or excess of estrogen the Zn level was getting low as compared to women before 40 year. The ratio Cu/Mn in women HE1 and 2 groups has been elevated significantly in comparison with groups with excess of androgens.

There was a tendency to raise the ratio Cu/Mn in women with elevated estrogen level as compared to control. The ratio Cu/Zn was significant lower in women any ages with abundant of androgens than in control. But, in case of abdominal obesity the values of this ratio were higher in comparison with control group.

4. Discussion

The hair follicle represents a unique, highly regenerative neuroectodermal – mesodermal interaction system. These transformations are controlled by changes in the expression/ activity

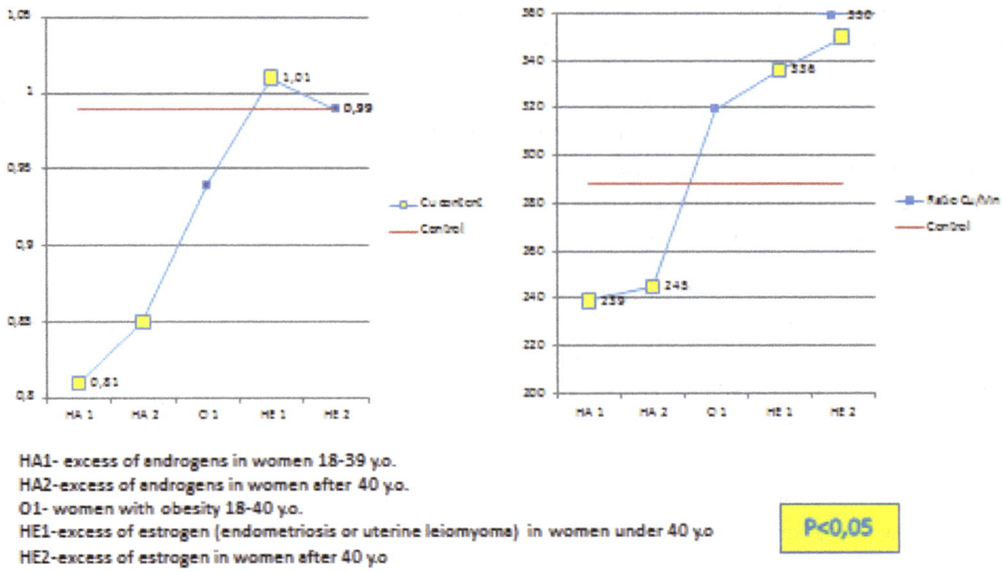

Figure 4. Cu content and ratio Cu/Mn in women with AA

of a numerous growing factors, cytokines, hormones, neurotransmitters, as well as transcription factors and enzymes.

Alopecia areata (AA) is the most common type of alopecia that the onset after puberty in both sexes. AA may affect up to 70 of men and 40% of women [8]. Male and female pattern hair loss are clinically distinct entities but pathogenically indistinguishable. The main role in the onset of AA in men is local disturbances in androgens metabolism which based on genetic predisposes to converse of terminal hair in vellus-like hair. AA is a polygenetic hereditary disease. A low number of CAG repeats in the androgen receptor gene implies increased risk factor for AA; prostate hyperplasia, coronary heart disease. But the role of sex hormones in females is less understood. Same of women suffering from AA are revealed androgens excess with other signs of elevated androgens such as hirsutism, acne, polycystic ovary syndrome. In women there is the appearance of AA combining with diffuse hair loss [9].

AA in men is due to implicate DNT production by 5 alpha-reductase type 2. The primary precursor of DHT in men is testosterone. The androgen receptor (AR) binding leads to increase production of cytokines such as TGFβ-1 and 2, which promote telogen, thinning and shortening hair. There is a low number of AR in occipital hair follicles that hair loss is mostly restricted to the scalp vertex and frontal and temporal areas. The using of a type 2 – selective inhibitor demonstrated the improvements in scalp hair growth in men. On stopping finasteride treatment, the balding process resumed. However, finasteride has been associated with depressive symptoms, persistent sexual side effects (loss of libido and erectile function). In contract to its beneficial effects of finasteride (5 alpha–reductase's inhibitor) in men; it didn't improve hair growth in women with AA. These findings suggested that the molecular mechanisms involved in the different metabolic ways in regulations hair growth in women.

Women with some markers of insulin resistant have increased risk of AA [9]. Several studies have analyzed the relationship between androgenetic alopecia and cardiovascular disease. Women with AGA showed higher significant mean values than non-alopecic women for all the parameters (triglyceridaemia, LDL-C, total cholesterol, total cholesterol/HDL-C and LDL-C/HDL-C) and lower significant HDL-C than controls.

Estrogens are indirect anti-androgens which increase SHMG production by binding to androgens and reducing their bioavailability. The production of estrogens from androgens via aromatase is of the importance in hair follicles. The comparison of scalp biopsies from men and women with AA revealed aromatase levels to be higher in hair follicles from occipital area in comparison to the frontal hair follicles. Furthermore, aromatase levels has found in six times higher in women when compared to men. Recent study has demonstrated that both dermal papilla and outer root sheath expressed aromatase activity. The levels of ER expression and aromatase activity may be modulated by steroid hormones in other tissues it would be important in the hair follicle. Likewise androgens have been reported to alter the ration of ERα to ERβ [2]. The alteration in the ratio of ERα to ERβ in dermal papilla cells could promote E2 signaling via ERβ in preference to ERα.

Since the hair follicles has been shown to express AR, glucocorticoid receptor, ERα, ERβ and progesterone receptors (PRα and PRβ). Both the dermal papilla cells and surrounding epithelial cells express ER. Additional local productions of E2 via conversion from A by aromatase may act in either an autocrine or paracrine manner to control lair growth and differentiation. In experimental studies PR inhibited the synthesis of DHT in dermal papilla by 75%. E2 was less able inhibit its production [6].

However, no direct effects of prolactin on hair growth have been reported [11]. Progesterone acts via PR receptors on cells to induce secretion of paracrine factor that in turn stimulate the expression 17β –hydroxysteroid dehydrogenase type 2 (HSD17β2). HSD17β2 metabolizes E2 to weak estrogenic estrone. The control of hair growth by E2 is much more complex than previously appreciated.

The E2 may modulate hair growth by interfering with androgen metabolism [12]. The estrogenic effects on dermal papilla cells are mediated via ERα.The role of ERβ may be to protect tissues from oxidative stress by inducing battery of antioxidative enzymes. Under hyperestrogenic conditions, the ratio PRβ to PRα is decreased but ratio ERβ to ERα is elevated in endometriosis and uterine leiomyoma. Serum Cu level is known to control by estrogens. Under excess of androgens Cu content in serum was decreased and associated with elevated DHT level which results of 5alpha-reductase type 2 activities. The pathogenic mechanism of AA is case of abundant of androgens doesn't differ in men and women with high androgens level. The development of AA shows up other clinical marks of androgens excess (hirsutism and acne) and reflect the interaction androgens and estrogen metabolism. Both AR and ERα are located into dermal papilla and influenced on hair growth [4]. In some studies have shown there was depressed ratio E2 to androgens [13].

We demonstrated the development of AA in women with endometriosis or /and uterine leiomyoma. These diseases have usually revealed of estrogens excess, high activity of aromatase and decreased level of progesterone. There was a high level of ratio ERβ to ERα against the background of changed ratio progesterone receptor (PRα/PRβ). The onset and development of AA in this group didn't link to abundant androgens level.

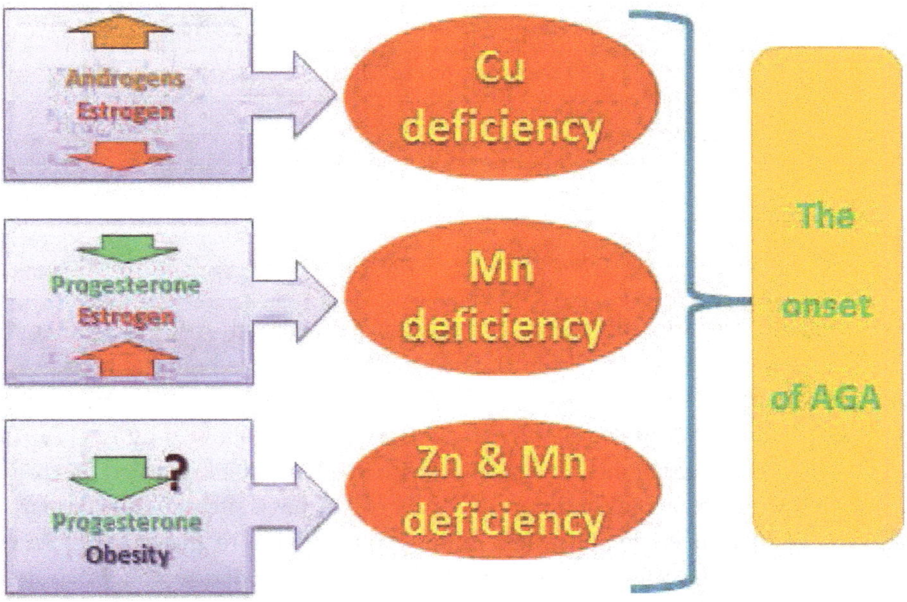

Figure 5. Proposed schema of TE dependent androgenetic alopecia

Normal or excess estrogens concentration and deficiency or resistant to progesterone were typical in these women. Cu content in serum and ratio Cu/Mn determined higher than in control. But, Mn level in these groups remains lower to compare with control. These data suggest that the important value in appearance of AA belongs to the relationship between E2 and PR and ratio of their receptors in peripheral tissues. About 15% from all examined women with AA have been detected the cut-off Mn level. Mn is known to impede the female and male reproductive function. In experimental studies the relationship Mn concentration and progesterone level have been shown. There is the high level of Mn-COD in lutein phase of menstrual cycle [14]. Manganese superoxide dismutase (Mn–COD), an antioxidant enzyme in the mitochondria, protects cells by scavenging superoxide radicals. Mn–COD increases by inducing progesterone. Experimental data suggests that Mn down-regulated steroidogenesis in Leydig cells [15]. Mn influences the receptor signaling pathways and contractile machinery of vascular smooth muscle cells [16]. The expression of Mn-COD was significantly increased by 17β–estrogen and testosterone in neutrophil granulocytes in healthy volunteers [17]. In our work we hypothesize that the assignment of low Mn content may reflect depressed value of PR, changed ratio PR receptors or cell's resistance to PR.

In women serum ferritin levels may also be assessed to determine hair loss. Appreciating the importance of iron as a factor in hair loss may be important in the therapy in a variety of etiologically distinct forms of hair loss. According to obtained findings there was no statistical difference in iron content between control and experimental groups [18].

Condition	excess of A	excess of estrogen
Hormonal status	↑ A→DHT	↑E, ↓Progesterone, ± A
Receptors	AR→ alteration ratio ERα/ERß	alteration ratio ERα/ERß and PRβ/PRα
Age	after puberty	middle age and premenopausal
Treatment	decrease level of A and modulation of ratio ER's	increase level of progesterone and modulation of ratio ER's

Table 3. The difference of the onset and development of AA under excess of androgen or estrogen.

In this hypothetic scenario, there were two groups' women with AA. One of them has been registered excess of A in serum (Table 3). The other demonstrated normal level of A but had the alteration of estrogen and progesterone contents in blood. A lot of hormones, growth's factors take part in development of AA. Many diseases have followed by AA. Typically, the excess of A in blood in both men and women with AA have been revealed. Surprisingly, in women with hyperestrogenic condition the onset of AA have shown. The comparable with control level of A has been demonstrated in this group. Therefore, the ratio of ERα to ERß in follicular dermal papilla cells may be important. The alteration of estrogen, progesterone and androgen receptors has the key of metabolic disturbances in dermal papilla cells and outer root sheath. That is why the typical approaches for treatment of AA which include in using hormonal replacement therapy, inhibitors of DHT production and others were not fruitful.

Author details

Margarita G. Skalnaya*

Address all correspondence to: skalnaya@yandex.ru

Center for Biotic Medicine, Moscow, Russia

References

[1] Jamin C. Androgenetic alopecia. //Ann. Dermato.l Venereol.-2002.-Vol. 129.-N.5 (Pt 2).-P.801-803.

[2] Thornton M.J. et al. The modulation of aromatase and estrogen receptor alpha in cultured human dermal papilla cells by dexamethasone: a novel mechanism for selective action of estrogen via estrogen receptor beta? //J. Investigative Dermatology.-2006.-Vol. 126.-P. 2010-2018.

[3] Ohnemus U. et al. The Hair Follicle as an Estrogen Target and Source. // Endocrine Reviews.-2006.-Vol. 27.-N. 6.-P. 677-706.

[4] Hoffmann R. Enzymology of the hair follicle. //European J. Dermatology.-2001.-Vol. 11.-N. 4.-P. 296-300.

[5] Hoffmann R. et al. 17alpha-estradiol induces aromatase activity in intact human anagen hair follicles ex vivo. //Exp. Dermatol. – 2002.-Vol.11.-N.4.-P. 376-380.

[6] Niiyama S, Happle R, Hoffmann R. //Influence of estrogens on the androgen metabolism in different subunits of human hair follicles. //Eur. J. Dermatol. – 2001.-Vol.11.-N.3.-P. 195-198.

[7] Chevronnay G.H.P. et al. Regulation of matrix metalloproteinases activity studied in human endometrium as a paradigm of cyclic tissue breakdown and regeneration. // Biochim. Biophys. Acta.-2012.-Vol. 1824.-N. 1.-P. 146-156.

[8] Kevin J. et al. Promising therapies for treating and /or preventing androgenic alopecia. //Skin Therapy Lett.-2012.-Vol. 17.-N. 6.-P.1-4.

[9] Arias-Santiago S. et al. A comparative study of dyslipidaemia in men and women with androgenic alopecia. //Acta Derm. Venereol.-2010.-Vol. 90.-P. 485-487.

[10] Niiyama R., Happle R. and Hoffmann R. Influence of estrogens on the androgen metabolism in different subunits of human hair follicles. //Eur. J. Dermatol.-2001.-Vol. 11.-N.3.-P. 195-198.

[11] Craven A.J. et al. Prolactin signaling influences the timing mechanism of the hair follicle: analysis of hair growth cycles in prolactin receptor knockout mice. //Endocrinology.-2001.-Vol. 142.-N. 6.-P. 2533-2539.

[12] Ohnemus U. et al. Hair cycle control by estrogens: catagen induction via estrogen receptor (ER)-α is checked by ER-β signaling. //Endocrinology.-2005.-Vol. 146.-N. 3.-P. 1214-1225.

[13] Matthew D. et al. Extra-adrenal glucocorticoids and mineralocorticoids: evidence for local synthesis, regulation and function. //Am. J. Physiol. Endocrinol. Metab.-2011.-Vol. 301.-P. 11-24.

[14] Sugino N. et al. Superoxide dismutase expression in the human corpus luteum during the menstrual cycle and in early pregnancy. //Mol. Hum. Reprod. – 2000. – Vol. 6. – N. 1. – P. 19-25.

[15] Cheng J., Fu J.L. and Zhou Z.C. The inhibitory effects of manganese on steroidogenesis in rat primary Leydig cells by disrupting steroidogenic acute regulatory (StAR) protein expression. // Toxicology.-2003.-Vol. 187.-N. 2-3.-P. 139-148.

[16] Kalea A.Z., Harris P.D. and Klimis-Zacas D.J. Dietary manganese suppresses alpha 1 adrenergic receptor-mediated vascular contraction. //J. Nutr. Biochem. – 2005.-Vol. 16.-N. 1.-P. 44-49.

[17] Adler I. et al. The effect of certain steroid hormones on the expression on genes involved in the metabolism of free radicals. //Gynecol. Endocrinol.-2012.-Vol.

[18] Kantor J.et al. Decreased serum ferritin is associated with alopecia in women. // J. Investigative Dermatology.-2003.-Vol.121.-P. 985–988.

5

Clinical and Hematological Profiles During Valproate Treatment of Epileptic Patients with Intellectual Disability

P. Kaipainen, T. Westermarck, F. Atroshi,
M. Kaski and M. Iivanainen

1. Introduction

Valproic acid or sodium valproate (VPA) is an antiepileptic drug commonly used for treatment of epilepsies [Aldenkamp et al. 2006; Ben-Menachem et al. 2006; Iivanainen & Alvarez 1998; Perucca et al. 2006). It affects the function of the neurotransmitter GABA in the human brain by enhancing the neurotransmission of GABA (Rosenberg, 2007). VPA is known to cause many harmful side effects such as hepatotoxicity (Koenig et al. 2006) and carnitine deficiency (Coppola et al. 2006). Carnitine as a healing agent has begun to play an important role in VPA-induced hepatotoxicity. When signs of hepatotoxicity occur, it is important to discontinue VPA immediately and substitute carnitine i.v (Koenig et al. 2006). Inhibitions of the β-oxidation, oxidative phoshorylation and urea synthesis and a decrease of intracellular carnitine are supposed to induce hepatopathy (Cotarlu & Zaldman 1988; Hjelm et al. 1987; Murakami et al. 1996). It has been reported that urinary concentration of a VPA metabolite, 4-en VPA, is markedly increased in acute VPA intoxication (Murakami et al. 1996). It is believed that this metabolite of VPA is responsible for developing hepatotoxicity. VPA metabolism returns to normal after L-carnitine supplementation (Murakami et al. 1996). Thurston & Hauhart 1993 reported that a reduction of intracellular CoA may be the central common pathway for VPA-induced hepatotoxicity.

The clinical relevance of coagulopathies, known as side effects of VPA, especially thrombocytopenia, von Willebrand disease and a decrease of factor XIII, is still unclear (Gerstner et al. 2006). The incidence of coagulation disorders related to VPA in children is estimated to be nearly 4% (Gerstner et al. 2006).

It has been reported that VPA may be associated with hyperammonemia and thrombocytopenia, but the aetiology of valproic acid-induced thrombocytopenia has not been elucidated (Mallet et al. 2004). In patients receiving long-term VPA VPA-induced hyperammonaemic encephalopathy may occur (Lheureux et al. 2005). It is suggested that this severe side-effect may be promoted by a pre-existing carnitine deficiency or by deficiency induced by VPA (Lheureux et al. 2005). Because the onset of the clinical symptoms of VPA-associated hepatotoxicity, especially in patients with intellectual disability, is sudden and unpredictable, the aim of our study was to find out suitable biochemical and haematological markers to prevent this state of illness.

2. Case presentation

Blood samples for assays of sodium (Na), potassium (K), aspartate aminotransferase (ASAT), alanine aminotranferase (ALAT), amylase, alkaline phosphatase, c-reactive protein (CRP), creatinine, haemoglobin, mean cell volume, haematocrit, erythrocytes, thrombocytes and leukocytes were obtained from ID patients with epilepsy and on VPA and from healthy persons of hospital staff after overnight fasting. All patients in this study used VPA as a monotherapy. Vacuette serum tubes were used to obtain serum samples and vacuette K_2EDTA tubes were used to obtain haematological samples. All assays were made immediately after sampling in the same day. The whole large patient material was from Rinnekoti hospital, Espoo-Finland. Sex and age varied in the VPA and control groups. Approximately 50% from the whole patient and control material was male. The mean ages for the VPA group and the control group were 37±15 years and 50±10 years, respectively. Laboratory determinations and reagents:Serum sodium (Na), potassium (K), aspartate aminotransferase (ASAT), alanine aminotransferase (ALAT), amylase, alkaline phosphatase, c-reactive protein (CRP) and creatinine were analyzed with Cobas Mira analyzer. Haemoglobin, mean cell volume (MCV), hematocrit, erythrocytes, thrombocytes and leukocytes were assayed with Sysmex KX-21N analyzer. All used reagents were reagent grade. All laboratory determinations were controlled with the control samples from Labquality Ltd, Helsinki, Finland.

3. Discussion and review

The levels of CRP and potassium (K) were higher while haematocrit and contents of thrombocytes and erythrocytes and the levels of sodium (Na), creatinine and haemoglobin were lower in the VPA group compared with the control group. All results of 14 clinical and haematological markers are shown in table 1. The results showed that thrombocyte and erythrocyte counts, haematocrit and the levels of sodium (Na), creatinine and hemoglobin were lower in the VPA group compared with the control group. Differences in haematocrit and thrombocyte and erythrocyte counts were statistically extremely significant so that these determinations besides assay of serum free carnitine can be used as markers to evaluate VPA toxicity. The haematological profile is the most common investigations patients undergo.

Many structural, biochemical and physiological changes take place in the brain following head trauma which in turn account for epileptogenesis (Katayama et al. 1990). For example, seizures occur in rats shortly after traumatic injury lead to increase in glutamate and aspartate levels which explain possible involvement in epileptogenesis (Nilson et al. 1994). Antiepileptic drugs affect hepatic enzyme levels in patients known to have a coexisting hepatic abnormality, those who develop symptoms of hepatic involvement while receiving AEDs, and perhaps those receiving bitherapy with high serum AED levels (Verma & Haidukewych, 1994). Rao et al. (1993) reported 72% of the AED-treated patients and 33% of the unmedicated patients showed an increase in one or several serum liver enzymes [alanine aminotransferase (ALT), aspartate aminotransferase (AST), and/or gamma-glutamyl transferase (gamma-GT)]; particularly gamma-GT.

The World Health Organisation defines anaemia as < 13 g Hb/dL for men and < 12 g Hb/dL for women (2001), accepting that women generally have lower haemoglobin concentrations than men. However, when ferritin levels (Waalen et al. 2002), is considered then the difference may be due to hormonal influences on red cell production (Shahidi, 1973), the do not support this (Waalen et al. 2002). Platelet counts have been found to be significantly higher in women (Butkiewicz et al.2006), with possible explanations of increased thrombopoietin in women being reported. Total leukocyte count showed to be significantly higher in women than men due to a highly significant difference in neutrophil count, with no significant correlation between monocytes, basophils and gender (Bain & England, 1975).

This study is in line with the earlier observations that VPA may induce thrombocytopenia (Koenig et al. 2006; Gerstner et al. 2006; Mallet et al. 2004). According to Gerstner et al. 2006 thrombocytopenia is the most common haematological adverse effect of VPA. An incidence varies from 5% to 60% (Gerstner et al. 2006; Zeller et al. 1999). It is suggested that there are two possible mechanisms inducing thrombocytopenia. First mechanism is that VPA have a direct toxic effect on bone marrow (Gertsner et al. 2006). Second mechanism is that VPA seems to induce the formation of autoantibody against platelets (Sandler et al. 1978). We found that contents of thrombocytes and erythrocytes lowered approximately 30 % and 10 %, respectively, in patients on VPA monotherapy. This observation supports the hypothesis that VPA seems to have a direct toxic effect on bone marrow (Gerstner et al. 2006).

To prevent severe hepatotoxicity in patients on long-term VPA therapy, it is important to control contents of thrombocytes and erythrocytes and to determine the level of serum free carnitine, regularly. If the level of serum free carnitine and the thrombocyte counts are lowered, addition of carnitine to long-term VPA regimen of epileptic patients may be indicated. Further investigations are needed to evaluate appropriate dosages of L-carnitine supplementation to epileptic patients on long-term VPA therapy.

Valproic acid (N-dipropylacetic acid, or 2-propylpentanoic acid) is one of the mainstays of therapy for epilepsy and bipolar mood disorders, due to its anticonvulsant and mood-stabilizing effects (Blaheta & Cinatl, 2002). It is a branched short-chain fatty acid with a half-life of 9 to 16 hours. Clinically, VPA is usually administered as uncoated tablets, but may also be administered in the form of syrup, capsules and enteric-coated tablets. Ninety per cent of VPA in the blood is bound to albumin (Cramer & Mattson, 1979), and despite its hydrophilic nature enters the CNS by crossing the blood brain barrier via passive diffusion and bidirectional carrier-mediated transport, such as an anion exchanger at the brain capillary endothelium (Perucca, 2002). VPA crosses into the brain parenchyma utilizing another set of transporters which results in higher neuronal and glial concentrations than interstitial fluid concentrations (Perucca, 2002). VPA, in addition to being an effective anticonvulsant and mood-stabilizing agent has been shown to be an effective anxiolytic (Lal et al., 1980), antidystonic and antinociceptive (Loscher, 1999), in animal studies. Clinically, VPA is effective in clinical depression (Delucchi & Calabrese, 1989), absence seizures (Coppola et al., 2004), tonic-clonic seizures, complex partial seizures (Dean & Penry, 1988), and juvenile myoclonic epilepsy (Calleja et al., 2001).

4. Haematological toxicity of valproic acid

Valproic acid has been shown to have some haematological toxicity. Acute toxicity is not common and the most adverse effects are nausea, vomiting, anorexia, thrombocytopenia, von Willebrand disease type 1, decreased factor XIII, abnormal platelet function, bleeding, haemolytic anaemia, leukopenia, leucocytosis, eosinophilia, thrombocytosis, prolonged prothrombin and thromboplastin times, fibrinogen and hematoma (Kreuz et al 1992; Gerstner et al. 2006; Gerstner et al, 2008; Pan et al 2007; Mazaira, 2008; Chen et al. 2013). However, some of these effects may lead to adverse effects and life-threatining complications such as bone marrow toxicity (Acharya & Bussel, 2000). Pharmacokinetics drug interaction involves a drug displacement from protein binding sites causing drug redistribution (McQueen & Wardell, 1971). Valproic acid is commonly used in the treatment of seizures and as a mood stabilizer in the treatment of manic depression.

Our study presents interesting clinical findings. Laboratory tests confirmed macrocytic anaemia. Thrombocytes concentrations were decreased, but other biochemical measurements such as haemoglobin were within the normal range (Table1). However, Taher et al. (2009) reported an association between divalproex sodium (DVPX) therapy and total Hb level. It has been reported that in patients treated with VAP 18% experienced at least one episode of thrombocytopenia (Nasreddine &, Beydoun, 2008). However, Rahman et al. (2009) reported 26% of his patients experienced leukopenia. The haematological complications in patients treated with VAP appear to be heterogenic depending on the period of treatment, taking other anticonvulsants, or additional medications (Hemingway et al. 1999; Antoniou et al. 2004). Valporic acid is able to alter hematopoiesis by inhibition of erythroid differentiation in the experimental K562 cell linkage (Chateauvieux et al. 2011). Ladd et al (2009) reported that an elevated level of creatinine phosphokinase is not required for a DSM-IV diagnosis of neuroleptic malignant syndrome (Ladds et al.2009). In our study creatinine phosphokinase was at levels 70 U/I compared to 82 U/l in controls. A creatinine phosphokinase level of 800,000 U/l was reported for a patient who was being treated with a conventional antipsychotic (Sanai et al. 2006).

Determinations	Patients (M±SD) (n)	Controls (M±SD) (n)	p-value	
Thrombocytes (E9/l)	186±67 (141)	259±59 (367)	1.4×10^{-23}	↓↓
Erythrocytes (E12/l)	4.1±0.43 (140)	4.5±0.4 (217)	2.1×10^{-10}	↓↓
Hematocrit	0.38±0.04 (142)	0.4±0.03 (217)	4.0×10^{-7}	↓↓
Sodium (Na) (mmol/l)	136±5.5 (49)	140±1.4 (49)	0.000016	↓
Potassium (K) (mmol/l)	4.4±0.4 (49)	4.1±0.3 (49)	0.000038	↑
Hemoglobin (g/l)	132±15 (142)	138±12 (217)	0.000100	↓
C-reactive protein (CRP) (mg/l)	28±32 (64)	10±18 (136)	0.000130	↑
Creatinine (μmol/l)	70±13 (13)	82±14 (50)	0.007600	↓
Mean cell volume (MCV) (fl)	92±3.9 (142)	91±5.0 (217)	0.028500	↑
Alanine aminotransferase (ALAT) (U/L)	21±18 (65)	41±90 (86)	0.044850	↓
Alkaline phosphatase (AFOS) (U/L)	150±53 (16)	125±41 (25)	0.134720	↑
Leukocytes (E9/l)	6.2±2.5 (140)	6.5±2.5 (217)	0.197680	↓
Aspartate aminotransferase (ASAT) (U/L)	26±14 (38)	31±22 (29)	0.330570	↓
Amylase (U/L)	205±45 (42)	192±75 (29)	0.399700	↑

M=mean value

SD=standard deviation

n=number of observations

Table 1. The levels of eight clinical and six hematological markers in patients on VPA and in control

Author details

P. Kaipainen[1], T. Westermarck[1], F. Atroshi[2], M. Kaski[1] and M. Iivanainen[1,3]

1 Rinnekoti Research Centre, FIN Espoo, Finland

2 Department of Clinical Sciences, Pharmacology & Toxicology, University of Helsinki, Finland

3 Department of Child Neurology, University of Helsinki, Finland

References

[1] Acharya S, Bussel JB. Hematologic toxicity of sodium valproate. J Pediatr Hematol Oncol. 2000 ;22(1):62-5.

[2] Aldenkamp A., Vigevano F., Arzimanoglou A & Covanis A. Role of valproate across the ages.Treatment of epilepsy in children. Acta neurological Scandinavica Supplementum;2006,184,1-13.

[3] Antoniou T, Gough K, Yoong D, Arbess G. Severe anemia secondary to a probable drug interaction between zidovudine and valproic acid.Clin Infect Dis. 2004,1;38(5): 38-40.

[4] Bain B, England J: Normal haematological values: sex difference in neutrophil count. BMJ 1975, 1:306-309.

[5] Ben-Menachem E., Schmidt B., Tomson T & Vajda F. Role of valproate across the ages. Treatment of epilepsy in adults. Acta neurologica Scandinavica Supplementum; 2006,184: 14-27.

[6] Blaheta, R. A., & Cinatl, J.,Jr. Anti-tumor mechanisms of valproate: A novel role for an old drug. Medicinal Research Reviews,2002; 22(5), 492-511.

[7] Butkiewicz AM, Kemona H, Dymicka-Piekarska V, Matowicka-Karna J, Radziwon P, Lipska A: Platelet count, mean platelet volume and thrombopoietic indices in healthy women and men. Thrombosis Res 2006, 118:199-204.

[8] Calleja, S., Salas-Puig, J., Ribacoba, R., & Lahoz, C. H. Evolution of juvenile myoclonic epilepsy treated from the outset with sodium valproate. Seizure: The Journal of the British Epilepsy Association,2001; 10(6), 424-427.

[9] Chateauvieux S, Eifes S, Morceau F, Grigorakaki C, Schnekenburger M, Henry E, Dicato M, Diederich M. Valproic acid perturbs hematopoietic homeostasis by inhibition of erythroid differentiation and activation of the myelo-monocytic pathway.Biochem Pharmacol. 2011,15;81(4):498-509.

[10] Chen HF, Xu LP, Luo ZY, Yu ZQ, Li ZY, Cui QY, Qin LM, Ren YY, Shen HS, Tang JQ, Jin LJ, Zhu JJ, Wang J, Wang KY, Wu TQ, Wang ZY. Valproic acid-associated low fibrinogen and delayed intracranial hemorrhage: case report and mini literature review. Drug Des Devel Ther. 2013,13;7:767-70.

[11] Coppola G, Auricchio G, Federico R, Carotenuto M, Pascotto A. Lamotrigine versus valproic acid as first-line monotherapy in newly diagnosed typical absence seizures: an open-label, randomized, parallel-group study.Epilepsia. 2004 ;45(9):1049-53.

[12] Coppola G., Epifanio G., Auricchio G., Federico RR., Resicato G & Pascotto A. Plasma free carnitine in epilepsy children, adolescents and young adults treated with old and new antiepileptic drugs with or without ketogenic diet. Brain & Development. 2006; 28: 358-65.

[13] Cotarlu D & Zaldman L. Valproic acid and the liver. Clinical chemistry. 1988; 34:890-897.

[14] Cramer, J. A., & Mattson, R. H. Valproic acid: In vitro plasma protein binding and interaction with phenytoin. Therapeutic Drug Monitoring,1979; 1(1), 105-116.

[15] Dean, J. C., & Penry, J. K. Valproate monotherapy in 30 patients with partial seizures. Epilepsia, 1988; 29(2): 140-144.

[16] Delucchi, G. A., & Calabrese, J. R. Anticonvulsants for treatment of manic depression. Cleveland Clinic Journal of Medicine,1989; 56(8): 756-761.

[17] Gerstner T, Bell N, Koenig SA. Valproate-associated reversible encephalopathy in a 3-year-old girl with Pallister-Killian syndrome. Ther Clin Risk Manag. 2008 ;4(3): 645-7.

[18] Gerstner T, Buesing D, Longin E, Bendl C, Wenzel D, Scheid B, Goetze G, Macke A, Lippert G, Klostermann W, Mayer G, Augspach-Hofmann R, Fitzek S, Haensch CA, Reuland M, Koenig SA. Valproic acid induced encephalopathy--19 new cases in Germany from 1994 to 2003--a side effect associated to VPA-therapy not only in young children. Seizure. 2006 ;15(6):443-8.

[19] Gerstner T., Teich M., Bell N., Longin E., Dempfle CE., Brand J & König S. Valproate-associated coagulopathies are frequent and variable in children. Epilepsia, 2006; 47, 1136-43.

[20] Hartwig A. Cadmium and cancer. Met Ions Life Sci. 2013;11:491-507.

[21] Hemingway C, Leary M, Riordan G, Schlegal B, Walker K. The effect of carbamazepine and sodium valproate on the blood and serum values of children from a third-world environment.J Child Neurol. 1999 Nov;14(11):751-3.

[22] Hjelm M., Oberholzer V., Seakins J., Thomas S & Kay JDS. Valproate inhibiton of urea cycle. Lancet. 1987; 923.

[23] Iivanainen M & Alvarez N. (eds). Drug treatment of epilepsy in people with intellectual disability. Journal of Intellectual Disability Research. 1998; 42 (suppl. 1), 1-92.

[24] Katayama Y, Becker DP, Tamura T, Hovda DA. Massive increases in extracellular potassium and the indiscriminate release of glutamate following concussive brain injury. J Neurosurg. 1990 ;73(6):889-900.

[25] Koenig SA, Buesing D, Longin E, Oehring R, Häussermann P, Kluger G, Lindmayer F, Hanusch R, Degen I, Kuhn H, Samii K, Jungck A, Brückner R, Seitz R, Boxtermann W, Weber Y, Knapp R, Richard HH, Weidner B, Kasper JM, Haensch CA, Fitzek S, Hartmann M, Borusiak P, Müller-Deile A, Degenhardt V, Korenke GC, Hoppen T, Specht U, Gerstner T. Valproic acid-induced hepatopathy: nine new fatalities in German from 1994 to 2003. Epilepsia. 2006;47, 2027-31.

[26] Kreuz W, Linde R, Funk M, Meyer-Schrod R, Föll E, Nowak-Göttl U, Jacobi G, Vigh Z, Scharrer I. Valproate therapy induces von Willebrand disease type I. Epilepsia. 1992;33(1):178-84.

[27] Ladds B, Thomas P, Mejia C, Hauser D. Extreme elevation of creatinine phosphokinase levels in neuroleptic malignant syndrome associated with atypical antipsychotics. Am J Psychiatry. 2009;166(1):114-5.

[28] Lal, H., Shearman, G. T., Fielding, S., Dunn, R., Kruse, H., & Theurer, K. Evidence that GABA mechanisms mediate the anxiolytic action of benzodiazepines:A study with valproic acid. Neuropharmacology,1980;19(8), 785-789.

[29] Lheureux PHR., Penaloza A., Zahir S & Gris Mireille. Science review:Carnitine in the treatment of valproic acid-induced toxicity-what is the evidence? Critical Care.2005; 9, 431-440.

[30] Loscher, W. Valproate: A reappraisal of its pharmacodynamic properties and mechanisms of action. Progress in Neurobiology,1999; 58(1), 31-59.

[31] Mallet L., Babin S & Morais JA. Valproic acid-induced hyperammonemia and thrombocytopenia in an elderly woman. The Annals of Pharmacotherapy. 2004; 38, 1643-7.

[32] Mazaira S. Haematological adverse effects caused by psychiatric drugs. Vertex, 2008; 19(82):378-86.

[33] McQueen EG, Wardell WM. Drug displacement from protein binding: isolation of a redistributional drug interaction in vivo.Br J Pharmacol. 1971;43(2):312-24.

[34] Murakami K., Sugimoto T., Woo M., Nishida N & Muro H. Effect of L-carnitine supplementation on acute valproate intoxication. Epilepsia,1996; 37, 687-689.

[35] Nasreddine W, Beydoun A. Valproate-induced thrombocytopenia: a prospective monotherapy study. Epilepsia. 2008;49(3):438-45.

[36] Nilsson P, Ronne-Engstrom E, Flink R, Ungerstedt U, Carlson H, Hillered L. Epileptic seizure activity in the acute phase following cortical impact trauma in rat. Brain Res. 1994; 637: 227–232.

[37] Pan CF, Shen MY, Wu CJ, Hsiao G, Chou DS, Sheu JR. Inhibitory mechanisms of gabapentin, an antiseizure drug, on platelet aggregation. J Pharm Pharmacol. 2007;59(9):1255-61.

[38] Perucca E., Aldenkamp A., Tallis R & Kramer G. Role of valproate across the ages. Treatment of epilepsy in the elderly. Acta neurologica Scandinavica Supplementum. 2006; 184, 28-37.

[39] Perucca, E. Pharmacological and therapeutic properties of valproate: A summary after 35 years of clinical experience. CNS Drugs,2002; 16(10), 695-714.

[40] Rahman A, Mican LM, Fischer C, Campbell AH. Evaluating the incidence of leukopenia and neutropenia with valproate, quetiapine, or the combination in children and adolescents. Ann Pharmacother. 2009 ;43(5):822-30.

[41] Rao ML, Stefan H, Scheid C, Kuttler AD, Fröscher W. Serum amino acids, liver status, and antiepileptic drug therapy in epilepsy. Epilepsia. 1993 ;34(2):347-54

[42] Rosenberg, G. "The mechanisms of action of valproate in neuropsychiatric disorders: Can we see the forest for the trees?". Cellular and Molecular Life Sciences; 2007, 64 (16): 2090–2103.

[43] Sanai T, Matsui R, Hirano T, Torichigai S, Yotsueda H, Higashi H, Hirakata H, Iida M. Successful treatment of six patients with neuroleptic malignant syndrome associated with myoglobulinemic acute renal failure.Ren Fail. 2006;28(1):51-5.

[44] Sandler RM., Emberson C., Roberts GE, Voak D., Darnborough J & Heeley AF. IgM platelet autoantibody due to sodium valproate. British Journal of Medicine.1978; 2, 1683-4.

[45] Shahidi N: Androgens and erythropoesis. NEJM 1973, 289:72.

[46] Taher AT, Musallam KM, Nasreddine W, Perrine SP, El-Hajj TI, Beydoun A. Effects of divalproex sodium on hemoglobin level.Blood Cells Mol Dis. 2009;43(1):49-52.

[47] Thurston JH & Hauhart RE. Reversal of the adverse chronic effects of the unsaturated derivative of valproic acid - 2-n-propyl-4-pentenoic acid - on ketogenesis and liver coenzyme A metabolism by a single injection of pantothenate, carnitine and acetylcysteine in developing mice. Pediatric Research.1993; 33, 72-76.

[48] Verma NP, Haidukewych D. Differential but infrequent alterations of hepatic enzyme levels and thyroid hormone levels by anticonvulsant drugs. Arch Neurol. 1994 ;51(4):381-4.

[49] Waalen J, Felitti V, Beutler E: Haemoglobin and ferritin concentrations in men and women: cross sectional study. BMJ 2002, 325:137.

[50] World Health Organization: Iron deficiency anaemia: assessment, prevention, and control; A guide for programme manager; 2001.

[51] Zeller JA., Schlesinger S., Runge U & Kessler C. Influence of valproate monotherapy on platelet activation and hematologic values. Epilepsia, 1999; 40,186-9.

6

Pharmacological Interventions of Selenium in Duchene Muscular Dystrophy: The Role of Reactive Oxygen Species in Mediating Lipid Peroxide Formation

Tuomas Westermarck, Shirly Ekvall and
Kaski Markus

1. Introduction

The muscular dystrophies are a group of muscle diseases which have three features in common: they are hereditary; they are progressive; and each causes a characteristic, selective pattern of weakness. Duchenne muscular dystrophy (DMD) is the most common inherited muscular disease, affecting one in 3,500 male births. DMD is characterized by rapid, progressive muscle wasting that typically kills patients in their twenties. Complete muscle dystrophin deficiency is a common mechanism for DMD.

Duchenne muscular dystrophy (DMD) is a severe X-linked recessive, progressive muscle-wasting disease affecting one in 3500 boys (Emery AEH, 1993). Patients are usually confined to a wheelchair before the age of 12 and die in their late teens or early twenties usually of respiratory failure. A milder form of the disease, Becker muscular dystrophy (BMD), has a later onset and a much longer survival.

The most widely studied dystrophies are those due to mutations in the dystrophin gene. In humans, dystrophin deficiency leads to the severe disease, Duchenne muscular dystrophy, whereas reductions or truncations of dystrophin lead to a milder disease, Becker muscular dystrophy. Numerous animal models of dystrophin deficiency are actively studied, but none more so than the *mdx* mouse. Despite over a decade of study of dystrophin and its associated proteins, some of which themselves cause muscular dystrophies when deficient or defective, the mechanisms by which the primary biochemical defects lead to muscle cell death remain to be determined.

Both disorders are caused by mutations in the DMS gene that encodes a 427-kDa cytoskeletal protein called dystrophin. The vast majority of DMD mutations result in the complete absence of dystrophin, whereas the presence of low levels of a truncated protein is seen in BMD patients. The defected gene causes a shortage or absence of the structural protein dystrophin, which is near the sites of Ca^{2+} release from sarcoplasmic reticulum and uptake of intracellular Ca^{2+}. The genetic alteration produces an abnormality in the membrane of muscular fibers that consists of a disturbance in the calcium transport (Ca^{++}), inside the muscular fibers, which is the base mechanism of cellular degeneration, necrosis, and apoptosis (Simonian and Coyle 1996). A nucleotide degeneration and decreased muscle AP and ADP content has been reported. Of the total body selenium reserves consists of muscle selenium supply. Selenium is gradually wasted out by the kidneys during the proceeding of the dystrophy of the legs (Westermarck et al 1982). Open follow-up trials with antioxidants are indicating positive clinical response (Gebre-Medhin et al 1985; Timberg 1989; Westermarck et al 1997).

2. Description and clinical features of Duchenne

Typically, DMD patients are clinically normal at birth, although serum levels of muscle isoform of creatine kinase are elevated. The onset of pseudohypertrophy of the calf muscles, proximal limb muscle weakness suggests DMD. Weakness of the arms occurs later along with progressive kyphoscoliosis (Dubowitz. Major Probl Clin Pediatr 1978).

Most patients die in their early twenties as a result of respiratory complications due to intercostal muscle weakness and respiratory infection. Death can also be the result of cardiac dysfunction with cardiomyopathy. BMD and DMD patients also present with mild cognitive impairment, indicating that brain function is also abnormal in these disorders (Blak and Martin-Rendon, 2002).

Fetal DMD is histologically normal except for occasional eosinophilic hypercontracted fibers (Bertorini et al. 1984). Necrotic or degenerating muscle fibers are seen in all postnatal DMD muscle biopsies even before muscle weakness is clinically seen. The necrotic fibers are phagocytized, and muscle biopsies from DMD patients reveal the presence of inflammatory cells at perimysial and endomysiel sites (Arahata and Engel 1984). The regenerative capacity of the muscle is lost and muscle fibers are gradually replaced by adipose and fibrous connective tissue, giving rise to the clinical appearance of pseudohypertrophy followed by atrophy (Emery 1993), resulting in muscle wasting and ultimately muscle weakness (Blake et al 2002). Most patients die in their early twenties as a result of respiratory complications due to intercostal muscle weakness and respiratory infection. Death can also be the result of cardiac dysfunction with cardiomyopathy. BMD and DMD patients also present with mild cognitive impairment, indicating that brain function is also abnormal in these disorders (Blake and Kroger 2000).

DMD muscle shows signs of oxidative damage (Murphy and Kehrer 1989). Muscle diseases in which oxidative damage may play a primary role show features in common with DMD (Mendell Et al 1971). Moreover, muscle cells from mdx mice have an increased susceptibility to oxidative stress (Rando et al 1998). The lack of neuronal-type nitric oxide synthase (nNOS) seen in DMD causes disregulation of vascular tone, and ischemia (Crosbie 2001, Blake et al 2002). This henomenon may increase the generation of free radicals. Open follow-up trials with antioxidants are indicating positive clinical response (Gebre-Medhin et al 1985; Timber 1989; Westermarck et al 1997).

A low blood selenium level has previously been observed in healthy inhabitants of Finland (WESTERMARCK, 1977). In this study even lower blood selenium values were observed in patients with acrodermatitis enteropathica, dystrophia musculorum progressiva (Duchenne), infantile and juvenile type of neuronal ceroid lipofuscinosis (NCL), severe mental retardation caused by various factors, and myocardial infarction. The selenium content of the brain, heart, kidney and liver in patients of different ages was also determined. The highest selenium level was found in the kidney. The mean liver selenium concentrations in stillborn, premature and full-term neonates were 1.11 +/- 0.23 (8), 1.21 +/- 0.17 (12) and 0.93 +/- 0.16 microgram/g dry weight (12) respectively (the number of subjects in parentheses). The selenium values are considerably higher than those in infants of from one to nine months of age and adults, whose liver selenium values were 0.58 +/- 0.21 (8) and 0.67 +/- 0.08 microgram/g dry weight (8) respectively. The vitamin E levels of serum in patients with NCL, as well as in subjects with severe mental retardation (controls), were low compared with values in healthy normal subjects. Sodium selenite supplementation in patients with NCL produced at least a transitory improvement without causing any toxic effects during one year of administration. In Duchenne muscular dystrophy we found that ^{75}Se-selenite was not absorbed in the lower extremities in the equal level compared to healthy ones.

3. Oxidative stress

Oxidative stress is often defined as an imbalance between the generation of reactive oxygen species and the removal of such species by enzymatic and nonenzymatic cellular defense systems (Figure 1). This imbalance could arise from overproduction of reactive species, as occurs under certain pathologic conditions and in association with inflammation, or from an impairment of the defense mechanisms, as occurs in certain genetic loss-of-function disorders and deficiency states. Implicit in this definition is the notion that such an imbalance is sufficient to lead to the oxidation of various cellular constituents and to cause cellular dysfunction and injury. As such, oxidative stress may also be viewed as a condition in which the production of oxidative products exceeds their removal by cellular repair mechanisms. Such conditions may lead to acute cellular dysfunction or cell death, and chronic tissue degeneration, if such changes accumulate.

During normal cellular metabolism, the primary generation of reactive oxygen species comes from the leakage of superoxide anions from the electron transport chain. A series of linked enzymatic reactions are responsible for the detoxification of superoxide. Superoxide is converted to hydrogen peroxide by the action of superoxide dismutase (SOD). Most animal cells contain two forms of SOD, a cytoplasmic Cu,Zn-SOD and a mitochondrial Mn-SOD. In addition, there is an extracellular form of the enzyme. Hydrogen peroxide is subsequently metabolized to oxygen and water by the selenium-containing enzyme glutathione peroxidase, which uses glutathione (GSH) as a cofactor in the reaction. Glutathione peroxidase converts most of the hydrogen peroxide in the cytoplasm. At sites of relatively high concentrations of hydrogen peroxide, such as peroxisomes, catalase is an important antioxidant enzyme that also converts hydrogen peroxide to water. Hydrogen peroxide can react with metal ions in the cell to produce the highly reactive hydroxyl radical, and superoxide can react with nitric oxide (NO•) to produce peroxynitrite. Hydroxyl radical and peroxynitrite are among the most reactive species present in biological systems and are capable of oxidizing nucleic acids, proteins, lipids, and carbohydrate moieties in the cell.

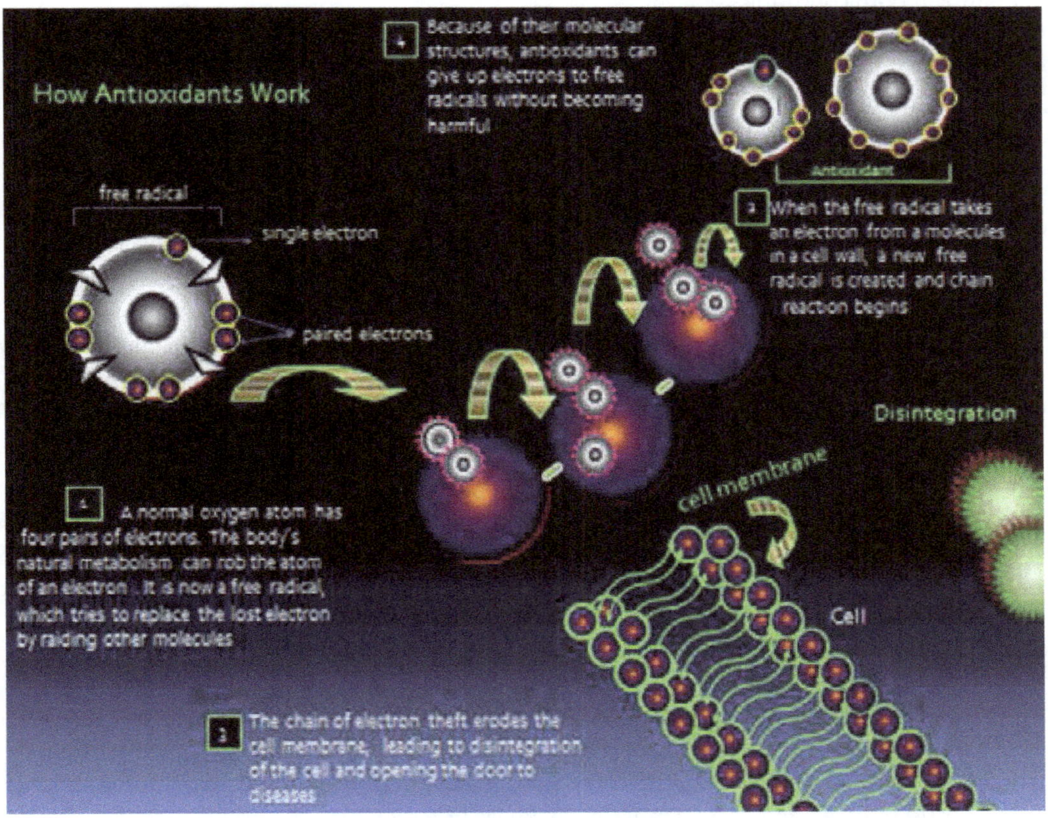

Figure 1. The role of free radical in inflammation

4. Oxidative stress cause dystrophic changes

One of the first observations that led to the oxidative stress hypothesis was the finding that vitamin E deficiency in animals leads to muscle degeneration with pathologic characteristics very similar to those of the muscular dystrophies. The similarities are most striking in avian species in which vitamin E deficiency myopathies closely mimic the hereditary dystrophies both anatomically and biochemically. In humans, vitamin E deficiency is associated with myopathic changes, and in these disorders, there is selective involvement of type IIB fibers as in the inherited muscular dystrophies. Vitamin E refers to a group of compounds of which [alpha]-tocopherol is the most potent and most prevalent in animal tissues as the major lipid-soluble antioxidant in the cell. Deficiencies of vitamin E are associated with increases in lipid peroxidation and decreases in polyunsaturated fatty acids in muscle and compensatory increases in muscle antioxidant enzymes and GSH levels. Although it is clear that inherited muscular dystrophies are not due to primary deficiencies in vitamin E, as was once proposed, the cumulative data strongly support the proposition that the mechanism of muscle injury is the same in both conditions.

5. Can antioxidant treatment ameliorate muscular dystrophy

In addition to evidence of oxidative damage preceding pathologic changes, amelioration of the pathology of a muscular dystrophy by antioxidant treatment would be strong support for the hypothesis that oxidative stress is a primary pathogenetic process. Various antioxidant treatments have been tried in humans and animals with muscular dystrophy. However, the benefit from any individual antioxidant treatment would depend on the actual nature of the oxidative stress that is occurring in the muscle tissue. For example, supplementation of vitamin E–deficient animals with the most prevalent cellular soluble antioxidant, ascorbic acid (vitamin C), does not significantly improve the myopathy. Different susceptibilities to oxidative stress are not identical. Even if oxidative stress is indeed the primary pathophysiologic process leading to muscle cell death in the dystrophies, effective treatment will need to be targeted to the specific deficit in antioxidant defense in the dystrophic muscle and thus will depend on a detailed understanding of the nature of that susceptibility.

Antioxidant treatments in animals with hereditary muscular dystrophies have provided modest benefits. Penicillamine, a sulfhydryl compound with antioxidant properties, and vitamin E slowed the degenerative process in avian dystrophy. Research showed that iron deprivation resulted in a significant reduction of necrosis in the mdx mouse, presumably by a decrease in the production of hydroxyl radical. Dietary supplementation rich in antioxidants significantly reduced an index of muscle weakness in mdx mice.

Clinical trials of antioxidant therapy in humans with Duchenne muscular dystrophy have included treatments with tocopherols, ascorbate, penicillamine, and SOD. No clear benefit has been found from any of these treatments. However, these trials have been very limited in duration and size. Furthermore, in no human study has antioxidant treatment begun early in the course of the disease. In fact, all of these studies involved boys with advanced disease (average age, >=10 yr). Based on the notion that oxidative injury is critical to the pathogenesis of muscle cell death and that antioxidant treatment might be effective to prevent such death, trials in humans would need to be initiated early in the course of the disease, and efficacy would need to be assessed primarily as the slowing, not a reversal, of muscle loss. The difficulties and pitfalls of clinical trials for new treatments of muscular dystrophies are well known. Thus, based on both statistical power and theoretical benefit, none of these human trials would even be predicted to demonstrate any benefit, and the negative results do not in any way refute the oxidative stress hypothesis.

6. Selenium in the brain and brain diseases

Oxidative stress and generation of reactive oxygen species (ROS) are strongly implicated in a number of neuronal and neuromuscular disorders, including stroke and cerebrovascular disease, Alzheimer's disease, Parkinson's disease, familial amyotrophic lateral sclerosis, and Duchenne muscular dystrophy (Dexter et al. 1989a,b; Smith et al. 1991; Ragusa et al. 1997; Cornett et al. 1998b; Facchinetti et al. 1998; Sagara et al. 1998; Tan et al. 1998). Selenium is known to provide protection from ROS-induced cell damage, and the proposed mechanisms mainly invoke the functions of glutathione peroxidases (GPxs) and selenoprotein P (SelP).

Considerable evidence exists linking heavy metals to neurodegenerative diseases (Thompson et al. 1988; Deibel et al. 1996; Cuajungco and Lees 1997; Schionning et al. 1997; Cornett et al. 1998b; Ely 2001). Heavy metals trigger the conversion of hydrogen peroxide to hydroxyl radical through Fenton reaction. Selenium has long been known to function as an antidote to toxicity of heavy metals. Co-administration of selenium was reported to play a role in reducing the toxic effects of mercury as early as the 1970s (Koelman et al. 1973; Kosta et al. 1975). Among the selenoproteins, SelP has been reported in several studies to possess metal-binding function (see below). The GPxs might also detoxify heavy metals through their well-known function of eliminating peroxides (Figure 2).

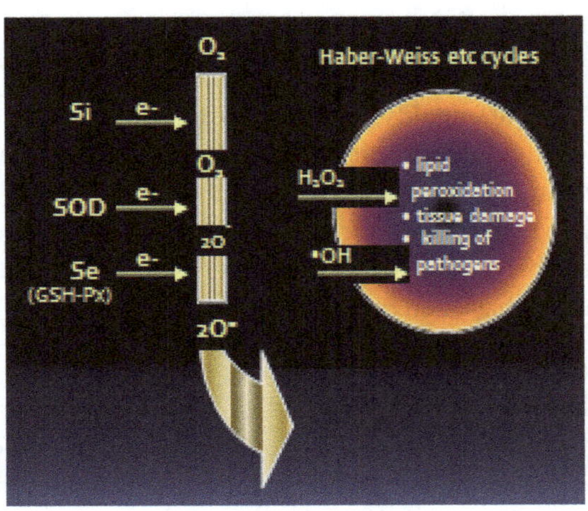

Figure 2. Complementary actions of selenium (GSH-Px) in free radical formation and lipid peroxidation (from Parantainen et al., 1987)

7. Treatment of brain diseases with selenium

Two children with severe neurodevelopmental retardation and elevated liver function tests developed intractable seizures during the first years of life. They were found systemically selenium deficient. Oral substitution with selenium supplements in both children (3–5 μg/kg body weight) resulted in reduction of seizures, improvement of the electroencephalogram (EEG) recordings, and return of normal liver function after 2 weeks (Ramaekers et al. 1994). It is unknown if selenium deficiency is a direct factor for the neurodevelopmental retardation or it affected the brain via abnormal liver function.

Methamphetamine (MA) exposure of animals results in enhanced formation of superoxide radical ($O2^-$) and nitric oxide (NO), which interact to produce peroxynitrite ($OONO^-$). Peroxynitrite is a potent oxidant, leading to dopaminergic damage (Imam and Ali 2000). Thus, multiple dose administration of MA to mice results in long-lasting toxic effects in the nigrostriatal dopaminergic system, which is a relevant model of PD. In selenium-replete mice, this dopaminergic toxicity was significantly attenuated, compared with selenium-deficient mice (Kim et al. 1999; Kim et al. 2000). Pre-treatment of animals with selenium and melatonin can completely protect against the depletion of striatal dopamine induced by MA exposure (Imam et al. 2001). The reason for the protective effects of selenium against MA was reported to be the efficient scavenging of peroxynitrite by selenoproteins (Sies and Arteel 2000).

6-hydroxydopamine (6-OHDA) is a neurotoxin specific for catecholamine neurons in both the central and peripheral nervous system. PD induced by this compound in rats was prevented by selenium in a dose-dependent manner, through up-regulating the antioxidant status and lowering the dopamine loss. This study revealed that selenium may be helpful in slowing down the progression of neurodegeneration in Parkinsonism (Zafar et al. 2003).

8. Hypotesis and intervention

It is possible to improve the life quality of Duchenne patients by biological active substances (antioxidants), and psychotherapeutic intervention. Therapy of DMD has been an elusive goal. Studies with isolated myocytes have shown that lipid peroxidation with an enhanced free radical production can be activated by increasing Ca concentration. No wonder that several kinds of antioxidants have been proposed as a treatment since increased levels of thiobarbituric acid (TBA) reactive material has been found in the muscles and blood of patients with DMD.

Vitamin E has been observed to decrease the amount of TBA reactive material in dystrophic muscle. Previously we have reported that the biological half-life of selenium -75 (75Se) in DMD patients is significantly shorter than in healthy controls (Westermarck et al 1982). On the basis of these facts we started to treat some DMD patients with selenium and other antioxidants. Selenium is activating a well-known antioxidative enzyme glutathione peroxidase (GSH-Px, iodothyronine desiodinase, selenoprotein P, thioredoxin reductase and the selenoprotein W, that all contain selenocystein. Beside iodothyronine desiodinase that facilitates the activation of thyroid hormones; all other selenoproteins have a role in the metabolisation and detoxification of reactive oxygen species and in the maintenance of the antioxidant defense of cells.

For example, in 1981 the antioxidant treatment of two siblings with DMD, aged six and ten years, was started. At that time the older brother was wheel-chair bound and was not able to walk since eight years of age, the younger one was still able to walk almost normally. The condition of the older brother, who practically had not got carnitine or coenzyme Q^{10} supplementation, was gradually deteriorated, and he deceased at 17 years of age. However, at the age of 15 years the younger brother was still able to walk without any assistance. Six months later he became wheel-chair bound. The younger brother was one of the most talented graduated students in his high-school. The mean IQ of DMD patients is without treatment 15-20 points lower than that of normal populations. Anyway for some years he was able to study at the University of Joensuu. Now he is 31 years old and still able to swim some meters, and to produce computer art. Actually he had his first art-show in 2003 in Helsinki. Moreover, only during the nights it is necessary to give him non-invasive breathing assistance.

The present daily megadoses of nutrients supplements (vitamin E 1200mg; sodium selenite 8mg; riboflavin 3mg; pyridoxine 75mg; carnitine 600mg; and coenzyme Q10 180mg) have been well tolerated and no side effects have observed in our open controlled trial (Westermarck et al 1997). The long-term pilot study speaks in favor for a larger study. Dr. Anders Erikson from Sweden (personal communication) has made the same observations with two Swedish siblings suffering from DMD, as we have also made with two 13- and 14-year old cousins 2with DMD.

Author details

Tuomas Westermarck[1], Shirly Ekvall[2,3] and Kaski Markus[1]

1 Rinnekoti Foundation, Espoo, Finland

2 University Affiliated Cincinnati Center for Developmental Disabilities, Children's Hospital Medical Center, Cincinnati, Ohio, USA

3 University of Cincinnati, Cincinnati, Ohio, USA

References

[1] Arahata K, Engel AG: Monoclonal antibody analysis of mononuclear cells in myopathies. I. Quantitation of subsets according to diagnosis and sites of accumulation and demonstration And counts of muscle fibers invaded by T cells. Ann Neurol 16: 193-208, 1984

[2] Blake DJ, Kroger S: The neurobiology of Duchenne muscular ystrophy: learning lessons From muscle? Trends Neurosci 23: 92-99, 2000

[3] Blake DJ, Weir A, Newey SE, Davies KE: Function and genetics of Dystrophin and Dystrophin-Related Proteins in Muscle: Physiol. Rev 82: 291-329, 2002.

[4] Blake DJ, Martin-Rendon E. Intermediate filaments and the function of the dystrophin-protein complex. Trends Cardiovasc Med 2002; 12:224-228.

[5] Dubowitz V: Muscle disorders in childhood. Major Probl Clin Pediatr 16: 1-282, 1978

[6] Emery AEH: Duchenne Muscular Dystrophy. Oxford Monographs on Medical Genetics (2nd ed. Oxford, UK: Oxford Univ Press, 1993, vol XV, p 392, 1993

[7] Gebre-Medhin M, Gustavson KH,Gamstorp I, Plantin LO: selenium supplementation in X-linked muscular Dystrophy. Effects on erythrocyte glutathione peroxidase activity. Acta Pediatr Scand 7:886-890, 1985

[8] Jackson MJ, Edwards RHT: Free radicals and trials of antioxidant therapy in muscle diseases. Adv Exp Med Biol 264:485-491, 1990

[9] Simonian NA, Coyle JT: Oxidative stress in neurodegenerative diseases. Annu Rev Pharmacol Toxical 36:83-106, 1996

[10] Timberg H: Progradu- studies. University of Helsinki 1989

[11] Westermarck T, Rahola T, Kallio A-K, Suomela M: Long turnover of selenite Se in children With motor disorders. Klin Pädiat 194:301-02, 1981

[12] Westermarck T, Antila E, Kaksonen S, Laakso J, Härkönen M, Atroshi F: Long-term follow-up Of two Duchenne muscle dystrophy patients treated with antioxidants. Publ.: Food and free radicals, Eds M. Hiramatsu, T. Yosikawa, M. Inoue. Plenum Press, New York 1997, pp 161-163.

[13] Basun H., Forssell L. G., Wetterberg L. and Winblad B. (1991) Metals and trace elements in plasma and cerebrospinal fluid in normal aging and Alzheimer's disease. *J. Neural. Transm. Park. Dis. Dement. Sect.* 3, 231–258.

[14] Behne D. and Kyriakopoulos A. (2001) Mammalian selenium-containing proteins. *Annu. Rev. Nutr.* 21, 453–473.

[15] Berr C., Nicole A., Godin J., Ceballos-Picot I., Thevenin M., Dartigues J. F. and Alperovitch A. (1993) Selenium and oxygen-metabolizing enzymes in elderly community residents: a pilot epidemiological study. *J. Am. Geriatr. Soc.* 41, 143–148.

[16] Burk R. F. (1991) Molecular biology of selenium with implications for its metabolism. *FASEB J.* 5, 2274–2299.

[17] Ceballos-Picot I., Merad-Boudia M., Nicole A., Thevenin M., Hellier G., Legrain S. and Berr C. (1996) Peripheral antioxidant enzyme activities and selenium in elderly

subjects and in dementia of Alzheimer's type – pace of the extracellular glutathione peroxidase. *Free Rad. Biol. Med.* 20, 579–587.

[18] Chanoine J. P., Braverman L. E., Farwell A. P., Safran M., Alex S., Dubord S. and Leonard J. L. (1993) The thyroid gland is a major source of circulating T3 in the rat. *J. Clin. Invest.* 91, 2709–2713.

[19] Clausen J., Jensen G. E. and Nielsen S. A. (1988) Selenium in chronic neurological diseases, multiple sclerosis and Batten's disease. *Biol. Trace Elem. Res.* 15, 179–203.

[20] Cornett C. R., Ehmann W. D., Wekstein D. R. and Markesbery W. R. (1998a) Trace elements in Alzheimer's disease pituitary glands. *Biol. Trace Elem. Res.* 62, 107–114.

[21] Covas M. I., Elosua R., Fito M., Alcantara M., Coca L. and Marrugat J. (2002) Relationship between physical activity and oxidative stress biomarkers in women. *Med. Sci. Sports Exerc.* 34, 814–819.

[22] Cuajungco M. P. and Lees G. J. (1997) Zinc metabolism in the brain: relevance to human neurodegenerative disorders. *Neurobiol. Dis.* 4, 137–169.

[23] Damier P., Hirsch E. C., Zhang P., Agid Y. and Javoy-Agid F. (1993) Glutathione peroxidase, glial cells and Parkinson's disease. *Neuroscience* 52, 1–6.

[24] Deibel M. A., Ehmann W. D. and Markesbury W. R. (1996) Copper, iron, and zinc imbalances in severely degenerated brain regions in Alzheimer's disease: possible relation to oxidative stress. *J. Neurol. Sci.* 143, 137–142.

[25] Dexter D. T., Carter C. J., Wells F. R., Javoy-Agid F., Agid Y., Lees A., Jenner P. and Marsden C. D. (1989a) Basal lipid peroxidation in substantia nigra is increased in Parkinson's disease. *J. Neurochem.* 52, 381–389.

[26] Dexter D. T., Wells F. R. and Lees A. (1989b) Increased nigra iron content and alterations in other metal ions occurring in brain in Parkinson's disease. *J. Neurochem.* 52, 1830–1836.

[27] Ely J. T. A. (2001) Mercury induced Alzheimer's disease: accelerating incidence? *Bull. Environ. Contam. Toxicol.* 67, 800–806.

[28] El-Yazigi A. A. L.,-Saleh I. and Al-Mefty O. (1984) Concentrations of Ag, Al, Au, Bi, Cd, Cu, Pb, Sb, and Se in cerebrospinal fluid of patients with cerebral neoplasms. *Clin. Chem.* 30, 1358–1360.

[29] Facchinetti F., Dawson V. L. and Dawson T. M. (1998) Free radicals as mediators of neuronal injury. *Cell Mol. Neurobiol.* 18, 667–682.

[30] Flentjar N. J., Crack P. J., Boyd R., Malin M., de Haan J. B., Hertzog P., Kola I. and Iannello R. (2002) Mice lacking glutathione peroxidase-1 activity show increased TUNEL staining and an accelerated inflammatory response in brain following a cold-induced injury. *Exp. Neurol.* 177, 9–20.

[31] Glauser T. A., Titanic-Schefft M. and Pippenger C. E. (1999) Racial differences in free radical scavenging enzyme activity in children. *J. Child Neurol.* 14, 382–387.

[32] Ho Y. S., Magnenat J. L., Bronson R. T., Cao J., Gargano M., Sugawara M. and Funk C. D. (1997) Mice deficient in celular glutathione peroxidases develop normally and show no increased sensitivity to hyperoxia. *J. Biol. Chem.* 272, 16644–16651. l

[33] Hock A., Demmel U., Schicha H., Kasperek K. and Feinendegen L. E. (1975) Trace element concentration in human brain. *Brain* 98, 49–64.

[34] Ip C. (1998) Lessons learned from basic research in selenium and cancer prevention. *J. Nutr.* 128, 1845–1854.

[35] Jeong D., Kim T. S., Chung Y. W., Lee B. J. and Kim I. Y. (2002) Selenoprotein W is a glutathione-dependent antioxidant *in vivo*. *FEBS Lett.* 517, 225–228.

[36] Johannsen P., Velander G., Mai J., Thorling E. B. and Dupont E. (1991) Glutathione peroxidase in early and advanced Parkinson's disease. *J. Neurol. Neurosurg. Psychiatry* 54, 679–682.

[37] Kalra J., Rajput A. H., Mantha S. V. and Prasad K. (1992) Serum antioxidant enzyme activity in Parkinson's disease. *Mol. Cell Biochem.* 110, 165–168.

[38] Kim H. C., Jhoo W. K., Choi D. Y., Im D. H., Shin E. J., Suh J. H., Floyd R. A. and Bing G. (1999) Protection of methamphetamine nigrostriatal toxicity by dietary selenium. *Brain Res.* 851, 76–86.

[39] Kim H. C., Jhoo W. K., Shin E. and Bing G. (2000) Selenium deficiency potentates methamphetamine-induced nigral neuronal loss; comparison with MPTP model. *Brain Res.* 862, 247–252.

[40] Kish S. J., Morito C. and Hornykiewicz O. (1985) Glutathione peroxidase activity in Parkinson's disease brain. *Neurosci. Lett.* 58, 343–346.

[41] Kosta L., Byrne A. R. and Zelenko V. (1975) Correlations between selenium and mercury in man following exposure to inorganic mercury. *Nature* 254, 238–239.

[42] Marttila R. J., Lorentz H. and Rinne U.K. (1988) Oxygen toxicity protecting enzymes in Parkinson's disease. *J. Neurol. Sci.* 86, 321–331.

[43] Meseguer I., Molina J. A., Jimenez-Jimenez F. J., Aguilar M. V., Mateos-Vega C. J., Gonzalez-Munoz M. J., de Bustos F., Orti-Pareja M., Zurdo M., Berbel A., Barrios E. and Martinez-Para M. C. (1999) Cerebrospinal fluid levels of selenium in patients with Alzheimer's disease. *J. Neural. Transm.* 106, 309–315.

[44] Oster O., Schmiedel G. and Prellwitz W. (1988) The organ distribution of selenium in German adults. *Biol. Trace Elem. Res.* 15, 23–45.

[45] Poirier J. and Barbeau A. (1987) Erythrocyte antioxidant activity in human patients with Parkinson's disease. *Neurosci. Lett.* 75, 345–348.

[46] Prohaska J. R. and Ganther H. E. (1976) Selenium and glutathione peroxidase in developing rat brain. *J. Neurochem.* 27, 1379–1387.

[47] Ramaekers V. T., Calomme M., Vanden Berghe D. and Makropoulos W. (1994) Selenium deficiency triggering intractable seizures. *Neuropediatrics* 25, 217–223.

[48] Rayman M. P. (2000) The importance of selenium to human health. *Lancet* 356, 233–241.

[49] Rotruck J. T., Pope A. L., Ganther H. E., Swanson A. B., Hafeman D. G. and Hoekstra W. G. (1973) Selenium: biological role as a component of glutathione peroxidase. *Science* 179, 588–590.

[50] Sagara Y., Tan S., Maher P. and Schubert D. (1998) Mechanisms of resistance to oxidative stress in Alzheimer's disease brain. *Neurotoxicology* 19, 339–345.

[51] Saito Y. and Takahashi K. (2002) Characterization of selenoprotein P as a selenium supply protein. *Eur. J. Biochem.* 269, 5746–5751.

[52] Saito Y., Hayashi T., Tanaka A., Watanabe Y., Suzuki M., Saito E. and Takahashi K. (1999) Selenoprotein P in human plasma as an extracellular phospholipids hydroperoxide glutathione peroxidase. *J. Biol. Chem.* 274, 2866–2871.

[53] Schomburg L., Schweizer U., Holtmann B., Flohe L., Sendtner M. and Kohrle J. (2003) Gene disruption discloses role of Selenoprotein P in selenium delivery to target tissues. *Biochem. J.* 370, 397–402.

[54] Sies H. and Arteel G. E. (2000) Interaction of peroxynitrite with selenoproteins and glutathione peroxidase mimics. *Free Rad. Biol. Med.* 28, 1451–1455.

[55] Smith C. D., Carney J. M., Starke-Reed P. E., Oliver C. N., Stadtman E. R., Floyd R. A. and Markesbery W. R. (1991) Excess brain protein oxidation and enzyme dysfunction in normal aging and in Alzheimer disease. *Proc. Natl Acad. Sci. USA* 88, 10540–10543.

[56] Stadtman T. C. (1996) Selenocysteine. *Ann. Rev. Biochem.* 65, 83–100.

[57] Syburra C. and Passi S. (1999) Oxidative stress in patients with multiple sclerosis. *Ukr. Biokhim. Zh.* 71, 112–115.

[58] Takizawa S., Matsushima K., Shinohara Y., Ogawa S., Komatsu N., Utsunomiya H. and Watanabe K. (1994) Immunohistochemical localization of glutathione peroxidase in infracted human brain. *J. Neurol. Sci.* 122, 66–73.

[59] Tan S., Wood M. and Maher P. (1998) Oxidative stress induces a form of programmed cell death with characteristics of both apoptosis and necrosis in neuronal cells. *J. Neurochem.* 71, 95–105.

[60] Thompson C. M., Markesbery W. R., Ehmann W. D., Mao X. Y. and Vance D. E. (1988) Regional brain trace-element studies in Alzheimer's disease. *Neurotoxicology* 9, 1–7.

[61] Torreilles F., Salman-Tabcheh S., Guerin M. C. and Torreilles J. (1999) Neurodegenerative disorders: the role of peroxynitrite. *Brain Res. Rev.* 30, 153–163.

[62] Turan B., Acan N. L., Ulusu N. N. and Tezcan E. F. (2001) A comparative study on effect of dietary selenium and vitamin E on some antioxidant enzyme activities of liver and brain tissues. *Biol. Trace Elem. Res.* 81, 141–152.

[63] Vahter M., Lutz E., Lind B., Herin P., Bui T. H. and Krakau I. (1997) Concentrations of copper, zinc and selenium in brain and kidney of second trimester fetus and infants. *J. Trace Elem. Med. Biol.* 11, 215–222.

[64] Vitorica J., Machado A. and Satrustegui J. (1984) Age-dependent variations in peroxide-utilizing enzymes from rat brain mitochondria and cytoplasm. *J. Neurochem.* 42, 351–356.

[65] Westermarck T. Selenium content of tissues in Finnish infants and adults with various diseases, and studies on the effects of selenium supplementation in neuronal ceroid lipofuscinosis patients. Acta Pharmacol Toxicol. 1977;41(2):121-8.

[66] Westermarck, T; Antila, E; Kaksonen, S; Laakso, J; Härkönen, M ; Atroshi, F. Long-term follow-up of two Duchenne muscle dystrophy patients treated with antioxidants. Food and free radicals (1997): 161-163.

[67] Whanger P. D. (2001) Selenium and the brain: a review. *Nutr. Neurosci.* 4, 81–97.

[68] Wilson D. S. and Tappel A. L. (1993) Binding of plasma selenoprotein P to cell membranes. *J. Inorg. Biochem.* 51, 707–714.

[69] Zachara B. A., Pawluk H., Bloch-Boguslawska E., Sliwka K. M., Korenkiewicz J., Skok Z. and Ryc K. (2001) Tissue level, distribution, and total body selenium content in healthy and diseased humans in Poland. *Arch. Environ. Health* 56, 461–466.

[70] Zafar K. S., Siddiqui A., Sayeed I., Ahmad M., Salim S. and Islam F. (2003) Dose-dependent protective effect of selenium in rat model of Parkinson's disease: neurobehavioral and neurochemical evidences. *J. Neurochem.* 84, 438–446.

[71] Zhang L., Maiorino M., Roveri A. and Ursini F. (1989) Phospholipid hydroperoxide glutathione peroxidase: specific activity in tissues of rats of different age and comparison with other glutathione peroxidase. *Biochim. Biophys. Acta* 1006, 140–143.

7

The Nutritional Status of Children with Suspected Abuse

Eileen Harper, Shirley Ekvall, Valli Ekvall and Wei Pan

1. Introduction

Child abuse is the willful infliction of injury to a child. Estimated at 2.8 million children affected per year, over 2,000 die from maltreatment [1]. In 1998 alone, 900,000 cases were reported [2] and from 1986-1993 cases doubled in the United States. Up to 10% of children seen in the emergency room (ER) under the age of 6 had a non-accidental injury accounting for nearly 25% of all hospital admissions for head injury in infancy, producing significant morbidity [3, 4]. Abuse is not limited to poor or racial minorities [5]. Physical and sexual abuse during childhood/adolescence was reported by 22% on a questionnaire [6]. Abused children frequently have moderate to severe malnutrition [7] due to withholding of food which may lead to compromised nutritional state and failure to thrive (FTT) [8]. Twenty-nine percent of 42 children with severe trauma had under nutrition resulting in growth retardation [9].

Bonnier et al. reported that all 13 children with whiplash shaken infant syndrome had a weight <50th percentile and 9 had a weight <10th percentile. Average birth weight was at the 30th percentile, but body weight at admission for shaking was below the 10th percentile [10]. Poor physical growth/nutrition are seen in 25-35% of abused children [11]. The most common chronic illness of childhood is lead poisoning [11]. Siblings in foster care, physically abused or neglected children are at high risk of lead poisoning and incurring a developmental disability [12-14]. Lead poisoning is caused by ingesting contaminated paint from window sills, furniture, Mexican terra cotta pottery, imported tamarind candy, hot-running water through lead soldered pipes or anything covered in lead-based paint [12-14]. The interaction between nutrition and toxic hazards depends on the baseline nutritional status of the individual as well as total food intake, percent dietary fat, calcium, iron, zinc, vitamin D and phosphorus [15, 16]. Food restriction increased lead retention in animals fed lead containing diets [16, 17]. Yet, one study found a positive association between total caloric intake and blood lead levels [18]. Low calcium diets elevate lead tissue concentrations as calcium functions as a chelating agent reducing lead absorption [17, 19]. Lead competes with calcium in enzyme systems, alters calcium metabolism regulation, modifies the calcium second messenger system, impairs normal modulation of intracellular calcium homeostasis, modifies induction of calcium-regulating proteins and interferes with energy metabolism [19-22, 23]. Zinc status has been found to be approximately 20% lower in children with substantially elevated blood lead concentration. Children may have increased lead absorption following shorter fasting time than adults because of rapid gastric emptying [24]. As dietary zinc intake increases, tissue lead levels and toxicity decrease. Research suggests that higher dietary iron intake might be protective against high blood lead levels [24-26]. Another study found anemia in 13% of the 5,181 abused/neglected children screened; potentially due to lead interfering with heme synthetase.[27] When examining dietary iron intake and H/H levels, the degree of anemia from iron-deficient/lead-intoxicated rats was greater than either condition alone [16]. Lead ia a divalent cation which can deplete iron and zinc. In abused/neglected children, poor nutritional status and lead toxicity can result in severe neurological effects [16]. Increased lead levels, malnutrition and iron deficiency have negative effects on growth and development. Diets adequate in zinc, calcium, iron, vitamin D, phosphorus and protein can reduce high blood lead levels [22, 28]. Lead leakage from outdated non zinc-lined soldering seams in canned vegetables and fruits should be avoided (usually found in underdeveloped countries); accordingly, for homemade baby foods only fresh or frozen fruits and vegetables are recommended [29]. Calcium in evaporated or canned milk is rarely a problem as calcium chelates lead for excretion. Itoh and Suyama report another problem regarding calcium retention, high dietary sodium intake produces greater loss of calcium in urine as sodium and calcium compete for the same recovery mechanism in the kidney [30]. The purpose of this study was to determine the nutritional status of children with suspected abuse since it relates to health risk.

2. Methods

When the child was admitted to the ER with suspected abuse, a social worker was notified, who informed the investigator of the admission. The dietary department was contacted by nursing staff to record the child's dietary intake while a medical resident/staff was notified to perform laboratory levels as determined from the medical/social history. Medical records provided the following information: age, sex, race, type of injury, family size and family characteristics. Nutritional status was assessed using anthropometric measures, biochemical values and dietary intakes. Height and weight were plotted on the growth charts and head circumference, upper arm circumference and triceps skinfold measurements were performed according to the standard methods [31-34]. Biochemical values were obtained by established standard laboratory procedures. A calorie count one to three-day food record was obtained for each child and calculated by the dietitian for calories, protein, zinc, vitamin A, calcium, magnesium, phosphorus, iron, thiamin, riboflavin, niacin, vitamin C and vitamin D from standard data; below two-thirds of the standard being deficient [35]. Due to confidentiality and legal issues with these families, only hospital dietary intakes could be obtained A t-test was performed from anthropometric, biochemical, and dietary values against the standard and further compared PA against SA children. The research proposal was accepted by the Children's Hospital Medical Center's Institutional Review Board. Fingerprick lead screening was performed on 14 of the 28 children, as determined by medical staff from the medical/social history, and thus are listed as an outgrowth of the study.

3. Results/Discussions

Twenty-eight children suspected victims of child abuse, aged 1.5 months to 8.75 years [10 Caucasians, 17 African American, 1 bi-racial child; 14 male, 14 female) were admitted to ER. Type of injury, number of cases, and size of family are shown in Table 1. Many of the families received financial assistance, which is not atypical (Table 1). Anthropometric results showed the majority of subjects (61%) below the 50th percentile; 32% above the 75th percentile for height-for-age and 64% below the 50th percentile for weight-for-age (Table 2). The majority had TSF values of 8-9 mm; below the standard of 10.6 mm. Weight was significantly below the mean for PA children (p=0.05) and PA significantly below the mean of SA children (p=0.019). TSF for PA children were significantly below national government standards (p=0.01). All SA children were in upper percentiles of height-for-age and weight-for-age, while the majority of PA children were below the 50th percentile for weight-for-age. Biochemical results (Table 2) revealed the average hemoglobin was 11.6 gm%; significantly below the average of 12.7 gm% (p=0.0005) and. the average hematocrit was 35.5%; significantly below the standard of 37.1% (p=0.025) although dietary iron was adequate. Of 14 children, 36% had lead levels above normal and 28% were borderline indicating that lead levels may be high in some children with suspected abuse. SA children (p=0.005) and PA children (0.025) had significantly higher lead levels with PA children having more variability within the group. Hematocrits of SA children were slightly higher. PA subjects show that weight (p=0.05) and TSF (p=0.01) were significantly below standards (Table 2). Although diets offered to the hospitalized children were nutritionally adequate, diets consumed by children with suspected abuse were significantly lower than standard data in vitamin D and zinc (p=0.0005). When comparing PA and SA children, height (p=0.033) and weight (p=0.019) were significantly different and lower in PA children. A history of PA was more often found in males, with SA occurring more often in females [36, 37]. The incidence of abuse is not limited to racial minorities [38]; many children with suspected PA were Caucasian. The decreased weight of PA children found in this study is consistent with other findings that underweight and poor physical growth accompany child abuse [11, 39-42]. Low TSF values are consistent with findings and further indicate poor nutritional status. Leung et al. suggested FTT in child abuse may be due to withholding of food or the child not eating (appetite loss) associated with abuse/neglect. Twenty-five of 50 abused children had hemoglobin concentrations of less than 10gm% [38], while 25% fell below 10 gm% in this study. Bithoney et al. stated that every FTT child is malnourished [13]. Thirty-six percent [5 of 14 children) had elevated blood lead levels with 28% borderline, while Flaherty found 64.7% of abused and neglected children had elevated levels [14]. Behavioral manifestations of elevated lead may be more noticeable than effects on intelligence (elevated tempers and mental retardation) [43]. Zinc and vitamin D, which enhances calcium absorption, were low; thus, nutrient chelators were not available to reduce lead absorption [44]. Reduced weight and triceps values often accompany abuse, possibly indicating inadequate availability of food. Due to confidentiality of being classified with suspected abuse, home visits were not available as is typical in other reports on dysfunctional families. PA children have a higher rate of malnutrition, reduced growth, low iron status and elevated blood levels. Each is interrelated increasing the effects of the other. Leung et al [8] claim that if children are suffering from malnutrition, it is essential to begin early intervention because of unknown prognosis. Adequate energy needs should be addressed immediately, followed by treatment of iron deficiency anemia and elevated lead levels [13]. Furthermore, early intervention is essential as children may develop significant long-term cognitive and developmental delay.

Age Range:		1.5 months to 8.75 years	
Age		**Number of Subjects**	
0-3 years		10	
1-3 years		8	
4-6 years		8	
Over age 6		2	
Total:		28	
Type of Abuse		**Number of Subjects**	
1. Sexual		7	
2. Bruises/lacerations		8	
Subdural hematomas/facial trauma		6	
3. Dehydration/severe neglect		1	
4. Burns		3	
5. Fractures		3	
Total:		28	
Cross-Tabulation for Type of Abuse with Socioeconomic Variables:			
		Sexually Abused (SA)	**Physically Abused (PA)**
Race	Caucasian	1 (14.3%)	10 (47.6%)
	Non-Caucasian	6 (85.7%)	11 (53.4%)
Parents	One	4 (57.1%)	15 (71.4%)
	Two	3 (42.9%)	6 (28.6 %)
Receiving Government Aid	Yes	3 (42.9%)	13 (61.9%)
	No	4 (57.1%)	8 (38.1%)

Table 1. Summary of Characteristics of Children with Suspected Abuse

Factor	Mean	Standard Values	Standard Deviation	*p
All Subjects:				
Height (cm)	84.6	86.1	24.0	NS
Weight (kg)	12.4	16.6	8.4	NS
Head Circumference (cm)	46.6	46.6	5.3	NS

Triceps (mm)	9.2	10.6	4.7	0.10
Hemoglobin (g/dL)	11.6	12.7	1.0	0.0005*
Hematocrit (%)	35.5	37.1	4.0	0.025*
Vitamin D (I.U.)	247.7	400.0	69.7	0.0005*
Calcium (mg)	761.6	671.0	264.1	0.10+
Protein (g)	48.8	21.7	24.87	0.005*+
Magnesium (mg)	122.4	141.4	58.0	0.10+
Zinc (mg)	5.8	7.9	2.8	0.0005*
Physically Abused:				
Height (cm)	79.1	79.0	21.3	NS
Weight (kg)	10.3	12.2	5.9	0.05*
Head Circumference (cm)	45.7	45.5	5.9	ND
Triceps (mm)	8.5	10.4	2.9	0.01*
Hemoglobin (g/dL)	11.6	12.5	1.1	0.001*
Hematocrit (%)	35.4	36.8	4.3	0.05*
Vitamin D (I.U.)	254.7	400.0	76.8	0.0005*
Calcium (mg)	699.0	628.6	269.8	NS+
Protein (g)	42.0	18.6	25.1	0.0005*+
Magnesium (mg)	102.7	119.5	53.8	0.10+
Zinc (mg)	5.3	7.3	2.8	0.0005*

	Mean		
All Subjects	**Sexually Abused (SA)**	**Physically Abused (PA)**	***p**
Height (cm)	101.1	79.1	0.0033*
Weight (kg)	18.7	10.3	0.019*
Head Circumference (cm)	49.6	45.7	0.09
Triceps (mm)	11.4	8.5	0.10
Hemoglobin (g/dL)	11.6	11.6	NS
Hematocrit (%)	35.7	35.4	NS
Vitamin D (% DRI)	55.1	65.2	0.185
Calcium (% DRI)	112.8	112.5	NS+
Protein (%DRI)	299.4	230.0	NS+
Magnesium (% DRI)	79.9	85.0	NS+
Zinc (% DRI)	74.4	82.5	NS
Lead Screen (14 subjects) (% std) high 5(36%) borderline 4(28%) SA p=0.005* PAp=0.025*			

*Statistically significant p<0.05 by "t" test

+Nutrient intake and dietary iron adequate

Table 2. Nutritional Status Evaluation of Children with Suspected Abuse

4. Conclusion

Research indicates that abused children may be at nutritional risk upon hospital admission. PA children are especially vulnerable; therefore, awareness of the child's nutritional status by the health care team should be increased. Interdisciplinary cooperation involving physicians, social workers, nurses, and dietitians are needed to provide the best health care for these children. Dietitians should be responsible for employing various nutritional assessment techniques and teamwork with other disciplines. Further studies concerning dietary patterns in the home environment and nutritional knowledge of the caretaker/parent(s) should be conducted to prevent reoccurrence.

5. Applications

Dietitians/nutritionists should be included as members of a child abuse team. Child abuse/neglect training materials for medical/health professionals should incorporate nutritional status and provide nutrition education to caretakers/parents through Parents Anonymous Groups and similar therapeutic sessions. Nutritional as well as other environmental toxins, such as lead and mercury, also should be discussed with the families. Cooking sessions with culturally diverse nutrition education materials, nutrition counseling, and teamwork may need to be conducted by dietitians with families who have minimal cooking and/or nutritional skills using some of the available resources [45-51].

Author details

Eileen Harper[1], Shirley Ekvall[2,3*], Valli Ekvall[2,3] and Wei Pan[3]

*Address all correspondence to: shirley.ekvall@uc.edu

1 Providence Everett Medical Center, Seattle, Washington, USA

2 University Affiliated Cincinnati Center for Developmental Disabilities, Children's Hospital Medical Center, Cincinnati, Ohio, USA

3 University of Cincinnati, Cincinnati, Ohio, USA

References

[1] Child abuse doubles: investigation lags. *Public Health Reports*. 1997; 112:4.

[2] Department of Health and Human Services, Administration for Families Fact Sheet. Washington, D.C.; September 22, 2002.

[3] Famularo, R., Fenton, T., Kinscherff, R. Medical developmental histories of maltreated children. *Clin Pediatr.* 1992; 31:536-541.

[4] Duhaine, A.C., Christian, C., Moss, E., Seidl, T. Long-term outcome in infants with the shaking infant syndrome. *Pediatr Neurosurg.* 1996; 24:292-298.

[5] Depanfilis, D. Rates, patterns and frequency of child maltreatment recurrences among families known to CPS. *Child Maltreat.* 1998; 3:27-42.

[6] McCauley, J. Kern, D.E., Kolodner, K., Dill, L., Schroeder, A.F., DeChant, K. Clinical characteristics of women with a history of childhood abuse: unhealed wounds. *JAMA.* 1997; 277(17):1362-1368.

[7] Helfer, R. Pollock, C. The Battered Child Syndrome. *Adv Pediatr.* 1968; 15:9-27.

[8] Leung, A. Robson, W., Fagan, J. Assessment of the child with failure to thrive. *Am Fam Physician.* 1993; 48:1432-1438.

[9] Birrell, R., Birrell, J. The maltreatment syndrome in children. *Med J Aust.* 1968; 2:1023-1029.

[10] Bonnier, C., Nassaqne, M.C., Evard, P. Outcome and prognosis of whiplash shaken infant syndrome: late consequences after a symptom-free interval. *Dev Med Child Neurol.* 1995; 37:943-956.

[11] Martin, H.P., Beezley, P., Conway, E.F., Kempe, C.H. The development of abused children. *Adv Pediatr.* 1974;1074:21-25.

[12] Chung, E.K., Webb, D., Clampet-Lundquist, S., Campbell, C. A comparison of elevated blood lead levels among children living in foster care, their siblings, and the general population. *Pediatrics.* 2001; 107:E81-82.

[13] Bithoney, W., Vandeven, A., Ryan, A. Elevated lead levels in reportedly abused children. *J Pediatr.* 1993; 122:719-720.

[14] Flaherty, R. Risk of lead poisoning in abused and neglected children. *Clin Pediatr.* 1995; 34:128-132.

[15] Hu, H., Kotha, S., Brennan, T. The role of nutrition in mitigating environmental insults: policy and ethical issues. *Environmental Health Perspect.* 1995; 103(6):185-189.

[16] Mahaffey, K.R. Nutritional factors and lead poisoning. *Nutr Rev.* 1981; 39:353-365.

[17] Ahrens, F.A. Effects of lead on glucose metabolism, ion flux, and collagen synthesis in cerebral capillaries of calves. *Am J Vet Res.* 1993; 54:808-812.

[18] Lucas, S. Sexton, M., Langenburg, P. The relationship between blood lead levels and nutrition factors in preschool children: a cross-sectional study. *Pediatrics*. 1996; 97:74-78.

[19] Mahaffey, K.R., Garthside, P.S., Glueck, C.J. Blood lead and dietary calcium in 2926 1-through 11 year-old black and white children: The second national health and nutrition examination survey,. *Pediatrics*. 1986; 78:257-262.

[20] Schanne, F.A., Gupta, R.K., Rosen, J.F. lead inhibits 1, 25 dihydrovitamin D-3 regulation of calcium metabolis, in osteoblastic osteosarcoma cells (ROS 17/2.8). *Biochem Biophys Acta*. 1992; 1180:187-194.

[21] Long, G.J., Pounds, J.G., Rosen, J.F. Lead intoxication alters basal and parathyroid hormone-regulated cellular calcium homoeostasis in rat osteosarcoma (ROS 17/2.8) cells. *Calcif Tissue Int*. 1992; 50:451-458.

[22] Long, G.J., Rosen, J.F. Lead perturbs epidermal growth factor (EGF) modulation of intracellular calcium metabolism and collagen synthesis in clonal rat osteoblastic (ROS 17/2.8) cells. *Toxicol Appl Pharmacol*. 1992; 114:63-70.

[23] Bogden, J.D., Gertner, S.B., Christakos, S. Kemp, F.W., Yang, Z., Katz, S.R. Dietary calcium modified concentrations of lead and other metals and renal calbindin in rats. *J Nutr*. 1992; 122:1351-1360.

[24] Mahaffey, K.R. Nutrition and lead: Strategies for public health. *Environ Health Perspect*. 1995;103(S6):191-196.

[25] Lanphear, B.P., Hornung, R., Ho, M., Howard, C.R., Eberle, S., Knauf, B.S. Environmental lead exposure during early childhood. *J Pediatr*. 2002; 140:40-47.

[26] Hammand, T.A., Sexton, M., Langenberg, P. Relationship between blood lead and dietary iron intake in preschool children. *Ann Epidemiol*. 1996; 6(1):30-33.

[27] Flaherty, E., Weiss, H. Medical evaluation of abused and neglected children. *Am J Dis Child*. 1990; 144:330-334.

[28] Mushal, P. Cronenti, A.F. Lead and nutrition: biologic interactions of lead with nutrients. *Nutr Today*. 1996; 31:12-18.

[29] Ziegler, E.E., Edward, B.B., Jensen, R.I., Mahaffey, K.R., Fomon, S.J. Absorption and retention of lead by infants. *Pediatr Res*. 1978; 12:29-34.

[30] Itoh, R., Suyama, Y. Sodium excretion in relation to calcium and hydroxyproline excretion in a healthy Japanese population. *Am J Clin Nutr*. 1996; 63:735-740.

[31] Ekvall, S.W., Ekvall V.K., Nehring, W., Walberg-Wolfe, J.Nutritional Assessment, All Ages and Levels,In: Ekvall, S. W., Ekvall, V.K.eds. *Pediatric Nutrition in Chronic Diseases and Developmental Disabilities*. 2nd ed. New York: Oxford University Press; 2005:50-80.

[32] Owen, C. The assessment and recording of measurements of growth of children: report of a small conference. *Pediatrics*. 1973; 51:461-466.

[33] Lohman, T., Roche, A. Martorell, R. *Anthropmetry standardization reference manual*. Champaign, IL: Herman Kinetics Books; 1988.

[34] *National Center for Health Statistics: Growth Charts*. Rockville, MD: Health Resources Administration, Monthly Vital Statistics Report. 25(3), Suppl. (HRA), 76-1120.

[35] Bowes and Church. *Food Values of Portions Commonly Used*, 16th ed., Philadelphia, PA: JB Lippincott Co.; 1994 (incorporated into computer values).

[36] Sobsey, D., Randall, W. Parrilla, P.K. Gender differences in abused children with and without disabilities. *Child Abuse Negl*. 1997; 21:707-720.

[37] MacMillan, H.L., Fleming, J.E., Trocme, N, Boyle, M.H., Wong, M., Racine, Y.A., Beardslee, W.R., Offord, D.R. Prevalence of child physical and sexual abuse in the community. *JAMA*. 1997; 278:131-135.

[38] Ebbin, A.J., Gollub, M.H., Stein, A.M., Wilson, M.G. Battered child syndrome at Los Angeles County General Hospital. *Am J Dis Child*. 1969; 118:660-667.

[39] Elmer, E. *Children in Jeopardy*. Pittsburgh: University of Pittsburgh Press; 1974.

[40] Wehner, F. Schieffer, M.C., Wehner, H.D., Percentile charts to determine the duration of child abuse by chronic malnutrition. *Forensic Sci Int*. 1999; 105(3):191-194.

[41] Rao, N,K,, Begum, S., Benkataramana,V., Gangadharappa, N. Nutritional neglect and physical abuse in children of alcoholics. *Indian J Pediatr*. 2001; 68(9):843-845.

[42] Bonet Alcaina, M., Martinez Roig, A, Pujals Ferrer, J.M., Vall combelles, O. Kwashiorkor as a symptom of abuse and neglect in Barcelona. *An Esp Pediatr*. 2001; 54(4): 405-408.

[43] Glotzer, D.E., Weitzman, M. Commonly asked questions about childhood lead poisoning. *Pediatr Ann*. 1995;24(12):631-639.

[44] Hutchinson, J., Langlykke, K. *Adolescent Maltreatment: Youth as Victims of Abuse and Neglect* (Maternal and Child Health Technical Information Bulletin), Arlington, VA: National Center for Education in Maternal and Child Health; 1998.

[45] Huber, A., Ekvall,S. Lead Toxicity and Pica. In Ekvall, S.W., Ekvall, V.K.eds. *Pediatric Nutrition in Chronic Diseases and Developmental Disorders*. 2nd edition, New York, Oxford University Press, 2005; 168-170.

[46] Stevens, F., Ekvall, S. *Empowering Children with Good Nutrition and Early Intervention :Focusing on Culturally Diverse Children with Special Health Care Needs*. Maternal and Child Health Manual 4, Cincinnati, University of Cincinnati, 2002.

[47] Rokusek, C, Jarka, E., Hanley, B., Earle-Hahn, J. Community Based Services and Resources. In *Pediatric Nutrition in Chronic Diseases and Developmental Disorders*. 2nd edition, New York, Oxford University Press, 2005, 63-69.

[48] Graff. C., Murthy, L., Ekvall, S. Magnon, M. In home toxic chemical exposures and children with developmental disabilities. *Pediatr. Nursing*. November/December, 2006;32(6):597-602.

[49] American Dietetic Association (Diabetic Care and Education Practice Group), American Diabetes Association. *Ethnic and Regional Food Practices*. Chicago, American Dietetic Association, 1998.

[50] Ekvall S.,EkvallV. Nutrition Support for Children with Developmental Disabilities. In Baker,S, Baker,R, Davis,A. *Pediatric Nutrition Support*, Sudbury, Mass., Jones and Bartlett Publishers, 2007.

[51] Tyler,C,White-Scott,S, Ekvall, S, Abulafa, L. Environmental Health and Developmental Disabliltities: A Life Span Approach, *Family and Community Health*. 2008:31(4)28:287.

8

Pharmacological and Clinical Effectiveness of *Zingiber officinale* and *Alpinia galanga* in Patients with Osteoarthritis

Guntars Selga, M. Sauka, L. Aboltina, A. Davidova, P. Kaipainen, D. Kheder, T. Westermarck and F. Atroshi

1. Introduction

Osteoarthritis (OA) is a progressive degenerative joint disease that has a major impact on joint function and quality of life. OA is a painful condition caused by a gradual loss of cartilage from the joints and, in some people, joint inflammation [1]. Pain, stiffness, and difficulty moving the joint easily are common symptoms of OA. Non-drug treatments for osteoarthritis have gained popularity according to the American College of Rheumatology (ACR) [2] and can often reduce the symptoms. Therefore, there is a significant need to improve current osteoarthritis therapies and to search for novel therapies. Nutraceuticals and dietary supplements derived from herbs have long been used in traditional medicine. Though they aren't recognized as drugs, herbal and natural remedies are used for a drug-like effect, and they can potentially cause the same reactions and complications prescription drugs can cause. There is considerable evidence that nutraceuticals may play an important role in inflammation and joint destruction in OA. The World Health Organization (WHO) [3] has taken an interest in the indigenous system of medicine; particularly, plant remedies. Ginger is widely used as a spice, an antiemetic and carminative agent, and for its essential oils. Gingerols, in particular 6-gingerol, are the active components of ginger. Proposed mechanisms include direct stimulation of the gastro-intestinal tract, or serotonin antagonism in the gut or central nervous system [4, 5]. A study on 6-gingerol was shown to significantly inhibit the production of nitric oxide, a highly reactive nitrogen molecule that quickly forms a very damaging free radical called peroxynitrite and greatly lessened depletion of glutathione [6]. Other reports suggest that ginger produces its anti-inflammatory effect by inhibiting arachidonic acid metabolism [4, 7], induce apoptosis in HL-60 leukemia [8], non-small cell lung cancer cells [9] and against acute monocytic leukemia [10]. It is also reported to be chemopreventive and anti-inflammatory [11, 12]. The antioxidant, antimicrobial and cytotoxic activities of Zingiber officinale displayed specific inhibition on Escherichia coli was also studied [13]. Gingerols also promoted significant reduction in mRNA transcription of TNF-α, IL-2 and INF-γ [14]. Ginsenoside Rg5 (Rg5), an abundant natural compound in Panax ginseng, has been found to be beneficial in treating AD [15]. Pharmacologic studies in the last decades have shown that ginsenosides (ginseng saponins) are primarily responsible for the actions of ginseng [16]. In diabetes ginger supplementation in oral administration reduced inflammation in type 2 diabetic patients [17]. Other studies have shown that ginger may benefits musculoskeletal disorder treatment [18] nausea and vomiting [19], inflammation or inflammatory states [20, 21] such as osteoarthritis [20-22], migraine [23], cancer [24], hyperlipidemia and hyperglycemia [25, 26]. In vitro studies suggest that ginger produces its anti-inflammatory effect by inhibiting arachidonic acid metabolism[4], [7]. This chapter intends to give a brief outline of ginger health benefit and to investigate the ability of ginger tablets to reduce postoperative pain in patients with osteoarthritis.

1.1. History

The earliest evidence of humans' use of plants for healing dates back to the Neanderthal period [27]. In the 16th century, botanical gardens were created to grow medicinal plants for medical schools [28]. Herbal medicine practice flourished until the 17th century when more "scientific" pharmacological remedies were favoured [29]. The use of plants for healing purposes predates human history and forms the origin of much modern medicine. Many conventional drugs originate from plant sources: a century ago, most of the few effective drugs were plant based. Examples include aspirin (from willow bark), digoxin (from foxglove), quinine (from cinchona bark), and morphine (from the opium poppy). The development of drugs from plants continues, with drug companies engaged in large scale pharmacological screening of herbs.

1.2. Therapeutic scope

Although herbal preparations are widely used as self-medication for acute conditions, practitioners of herbal medicine tend to concentrate on treating chronic conditions. A typical caseload might include asthma, eczema, premenstrual syndrome, rheumatoid arthritis, migraine, menopausal symptoms, chronic fatigue, irritable bowel syndrome and lately to treat mental or musculoskeletal disorders.

1.3. Safety

Many plants are highly toxic. Herbal medicine probably presents a greater risk of adverse effects and interactions than any other complementary therapy. There are case reports of serious adverse events after administration of herbal products. In most cases the herbs involved were self-prescribed and bought over the counter or obtained from a source other than a registered practitioner. In the most notorious instance, several women developed rapidly progressive interstitial renal fibrosis after taking Chinese herbs prescribed by a slimming clinic

2. Method and subjects

2.1. Method

Fourthly patients with OA of the knee and moderate-to-severe pain were enrolled in a randomised, double –blind, placebo-controlled, two-center, parallel group, 12-week study. The primary efficacy variable was the proportion of responders experiencing a reduction in "knee pain on standing" using a visual analog scale.

The study was approved by the ethics committee of the Latvian Institute of Cardiology for clinical and physiological research, drug and pharmaceutics product clinical investigation.

Only those willing to participate and after getting their informed consent will be involved in the investigation

2.2. Subjects

Elderly patients with clinical diagnosis of osteoarthritis (OA) of the knee, defined as knee (articular and not periarticular or referred) pain for most days of the prior month and radiographic osteophytes at the tibiofemoral joint margins were involved in the study. All involved patients had a baseline pain score > 40 mm and < 90 mm on a 100-mm Visual Analogue Scale (VAS) at the time of randomization, when evaluating pain on standing during the last 24 hours. Both men and women were included.

Exclusion Characteristics

- No NSAID's or other medication before intervention start-or consider including one week wash-out period.
- History of allergy to ginger;
- History of rheumatoid disease;
- History of asthma, if the patient needs treatment with steroids;
- Treatment with oral corticosteroids within four weeks prior to screening;
- Treatment with intra-articular corticosteroids;
- Treatment with intra-articular hyaluronic acid within 6 months prior screening;
- Prior treatment with immuno-suppressive drugs, cytostatic drugs, gold or peniciilamine;
- Other investigational drugs within one month prior to screening;
- History or clinical signs of impaired kidney function;

- Clinical signs of liver disorders;
- Severe neurological diseases;
- Increased oral temperature, (37,5 C) at the time of screening;
- Affection of the hip to an extent that would influence the ratings done at the visits";
- History of fibromyalgia;
- Gout;
- Recurrent or active pseudo-gout;

2.2.1. Study design

The study was 12 weeks, double blind, and placebo-controlled, parallel group trial performed in two social care centres for elderly people. The study was approved by the ethics committee of the Latvian Institute of Cardiology for clinical and physiological research, drug and pharmaceutics product clinical investigation. Only those willing to participate and after getting their informed consent will be involved in the investigation. Patients were randomised to receive treatment and both investigators and the patients were blind to treatment assignment.

2.2.2. Treatment

During the 12-week period, patients ingested 1 capsule twice daily, morning and evening. Each capsule contained 150 mg Ginger rhizome *(lat. Zingiberis officinale rhizome)* powdered extract and 125 mg Galangae rhizome (*Alpinia officinarum rhizome)* dry extract. 22 patients were got tablets with "A" and 18 patients got tablets with "B". Examination was done at the baseline, after 6 weeks and after 12 weeks.

2.2.3. Results

Characteristics of the subjects

Forty patients were included in the study (for group "A"-mean age ± SD 69±13,7 and for group "B"-mean age ± SD 75 ± 8,6). There were ten males (35 %) and thirty females (75%). The patients in both groups were generally overweight, since the average was >28 kg/m^2 (range 43 – 120 kg).

2.2.4. Assessments

The primary efficacy parameter was proportion of respondents experiencing at least a 15-mm reduction in pain between baseline and the final examination for knee pain on standing and walking during preceding 24 hours, as measured by a 100-mm, VAS.

The secondary measurement was mean ±SE of measurements for knee pain on standing and walking.

	" A" group (n=22)	"B "group (n=18)
Age, mean ± SD years	69 ± 13,7	75 ± 8,6
Sex %		
Men	23	28
Women	77	72
Body mass index ± SD kg/m²	29.31 ± 7,7	28 ± 7,0
Waste/hip ratio ± SD	0,88 ± 0,04	0,91 ± 0,04

Table 1. Demographic characteristics

	Baseline data		After 6 weeks		after 12 weeks	
	A	B	A	B	A	B
	n=22	n=18	n=20	n=18	n=20	n=18
Pain on standing and walking (%)						
> 15 mm	-	-	-	-	50	44
0 – 15 mm	-	-	-	-	41	50
≤ 0	-	-	-	-	9	6
Pain on standing, mean ± SE (mm)	62.95±2.2	57.11±+2.5	56.65±2.3	49.52±2.5	51.2±2.3	43.88±2.5
Pain on walking, mean ± SE (mm)	61.68±2.4	60.64±2.7	54.85±2.5	54±2.7	49.25±2.5	49.23±2.7

Table 2. Measurements for knee pain between group "A" and group "B"

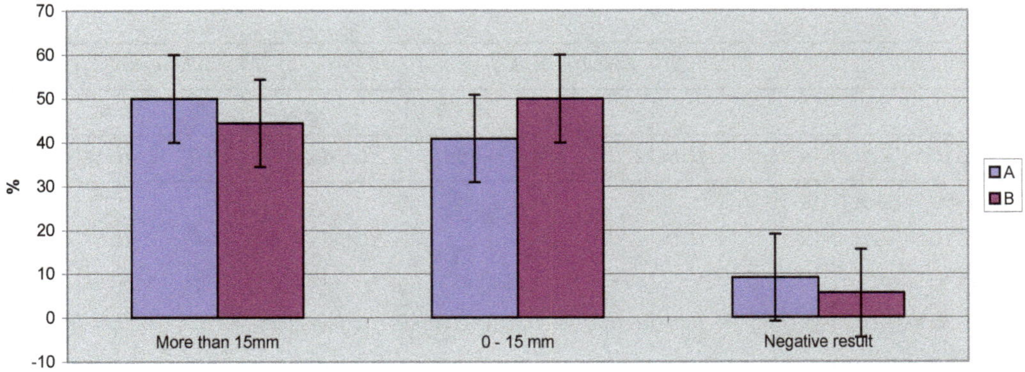

Figure 1. Pain on standing and walking after using of Ginger containg food supplements

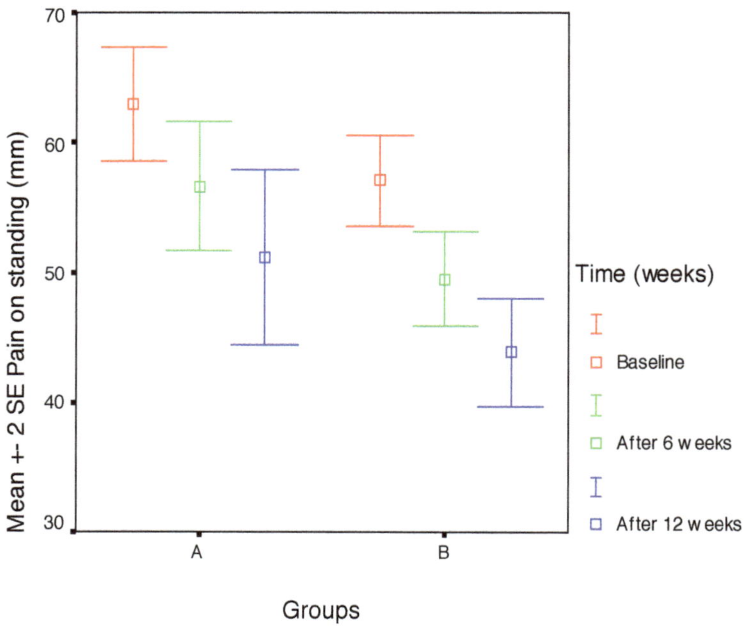

Figure 2. Knee pain on standing as measured by 100-mm visual analog scale at baseline and after 6 weeks and 12 weeks. Bars shows means with 2 SE (mm)

Additionally blood sample was checked in both groups. There were no statistically significant changes between groups.

	Baseline data		After 12 weeks	
	A	B	A	B
	n=22	n=18	n=20	n=18
Erytrocytes, Mean±SE, (10 [12]/L)	4.42±0.9	4.46±1	4.31±0,09	4.2±1
Hb Mean±SE, (g/L)	131.66±5.8	135.8±6.5	134.8+5.9	113.15±6.5
Hematocrit Mean±SE (%)	39.28±0.9	40.03±1.0	38.8±0.9	37.85±1.0
WBC Mean±SE (10^9/L)	7.7±0.5	6.4±0.5	6.38±0.5	5.6±0.5
ESR Mean±SE (mm/h)	23.77±3.6	20.06±4.0	19.31±3.8	18.76±4.1

Table 3. Comparison of blood samples between both groups in the study.

3. Discussion and conclusion

Ginger (Zingiber officinale Roscoe), a well-known spice plant, has been used traditionally in a wide variety of ailments including hypertension and osteoarthritis. Gingerol, the active components of ginger, derivatives are currently under investigation as potential drug therapy for disorders of platelet function, but the small amounts consumed in the diet are unlikely to influence platelet function. We report here the osteoarthritis effects of Zingiber officinale and Alpinia galanga tablets under controlled experimental conditions.

Osteoarthritis, the most common form of arthritis, is a debilitating progressive disease principally affecting the elderly. Osteoarthritis therapy has evolved in the past few decades from symptomatic treatment to possible disease-modifying solutions. Osteoarthritis continues to be a difficult disorder to treat, as there is no cure as such and current treatments focus mainly on relieving pain and maintaining joint function. The search nevertheless continues for management regimens that can slow, alter or reverse the degenerative processes of osteoarthritis. Experimental therapies that seek to modify the course of osteoarthritis. These include such medications as colchicine, bisphosphonates and hormones. Dietary therapeutics, such as ginger extract also has been suggested. Current approaches to treating osteoarthritis-i.e. medications; nonpharmacological modalities, such as physical therapy, exercise, weight management and orthotics; and (as a last resort) surgery-focus on reducing pain and improving (or at least maintaining) mobility

Musculoskeletal conditions are prevalent and their impact is pervasive. They are the most common cause of severe long-term pain and physical disability. The prevalence of many of these conditions increases markedly with age, and many are affected by lifestyle factors, such as obesity and lack of physical activity. The increasing number of older people and the changes in lifestyle throughout the world mean that the burden on people and society will increase dramatically. This has been recognized by the United Nations and WHO, with their endorsement of Bone and Joint Decade 2000–2010 [30]. Osteoarthritis was estimated to be the eighth leading non-fatal burden of disease in the world in 1990, accounting for 2.8% of total years of living with disability, around the same percentage as schizophrenia and congenital anomalies [31]. It was the sixth leading cause of years of living with disability at the global level, accounting for 3% of the total global years of living with disability [32], [33], [34]. According to the American Holistic Medical Association it is believed that the spiritual element should also be taken into account when assessing a person's overall well-being [35], [36]. Ginger is an herb which has been used for centuries in Ayurdevic medicine to relieve the pain of arthritis although few studies are available to demonstrate its benefits. There appears to be good evidence from epidemiological studies and clinical trials that Zingiber officinale and Alpinia galanga tablets lower osteoarthritis tendency. The mechanism of action is believed to be due to the inhibition of prostaglandin and leukotriene synthesis. Zingiber officinale and Alpinia galanga was also tested for antibacterial activities by evaluating growth delays using human strains of the genera Staphylococcus and Micrococcus. Staphylococcus aureus was found to be sensitive to the ginger extract. When the extract was tested for the haemolytic effect, no lytic effects on procaryotic cells were found. Patients suffering from such disorders reported relief in pain and associated symptoms on extract administration. No significant side effects of supplementation were noted, which may be considered as adjuvant therapy in patients with osteoarthritis of the knee. In this study ginger extract may have a beneficial effective in treatment for osteoarthritis. However, more observational studies, with a larger sample size, are needed to confirm the encouraging preliminary data on effectiveness and safety. The use of Zingiber officinale and Alpinia galanga in osteoarthritis will reduce the symptoms to an equivalent extent in elderly people with osteoarthritis.

Author details

Guntars Selga[1], M. Sauka[1], L. Aboltina[1], A. Davidova[1], P. Kaipainen[2], D. Kheder[1], T. Westermarck[2] and F. Atroshi[3]

1 Department of Oral and Maxillofacial Surgery, Faculty of Dentistry, Rīga Stradiņš University, Rīga, Latvia

2 Rinnekoti Research Center, Espoo, Finland

3 Pharmacology &Toxicology, University of Helsinki, Finland

References

[1] Kraus JF, D'Ambrosia RD, Smith EG, Van Meter J, Borhani NO, Franti CE, Lipscomb PR. An epidemiological study of severe osteoarthritis. Orthopedics. 1978 Jan-Feb; 1(1):37-42.

[2] ACR, Recommendations for the medical management of osteoarthritis of the hip and knee: 2000 update. American College of Rheumatology Subcommittee on Osteoarthritis Guidelines. Arthritis Rheum. 2000;43(9):1905.

[3] WHO. "Fact sheet no. 134: Traditional medicine". World Health Organization. 2008-12-01. Retrieved 2009-05-02.

[4] Grant KL, Lutz RB. Ginger. American Journal of Health-System Pharmacy 2000; 57: 945–7.

[5] Ernst E, Pittler MH. Efficacy of ginger for nausea and vomiting: a systematic review of randomised controlled clinical trials. British Journal of Anaesthesia 2000; 84: 367–71.

[6] Jagetia GC, Baliga MS, Venkatesh P, Ulloor JN. Influence of ginger rhizome (Zingiber officinale Rosc) on survival, glutathione and lipid peroxidation in mice after whole-body exposure to gamma radiation. Radiat Res. 2003 Nov;160(5):584-92. 2003

[7] Koo KL, Ammit AJ, Tran VH, Duke CC, Roufogalis BD. Gingerols and related analogues inhibit arachidonic acid-induced human platelet serotonin release and aggregation. Thrombosis Research 2001; 103: 387–97.

[8] Lee E, Surh YJ: Induction of apoptosis in HL-60 cells by pungent vanilloids, [6]-gingerol and [6]-paradol. Cancer Lett 1998;134:163–168.

[9] Wang G, Li X, Huang F, Zhao J, Ding H, Cunningham C, Coad JE, Flynn DC, Reed E, Li QQ: Antitumor effect of β-elemene in non-small cell lung cancer cells is mediated via induction of cell cycle arrest and apoptotic cell death. Cell Mol Life Sci 2005;62:881–893.

[10] Omoregie SN, Omoruyi FO, Wright VF, Jones L, Zimba PV. Antiproliferative activities of lesser galangal (Alpinia officinarum Hance Jam1), turmeric (Curcuma longa L.), and ginger (Zingiber officinale Rosc.) against acute monocytic leukemia. J Med Food. 2013 Jul;16(7):647-55.

[11] Nonn L, Duong D, Peehl, DM: Chemopreventive anti-inflammatory activities of curcumin and other phytochemicals mediated by MAP kinase phosphatase-5 in prostate cells. Carcinogenesis 2007;28:1188–1196.

[12] Zick SM, Djuric Z, Ruffin MT, Litzinger AJ, Normolle DP, Alrawi S, Feng MR, Brenner DE: Pharmacokinetics of 6-gingerol, 8-gingerol, 10-gingerol, and 6-shogaol and conjugate metabolites in healthy human subjects. Cancer Epidemiol Biomarkers Prev 2008;17:1930–1936.

[13] Lu CL, Zhao HY, Jiang JG. Evaluation of multi-activities of 14 edible species from Zingiberaceae. Int J Food Sci Nutr. 2013 Feb;64(1):28-35.

[14] Rodrigues FA, Prata MM, Oliveira IC, Alves NT, Freitas RE, Monteiro HS, Silva JA, Vieira PC, Viana DA, Libório AB, Havt A. Gingerol Fraction from Zingiber officinale Protects Against Gentamicin-Induced Nephrotoxicity. Antimicrob Agents Chemother. 2014 Jan 6. (Epub ahead of print).

[15] Chu S, Gu J, Feng L, Liu J, Zhang M, Jia X, Yao D, Liu M. Ginsenoside Rg5 improves cognitive dysfunction and beta-amyloid deposition in STZ-induced memory impaired rats via attenuating neuroinflammatory responses.Int Immunopharmacol. 2014 Feb 3. pii: S1567-5769(14)00032-0. doi: 10. 1016/j.intimp.2014. 01. 018.

[16] Im DS, Nah SY. Yin and Yang of ginseng pharmacology: ginsenosides vs gintonin. Acta Pharmacol Sin. 2013 Nov;34(11):1367-73.

[17] Mahluji S, Ostadrahimi A, Mobasseri M, Ebrahimzade Attari V, Payahoo L. Anti-inflammatory effects of zingiber officinale in type 2 diabetic patients. Adv Pharm Bull. 2013;3(2):273-6.

[18] Srivastava KC, Mustafa T. Ginger (zingiber officinale) in rheumatism and musculoskeletal disorders. Med Hypotheses. 1992;39(4):342–8.

[19] Bryer E. A literature review of the effectiveness of ginger in alleviating mild-to-moderate nausea and vomiting of pregnancy. J Midwifery Womens Health. 2005;50(1):e1–3.

[20] Leach MJ, Kumar S. The clinical effectiveness of ginger (zingiber officinale) in adults with osteoarthritis. Int J Evid Based Healthc. 2008;6(3):311–20.

[21] Altman RD, Marcussen KC. Effects of a ginger extract on knee pain in patients with osteoarthritis. Arthritis Rheum. 2001;44(11):2531–8.

[22] Therkleson T. Ginger Therapy for Osteoarthritis: A Typical Case. J Holist Nurs. 2014 Jan 29. [Epub ahead of print].

[23] Mustafa T, Srivastava KC. Ginger (Zingiber officinale) in migraine headache. J Ethnopharmacol. 1990;29(3):267–73.

[24] Shukla Y, Singh M. Cancer preventive properties of ginger: A brief review. Food Chem Toxicol. 2007;45(5):683–90.

[25] Ali BH, Blunden G, Tanira MO, Nemmar A. Some phytochemical, pharmacological and toxicological properties of ginger (Zingiber officinale Roscoe): a review of recent research. Food Chem Toxicol. 2008;46(2):409–20.

[26] White B. Ginger: An overview. Am Fam Physician. 2007;75(11):1689–91.

[27] Kleiner SM. The true nature of herbs. Phys Sports Med. 1995;23:13-14.

[28] Akerele O. Nature's medicinal bounty: don't throw it away. World Health Forum. 1993;14:390-395.

[29] Trevelyan J. Herbal medicine. Nurs Times. 1993;89:36-38.

[30] Woolf AD. The bone and joint decade 2000-2010. Ann Rheum Dis. 2000 Feb;59(2):81-2

[31] Murray CJ, Lopez AD. Evidence-based health policy--lessons from the Global Burden of Disease Study. Science. 1996 Nov 1;274(5288):740-3.

[32] Lau EM, Symmons DP, Croft P. The epidemiology of hip osteoarthritis and rheumatoid arthritis in the Orient. Clin Orthop Relat Res. 1996 Feb;(323):81-90.

[33] Symmons DP. Safety profile of low-dose aspirin. Lancet. 1996 Nov 23;348(9039): 1394-5.

[34] Akhtar N and Haqqi TM. Current nutraceuticals in the management of osteoarthritis: a review. Ther Adv Musculoskelet Dis. 2012 June; 4(3): 181–207.

[35] Roberts M, American Holistic Medical Association 02/05/2014.

[36] Strandberg, E; Ovhed, I; Borgquist, L; Wilhelmsson, S. "The perceived meaning of a (w) holistic view among general practitioners and district nurses in Swedish primary care: A qualitative study". BMC Family Practice, 2007, 8: 8. doi:10. 1186/1471-2296-8-8.

9

Adaptive Behavior Change and Health in Adults with Down Syndrome: A Prospective Clinical Follow-Up Study

T. Määttä, T. Tervo-Määttä, A. Taanila, M. Kaski and M. Iivanainen

1. Introduction

People with Down syndrome are prone to early ageing and Alzheimer's disease (Zigman & Lott 2007). The functional decline in adults with Down syndrome starts decades earlier, compared to the mainstream population and other people with intellectual disabilities (Zigman *et al.* 1996; Strydom *et al.* 2007). The coping skills necessary for daily life, social interactions and work are gradually lost during the progression of dementia (Margallo-Lana *et al.* 2007).

Typical neuropathology of Alzheimer's disease is seen in virtually all people with Down syndrome by the age of 40 (Wisniewski *et al.* 1985). Depending on diagnostic criteria, 17-55% of them develop clinical dementia after that age (Holland *et al.* 2000; Janicki & Dalton 2000; Coppus *et al.* 2006). Genetic factors modifying the risk of dementia in adults with Down syndrome have been identified (Zigman & Lott 2007; Prasher *et al.* 2008; Patel *et al.* 2010). The rates of dementia in adults with intellectual disability without Down syndrome aged 60 years and older are greater than expected (Strydom *et al.* 2007).

The cognitive impairment in adults with Down syndrome has similarities to early cognitive changes in Alzheimer's disease (Brugge *et al.*1994). Personality and behaviour changes (Ball *et al.* 2006), executive dysfunction (Ball *et al.* 2008) and selective attention deficits (Krinsky-McHale *et al.* 2008) are early signs of dementia in adults with Down syndrome. Frontal-like dementia can be diagnosed in 33% in their thirties (Holland *et al.* 2000). Maladaptive behaviour is often seen and includes aggression, fearfulness, sadness, sleep problems, social inadequacy, stealing and general regressive behaviour (Urv *et al.* 2008). Increasing age associates with decreasing cognitive and language abilities; the deterioration with the age is largely explained by the presence of Alzheimer's disease (Iacono *et al.* 2010).

Identification of persons with risk of early dementia remains a challenge (Shulz *et al.* 2004). Direct assessments of cognitive functions of people with intellectual disabilities may be difficult (Pyo *et al.* 2007). Informant-based assessments are useful as complementary or alternative methods in clinical work (Ball *et al.* 2004; Prasher *et al.* 2004; Niuwenhuis-Mark 2009).

The Adaptive Behavior Scale - Residential and Community (Nihira *et al.* 1993) and its earlier versions have been widely used in research. Cross-sectional studies have demonstrated lower scores on people with Down syndrome older than 40 years compared to younger participants with Down syndrome (Collacott 1992). The age-related decline of adaptive behaviour associates to dementia (Prasher & Chung 1996). Prospective studies have confirmed changes in adaptive behaviour (Rasmussen & Sobsey 1994; Prasher *et al.* 1998). Zigman *et al.* (2002) described the incidence and temporal patterns of adaptive behaviour changes in adults with intellectual disabilities. Rasmussen and Sobsey (1994) found stability of adaptive behaviour in adults with Down syndrome in the age groups younger than 40 years and a pattern of decline in self-help and communication skills in several individuals with Down syndrome older than 40, including declines in dressing, receptive language, vocational and domestic behaviour.

Relative preservation of cognitive and functional ability in persons with Down syndrome older than 45 associates with better survival whereas clinically, the most important disorders that are related to mortality are dementia, mobility restrictions, visual impairment, and epilepsy (Coppus *et al.* 2008).

Health co-morbidities in ageing persons with Down syndrome and Alzheimer's dementia are common (McCarron *et al.* 2005). Depression often precedes the onset of dementia in people with Down syndrome (Burt *et al.* 1992). Visual impairment and hearing loss are very common in elderly people with Down syndrome (van Splunder *et al.* 2006; Meuwese-Jongejeugd *et al.* 2006; Meuwese-Jongejeugd *et al.* 2008). Epilepsy is often seen at the same age with dementia (Collacott 1993). Hypothyroidism may also affect adaptive behaviour (Bhaumik *et al.* 1991). The absence of a medical illness predicts a higher level of adaptive behaviour, while dementia is a predictive factor for increased maladaptive behaviour (Prasher & Chung 1996) and psychiatric symptoms (Urv *et al.* 2010)

Medication for Alzheimer's disease might benefit many people with Down syndrome by slowing the progression of the disease (Prasher *et al.* 2002). Accurate measures are important for the follow-up and evaluation of treatments. It is necessary to find and use valid, reliable and sensitive methods for assessments of adults and ageing people with Down syndrome and Alzheimer's disease.

The aim of the present study was to explore the clinical usefulness of repeated assessments of adaptive behaviour in people with Down syndrome and suspected or confirmed dementia. Repeated assessments of adaptive behaviour in people at risk of functional decline might help to confirm the change and lead to necessary additional evaluations of the underlying reasons and help in follow-up.

2. Methods

Study population

The participating adults with Down syndrome were recruited to the study at a specialized service centre for people with intellectual disabilities serving a population of 79 690 (December 2008), among them 723 people with identified intellectual disability. These include 84 people with Down syndrome; 19 of them were 0-19 years old, 65 were 20 years old or older. Forty of the 65 adults belonged to the age group 40 years old or older.

Assessments of adaptive behaviour were conducted to 42 persons with Down syndrome (Table 1). Twenty five persons had repeated assessments. These persons' proxies had noticed a change of mood, behaviour or performance. At the time of the first evaluation, their age range was 24-61 years, with a mean of 45.8 and SD of +/- 8.4; at the time of the last evaluation, the corresponding figures were 25-65.5, 48.8, and +/- 8.4 years, respectively. The mean time of follow-up was, thus, 3.0 years (range 0-8 years). Five participants died during the follow up. Twenty participants (80%) of the 25 were 40 years or older at the time of the first evaluation. Most participants (17/25, 68%) resided at the beginning of the follow-up in small group homes, seven (28%) at home with parents or siblings and one in institution. Fourteen participants (56%) had organized weekly activities outside the home and two participants had part time supported work.

Methods

Repeated informant evaluations regarding observed changes in behaviour were recorded prospectively. Evaluations of adults with Down syndrome were performed over ten years, beginning in 2001. Adaptive behaviour assessments were performed by the closest relatives or carers who lived or worked with the participants and knew the persons and their daily skills for a long time.

The current coping skills for daily living were assessed using the Adaptive Behavior Scale - Residential and Community, ABS-RC: 2 1993, Part I (Nihira *et al.* 1993). The Adaptive Behavior Scale (ABS) was chosen because the reliability and validity of this method are well established. Earlier research supports its feasibility in the use of scientific studies of ageing and dementia in people with intellectual disabilities (Rasmussen & Sobsey 1994; Prasher *et al.* 1998; Zigman *et al.* 2002).

The first part of ABS is focused on personal independence and includes ten domains or subscales: Independent Functioning, Physical Development, Economic Activity, Language

Development, Numbers and Time, Domestic Activity, Prevocational/Vocational Activity, Self-Direction, Responsibility and Socialization. The ABS Manual reports that factor analysis has found three Part One factors: Personal Self-Sufficiency, Community Self-Sufficiency, and Personal–Social Responsibility.

Clinical evaluations were done by the principal investigator. These included interviews of the proxies, referrals for differential diagnostics and specialist consultations, and prescriptions and assessments of medications. Additional clinical data was drawn from the case records of the health centres, central hospital and service centre regarding all persons with Down syndrome in the region. The data of medical treatments for Alzheimer's disease, depression, behavioural problems, epilepsy, and other major health concerns possibly affecting adaptive behaviour were analyzed. The age at the time of the first observation of functional decline was calculated.

Informant ratings by ABS were scored and analysed. Total scores, scores for the ten subscales and three factors of ABS and changes of scores from the first to the last evaluation were counted. The ABS score changes as percentages per three years were calculated for subgroups of participants with and without Alzheimer's disease, depression, epilepsy, hypothyroidism, and antipsychotic medication use for challenging behaviour.

The ethical committee of the Kainuu Central Hospital approved the study and permission for combining data from medical and social records was given by the Ministry of Social and Health Affairs.

3. Results

The number of people with Down syndrome living in the area is well known and their morbidity data was available for comparison. The participants with repeated ABS assessments were older than participants with single assessments. Dementia, medication use for challenging behaviour, depression and epilepsy were more common among participants than among adults with Down syndrome living in the region.

Alzheimer's disease

Alzheimer's disease with dementia was diagnosed in 15 out of the 25 participants assessed repeatedly. Four of them died during the survey. The diagnosis was confirmed in ten participants by a neurologist and in five participants by the first author with competence in intellectual disability medicine. Other causes of dementia were excluded. Computerized tomographies of the brain were performed in ten of these participants. Eleven persons received medication for Alzheimer's disease (donepezile, galantamine or rivastigmine, in three participants combined with memantine). Early dementia was suspected in an additional four participants; they had increasing difficulties following instructions and performing their usual domestic work.

The number of living people with diagnosed and suspected dementia (fifteen persons among the participants and two not participating in this study) among adults with Down syndrome in the region gives prevalence's of dementia 38% (15 of 40 persons) in the age group 40 years and more, and 13% (two of 15 persons) in the age group 30-39 years. The prevalence estimate of dementia for the age group 30 years and more is thus 31% (17 of 55 persons).

Medical problems

Of the 25 participants eleven (44%) had experienced long periods of depression. Thirteen (52%) had received antipsychotic medication mainly for behavioural problems, six of them already during early adulthood and eight for behavioural problems with dementia. Eleven persons were treated for hypothyroidism. Varying degrees of visual impairment were common, and three had cataracts. Recurrent faints were seen in eight, with falls causing fractures in three persons. Epilepsy was diagnosed in eight persons.

Among participants with Alzheimer's disease (n=15), antipsychotic medication had been used for eleven (73%), depression had been diagnosed in ten (67%), thyroid disease in ten (67%), and epilepsy in seven (47%) participants. Among participants without Alzheimer's disease (n=10), antipsychotic medication had been used for two (20%), depression had been diagnosed in one (10%), thyroid disease in four (40%), and epilepsy in one participant (10%). Among eleven participants with depression (N=11), antipsychotic medication had been used for seven (64%), Alzheimer's disease had been diagnosed in ten (91%), thyroid disease in 6 (55%), and epilepsy in five (45%) participants.

Informant observations

A decline of daily functioning was observed by informants in regards to 19 of 25 persons, starting at the ages of 37-51 years with a mean of 44.9 and SD +/- 4 years in persons with full trisomy of chromosome 21. In addition, there was one participant with mosaic trisomy of chromosome 21 whose decline started only at the age of 60 (Figure 3, participant 2).

Adaptive Behavior Scale (ABS) scores

The mean ages, ABS total scores at first and last assessments and the calculated percentages of score changes per three years in subgroups of participants are presented in Table 1. The mean ABS total scores for the 25 participants with multiple assessments declined from 161 to 126 (21.8%) during the mean 3.0 years between the first and last assessments. The decline of ABS total scores associated very strongly to Alzheimer's disease: there was no decline in the mean ABS total scores in the group of participants with no suspected or confirmed Alzheimer's disease. The mean rates of ABS score change were higher in participant groups with Alzheimer's disease (33.6% in three years), and depression (32.0%) compared to participants without these conditions (0.6% and 13.9% respectively). The participants treated with medication for Alzheimer's disease had lower mean rates of score declines compared to untreated patients, 31% and 40% declines in three years respectively. The mean rates of change were almost similar in groups of persons with and without epilepsy, antipsychotic medication, and hypothyroidism. (Table 1)

Participants (number of persons)	Age of participants at first (last) assessment	ABS total scores, means at first (last) assessment	ABS score change percentage per three years, %
Participants with single assessments (17)	36.5 (36.5)	174 (174)	
males (10)	32.3 (32.3)	188 (188)	
females (7)	42.4 (42.4)	155 (155)	
Participants with repeated assessments (25)	45.8 (48.8)	161 (126)	-21.8
males (11)	43.8 (47.0)	135 (117)	-12.4
females (14)	48.4 (51.5)	193 (137)	-28.4
Alzheimer`s disease (AD, 15)	49.7 (52.9)	165 (106)	-33.6
AD, no medication (4)	47.8 (50.8)	155 (93)	-40.0
AD, medication (11)	50.6 (53.9)	170 (112)	-31.0
No AD (10)	40.0 (43.1)	154 (155)	+0.6
Depression (11)	47.6 (50.5)	159 (112)	-32.0
No depression (14)	44.4 (47.8)	162 (136)	-13.9
Epilepsy (8)	50.6 (54.5)	193 (141)	-23.0
No epilepsy (17)	43.5 (46.5)	145 (118)	-18.7
Antipsychotic medication (13)	49.0 (52.0)	168 (132)	-21.7
No antipsychotic medication (12)	42.3 (45.7)	152 (119)	-19.3
Hypothyroidism (11)	45.8 (48.7)	152 (125)	-19.4
No hypothyroidism (14)	45.8 (49.1)	166 (126)	-21.5

Table 1. Ages, ABS-RC:2 total scores and score changes in subgroups of participants with Down syndrome.

ABS-RC:2 subscale	Scores, first assessment Mean (SD)	Scores, last assessment Mean (SD)	Score change, %
Domestic Activity	9.6 (6.1)	5.8 (6.1)	-64.8
Responsibility	5.0 (3.0)	3.3 (3.1)	-51.2
Self-Direction	12.1 (5.9)	8.0 (6.9)	-50.3
Prevocational/Vocational Activity	5.8 (3.1)	4.0 (3.6)	-44.0
Numbers and Time	5.4 (3.4)	3.8 (3.8)	-41.1
Independent Functioning	64.8 (24.3)	52.3 (32.0)	-23.8
Language Development	21.0 (9.4)	17.2 (8.9)	-22.0
Economic Activity	3.6 (3.3)	3.2 (3.5)	-12.5
Physical Development	18.4 (3.5)	16.0 (5.5)	-15.0
Economic Activity	3.6 (3.3)	3.2 (3.5)	-12.5

Table 2. ABS-RC:2 subscale mean scores and their change during the prospective follow-up of 25 participants with Down syndrome.

The biggest mean declines were seen in the subscales Domestic Activity, Responsibility and Self-Direction, to 35.2, 48.8 and 49.7%, respectively. The slightest changes were seen in the domains of Economic Activity, Physical Development and Language Development (Table 2). The mean changes of scores for the ABS factors Personal Self-Sufficiency, Community Self-Sufficiency and Personal–Social Responsibility were 22.2, 27.9 and 36.8%, respectively.

Individual changes in ABS scores

The ABS scores remained stable in nine and improved in three persons. A progressive decline of ABS scores was seen in 13 of 25 (52%) participants after their early forties. The direction, amount and rate of change of ABS scores varied from an increase of 27% within a year in the youngest participant recovering from deep depression to 90% decline during seven years in an ageing participant.

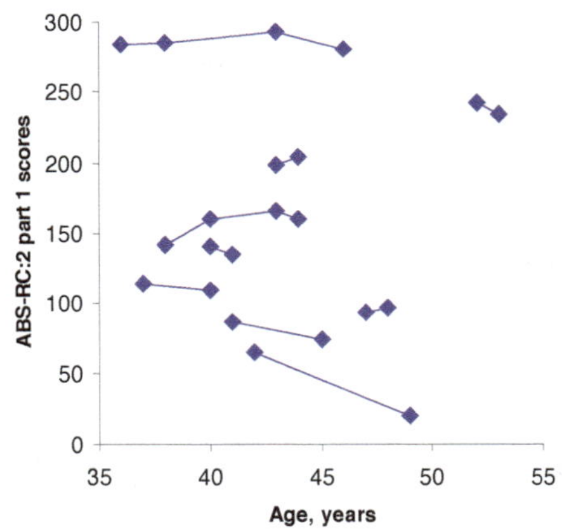

Figure 1. Adaptive behaviour in 9 participants without clinical Alzheimer's disease

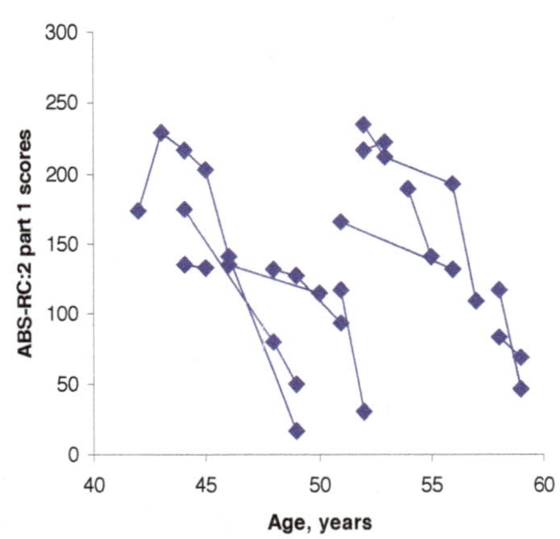

Figure 2. Adaptive behaviour in 12 participants with diagnosed Alzheimer's disease

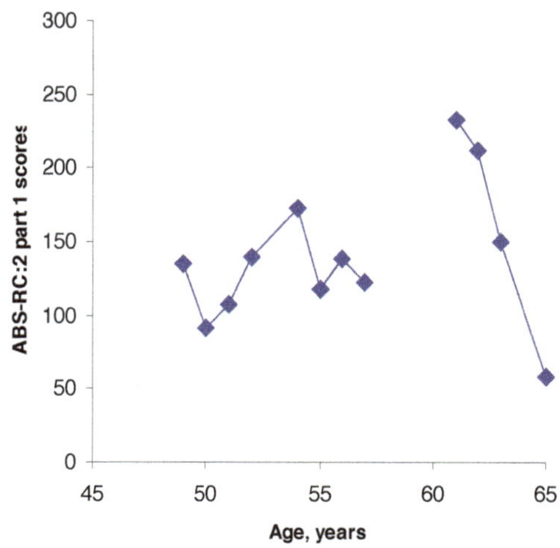

Figure 3. Adaptive behaviour in two participants with different clinical course of diagnosed Alzheimer's disease: participant 1 with slow progression of dementia (clinical case data given in text), participant 2 with mosaic trisomy of chromosome 21 and late onset of dementia

4. Late onset of dementia with mosaic trisomy of chromosome 21

For most of the younger and many of older participants too, changes in ABS scores were minimal (Figure 1). Slight improvement in scores at ages 38-40 was seen in an participant after a change of residence, coupled with increasing exercise, weight loss and improved fitness. The highest scores with slight improvement at ages 38-43 were seen in a participant in spite of many treated health problems, including a slight permanent visual impairment, hypothyroidism, fractures associated with osteoporosis and bronchial asthma.

The ABS scores declined in most participants with Alzheimer's disease (Figure 2). Improvements in ABS scores were seen in two elderly participants. In the first participant (Figure 2), the improvement at age 42 to 43 associated to the change of residence and medical treatment of Alzheimer's disease with response for two years before advancing deterioration later. Epilepsy and loss of mobility after a fall resulting in a hip fracture, and poor visual acuity contributed to the loss of independent functioning.

The improvement of the other participant (Figure 3) during the treatment of confirmed Alzheimer's disease, after a decline at age 48 to 49 lasted five years before further deterioration. Contributing factors to the functional improvement were the removal of cataracts resulting in improved visual acuity, active participation in activities with support of the carers, and stabilization of mood and behaviour. This participant had a long history of hypothyroidism, depression and challenging behaviour and he had long-term antidepressant and antipsychotic medication, and successful treatment of late onset epilepsy.

5. Discussion

We report experiences of a long term prospective clinical follow-up of adults with Down syndrome. The participants in this study were adults with Down syndrome and behavioural changes as perceived by carers. Adults without behavioural or mood changes observed by their proxies were not actively recruited and thus this group is not represented in this survey. The participants represent adults with Down syndrome with observed change of mood, behaviour or performance causing concern in their proxies.

Depression and, among participants in their forties and older, Alzheimer's dementia were the most common underlying reasons for the behavioural change. The number of participants with diagnosed and suspected dementia gave estimates of prevalence comparable to published epidemiological studies. Most people with Down syndrome and diagnosed Alzheimer's dementia in this population participated in this study. A change of behaviour or adjustment had been noticed by their proxies before the diagnosis of Alzheimer's dementia.

The current coping skills of the participants were assessed repeatedly using Adaptive Behaviour Scale - Residential and Community, Part I (Nihira *et al.* 1993). Earlier research supports its feasibility in scientific studies of ageing and dementia in people with intellectual disabilities. The clinical use of ABS to monitor ageing and dementia from the early non-symptomatic phase to the advanced stages at various levels of abilities proved to be possible and helpful for the clinician. A decline in ABS scores was seen in most participants after their early forties. This supported the suspicion of Alzheimer's disease, led to differential diagnostic assessments and also helped in monitoring the progression of the disease.

Adaptive behaviour can be assessed by ABS in adults with intellectual disability at all phases of ageing and dementia. This informant-based method overcame many of the problems of cognitive based measures. For example, no cooperation or communication skills of the person to be evaluated were needed for this assessment. Direct evaluations of cognitive functions were not possible in this study due to the limited neuropsychological resources available. Stable scores in clinically stable participants between repeated evaluations supported the reliability of ABS, when used by proxy informants. The informants with a close and long familiarity to their proxies observed and reported subtle changes in daily life and completed adaptive behaviour questionnaires without obvious difficulty.

A careful evaluation of the life situation and comprehensive assessment of physical and mental health is necessary when carers describe a decline in everyday functioning - that is a difficulty in accomplishing daily tasks which the individual would normally complete with ease (Ball et al. 2006). This is also needed in the elderly with established Alzheimer's disease because of common co-morbidities. In the case of a rapid deterioration of function, the underlying reasons should be assessed even when Alzheimer's disease has been diagnosed and treatment started. Visual acuity and hearing should be regularly monitored in all adults with Down syndrome because of high prevalence's of visual impairment and hearing loss. Alzheimer's disease does not protect from any other disease or disability. Other treatable conditions, including hypothyroidism, visual impairment and hearing loss, may be found.

The decline of the ABS total scores associated strongly to Alzheimer's disease; therefore the described declines in the ABS subscale scores probably reflect changes attributable to Alzheimer's disease. The relative rates of change among of the subscales of ABS differed. The scores of the domains Domestic Activity, Responsibility, Self-Direction and Vocational Activity declined more, as compared to other domains including Independent Functioning and Physical Activities. This may reflect the early impairment of frontal lobe functions among people with Down syndrome (Holland *et al.* 2000), including executive dysfunction in the development of Alzheimer's disease (Ball *et al.*2008).

Individual differences of the functional skills assessed by ABS scores were considerable. Decline of skills with ageing started at very different ages among participants in this study. The improvements of adaptive behaviour seen in several participants highlight the need for careful assessment of treatable medical conditions and possibilities for supporting the maintenance of functional independence. Stabilization of ABS scores was seen during medication for Alzheimer's disease in one participant for up to five years. Studies using population based representative larger samples would be needed to further analyse factors that represent potential confounders affecting adaptive behaviour more vigorously.

A considerable proportion of people with Down syndrome do not develop clinical dementia at all (Coppus et al. 2006). People with Down syndrome differ in their individual biological and genetic risk of dementia (Zigman & Lott 2007; Prasher et al. 2008; Patel et al. 2008). Better understanding of genetic and environmental influences and medical conditions contributing to these differences is needed.

Repeated prospective assessments overcome memory errors compared to retrospective evaluations. Short questionnaires of adaptive behaviour change may be sufficient for screening purposes (Prasher *et al.* 2004). However, repeated assessments are needed for the confirmation of dementia and evaluation of interventions. The possibility of performing an assessment in various settings without special professional expertise is a benefit of this approach.

The informant-based assessments of coping skills for daily living may prove practical and useful for the follow up of ageing and dementia from the early non-symptomatic phase to the advanced stages at various levels of abilities. The authors suggest repeated assessments of adaptive behaviour and careful clinical evaluations to detect treatable medical conditions in adults with Down syndrome.

Author details

T. Määttä[1*], T. Tervo-Määttä[2], A. Taanila[3,4], M. Kaski[5] and M. Iivanainen[5,6]

*Address all correspondence to: tuomo.maatta@kainuu.fi

1 Kainuu Social and Health Care Joint Authority, Finland

2 Department of Teacher Education, University of Oulu, Finland

3 Institute of Health Sciences, University of Oulu, Finland

4 Unit of General Practice, University Hospital of Oulu, Finland

5 The Rinnekoti Research Centre, Espoo, Finland

6 Department of Child Neurology, University of Helsinki, Finland

References

[1] Ball, S. L., Holland, A. J., Hon, J., Huppert, F. A., Treppner, P., & Watson, P. C. (2006). Personality and behaviour changes mark the early stages of Alzheimer's disease in adults with Down's syndrome: Findings from a prospective population-based study. *International Journal of Geriatric Psychiatry* 21, 661-673.

[2] Ball, S. L., Holland, A. J., Huppert, F. A., Treppner, P., Watson, P., & Hon, J. (2004). The modified CAMDEX informant interview is a valid and reliable tool for use in the diagnosis of dementia in adults with Down's syndrome. *Journal of Intellectual Disability Research* 48, 611-620.

[3] Ball, S. L., Holland, A. J., Treppner, P., Watson, P. C., & Huppert, F. A. (2008). Executive dysfunction and its association with personality and behaviour changes in the development of Alzheimer's disease in adults with Down syndrome and mild to moderate learning disabilities. *The British Journal of Clinical Psychology / the British Psychological Society* 47, 1-29.

[4] Bhaumik, S., Collacott, R. A., Garrick, P., & Mitchell, C. (1991). Effect of thyroid stimulating hormone on adaptive behaviour in Down's syndrome. *Journal of Mental Deficiency Research* 35, 512-520.

[5] Brugge, K. L., Nichols, S. L., Salmon, D. P., Hill, L. R., Delis, D. C., Aaron, L., et al. (1994). Cognitive impairment in adults with Down's syndrome: Similarities to early cognitive changes in Alzheimer's disease. *Neurology* 44, 232-238.

[6] Burt, D. B., Loveland, K. A., & Lewis, K. R. (1992). Depression and the onset of dementia in adults with mental retardation. *American Journal of Mental Retardation* 96, 502-511.

[7] Collacott, R. A. (1992). The effect of age and residential placement on adaptive behaviour of adults with Down's syndrome. *The British Journal of Psychiatry : The Journal of Mental Science* 161, 675-679.

[8] Collacott, R. A. (1993). Epilepsy, dementia and adaptive behaviour in Down's syndrome. *Journal of Intellectual Disability Research* 37, 153-160.

[9] Coppus, A., Evenhuis, H., Verberne, G. J., Visser, F., van Gool, P., Eikelenboom, P., et al. (2006). Dementia and mortality in persons with Down's syndrome. *Journal of Intellectual Disability Research* 50, 768-777.

[10] Coppus, A. M., Evenhuis, H. M., Verberne, G. J., Visser, F. E., Oostra, B. A., Eikelenboom, P., et al. (2008). Survival in elderly persons with Down syndrome. *Journal of the American Geriatrics Society* 56, 2311-2316.

[11] Holland, A. J., Hon, J., Huppert, F. A., & Stevens, F. (2000). Incidence and course of dementia in people with Down's syndrome: Findings from a population-based study. *Journal of Intellectual Disability Research* 44, 138-146.

[12] Iacono, T., Torr, J., & Wong, H. Y. (2010). Relationships amongst age, language and related skills in adults with Down syndrome. *Research in Developmental Disabilities* 31, 568-576.

[13] Janicki, M. P., & Dalton, A. J. (2000). Prevalence of dementia and impact on intellectual disability services. *Mental Retardation* 38, 276-288.

[14] Krinsky-McHale, S. J., Devenny, D. A., Kittler, P., & Silverman, W. (2008). Selective attention deficits associated with mild cognitive impairment and early stage Alzheimer's disease in adults with Down syndrome. *American Journal of Mental Retardation 113*, 369-386.

[15] Margallo-Lana, M. L., Moore, P. B., Kay, D. W., Perry, R. H., Reid, B. E., Berney, T. P., et al. (2007). Fifteen-year follow-up of 92 hospitalized adults with Down's syndrome: Incidence of cognitive decline, its relationship to age and neuropathology. *Journal of Intellectual Disability Research* 51, 463-477.

[16] McCarron, M., Gill, M., McCallion, P., & Begley, C. (2005). Health co-morbidities in ageing persons with Down syndrome and Alzheimer's dementia. *Journal of Intellectual Disability Research* 49, 560-566.

[17] Meuwese-Jongejeugd, A., van Splunder, J., Vink, M., Stilma, J. S., van Zanten, B., Verschuure, H., et al. (2008). Combined sensory impairment (deaf-blindness) in five percent of adults with intellectual disabilities. *American Journal of Mental Retardation* 113, 254-262.

[18] Meuwese-Jongejeugd, A., Vink, M., van Zanten, B., Verschuure, H., Eichhorn, E., Koopman, D., et al. (2006). Prevalence of hearing loss in 1598 adults with an intellectual disability: Cross-sectional population based study. *International Journal of Audiology* 45, 660-669.

[19] Nieuwenhuis-Mark, R. E. (2009). Diagnosing Alzheimer's dementia in Down syndrome: Problems and possible solutions. *Research in Developmental Disabilities* 30, 827-838.

[20] Nihira, K., Leland, H., & Lambert, N. (1993). *AAAMR adaptive behavior scales, residential and community edition (2nd ed), TX:Pro-ed.*

[21] Patel, A., Rees, S. D., Kelly, M. A., Bain, S. C., Barnett, A. H., Thalitaya, D., et al. (2010). Association of variants within APOE, SORL1, RUNX1, BACE1 and ALDH18A1 with dementia in Alzheimer's disease in subjects with Down syndrome. *Neuroscience Letters,*

[22] Prasher, V., Farooq, A., & Holder, R. (2004). The adaptive behaviour dementia questionnaire (ABDQ): Screening questionnaire for dementia in Alzheimer's disease in adults with Down syndrome. *Research in Developmental Disabilities* 25 385-397.

[23] Prasher, V. P., & Chung, M. C. (1996). Causes of age-related decline in adaptive behavior of adults with Down syndrome: Differential diagnoses of dementia. *American Journal of Mental Retardation* 101, 175-183.

[24] Prasher, V. P., Chung, M. C., & Haque, M. S. (1998). Longitudinal changes in adaptive behavior in adults with Down syndrome: Interim findings from a longitudinal study. *American Journal of Mental Retardation* 103, 40-46.

[25] Prasher, V. P., Huxley, A., Haque, M. S., & Down syndrome Ageing Study Group. (2002). A 24-week, double-blind, placebo-controlled trial of donepezil in patients with Down syndrome and Alzheimer's disease--pilot study. *International Journal of Geriatric Psychiatry* 17, 270-278.

[26] Prasher, V. P., Sajith, S. G., Rees, S. D., Patel, A., Tewari, S., Schupf, N., et al. (2008). Significant effect of APOE epsilon 4 genotype on the risk of dementia in Alzheimer's disease and mortality in persons with Down syndrome. *International Journal of Geriatric Psychiatry* 23, 1134-1140.

[27] Pyo, G., Kripakaran, K., Curtis, K., Curtis, R., & Markwell, S. (2007). A preliminary study of the validity of memory tests recommended by the working group for individuals with moderate to severe intellectual disability. *Journal of Intellectual Disability Research* 51, 377-386.

[28] Rasmussen, D. E., & Sobsey, D. (1994). Age, adaptive behavior, and Alzheimer disease in Down syndrome: Cross-sectional and longitudinal analyses. *American Journal of Mental Retardation* 99, 151-165.

[29] Shultz, J., Aman, M., Kelbley, T., LeClear Wallace, C., Burt, D. B., Primeaux-Hart, S., et al. (2004). Evaluation of screening tools for dementia in older adults with mental retardation. *American Journal of Mental Retardation* 109, 98-110.

[30] Strydom, A., Livingston, G., King, M., & Hassiotis, A. (2007). Prevalence of dementia in intellectual disability using different diagnostic criteria. *The British Journal of Psychiatry : The Journal of Mental Science* 191, 150-157.

[31] Urv, T. K., Zigman, W. B., & Silverman, W. (2008). Maladaptive behaviors related to dementia status in adults with Down syndrome. *American Journal of Mental Retardation* 113, 73-86.

[32] Urv, T. K., Zigman, W. B., & Silverman, W. (2010). Psychiatric symptoms in adults with Down syndrome and Alzheimer's disease. *American Journal on Intellectual and Developmental Disabilities, 115*(4), 265-276.

[33] van Splunder, J., Stilma, J. S., Bernsen, R. M., & Evenhuis, H. M. (2006). Prevalence of visual impairment in adults with intellectual disabilities in the netherlands: Cross-sectional study. *Eye (London, England), 20*(9), 1004-1010.

[34] Wisniewski, K. E., Wisniewski, H. M., & Wen, G. Y. (1985). Occurrence of neuropathological changes and dementia of Alzheimer's disease in Down's syndrome. *Annals of Neurology, 17*(3), 278-282.

[35] Zigman, W. B., & Lott, I. T. (2007). Alzheimer's disease in Down syndrome: Neurobiology and risk. *Mental Retardation and Developmental Disabilities Research Reviews, 13*(3), 237-246.

[36] Zigman, W. B., Schupf, N., Sersen, E., & Silverman, W. (1996). Prevalence of dementia in adults with and without Down syndrome. *American Journal of Mental Retardation : AJMR, 100*(4), 403-412.

[37] Zigman, W. B., Schupf, N., Urv, T., Zigman, A., & Silverman, W. (2002). Incidence and temporal patterns of adaptive behavior change in adults with mental retardation. American Journal of Mental Retardation : AJMR, 107(3), 161-174.

10

Possible Relation Between Trace Element Status and Clinical Outcomes in Parkinson Syndrome

Erland Johansson, Tuomas Westermarck and
Faik Atroshi

1. Introduction

Parkinson disease (PD) is a degenerative disorder of the central nervous system and one of the most common neurologic disorders, affecting approximately 1% of individuals older than 60 years and causing progressive disability that can be slowed, but not halted, by treatment (Poewe, 2006; DeLong & Juncos, 2008). The epidemiology of Parkinson disease is not genetically predetermined, but influenced by environmental factors which may be geographically heterogeneousn (Tanner & Langston, 1990). Major gene mutations cause only a small proportion of all cases and that in most cases; non-genetic factors play a part, probably in interaction with susceptibility genes (de Lau & Breteler, 2006). A number of environmental factors have been associated with an increased risk of Parkinson's including: pesticide exposure, head injuries, and living in the country or farming (Noyce et al. 2012; Van Maele-Fabry et al. 2012). Parkinson disease is characterised by focal loss of melanin –containing neurons of the central and caudal parts of the zona compacta of the substantia nigra (Jellinger 1987). Dopamine deficiency of the nigrostrial system is the hallmark of PD disorder. The cause of the degeneration of the dopamine containing neurons in the substantia nigra of patients with PD is nknown. Excessive free radical production has been suggested as a consequence of the catabolism of the monoamines (Dexter et al 1989). It has been shown those catalase and glutathione peroxidases are reduced in the substantia nigra of PD patients (Sofic et al. 1992). It has therefore been suggested that additional antioxidant therapy ncluding vitamins-E and C may be helpful to slowing the progression of PD. Increasing evidence indicates that PD is primarly a Mitochondrial disorder and thus the use of compounds With good mitochondrial penetrance, (CoQ10), could Potentially be of benefit in this disease (Matthews et al 1998).

2. Current treatment pathways

Parkinson's disease is a degenerative disease of the nervous system. The exact cause for Parkinson's disease is not well understood. There is no definitive test for PD – diagnosis is often based on medical history and the presence of the classic symptoms and signs of PD (Samii et al. 2004; Tolosa & Katzenschlager, 2007). Sometimes people are given anti-PD drugs to see if they respond, or other tests may be performed, such as MRI and CAT scans, to rule out other disorders with similar symptoms (Gelb et al. 1999; Hughes et al. 2002). The presence of other diseases, such as dementia and general ageing can obscure PD symptoms and reduce the chance of an accurate diagnosis. Certain drugs, when taken for long periods of time or in amounts greater than recommended, can cause Parkinsonism (Di Fabio et al. 2013) and have side effects. These medications do not result in Parkinson's disease, however, and symptoms resolve when the medications are no longer used.

3. Environmental and nutritional factors in Parkinson disease

Environmental factors and nutrients may play an important role in early life. In people who are genetically predisposed to Parkinson's disease, many experts believe that environmental exposures, such as unusual exposure to herbicides and pesticides, increase a person's risk of developing Parkinson's disease (Tanner & Langston, 1990; Van Maele-Fabry et al. 2012).

Numerous epidemiological studies and interventional trials have suggested a link, in aging, between an adequate nutritional status and health (de Lau & Breteler, 2006; Barichella et al. 2009). Nutrient deficiencies and constipation may also play a role (Dan Beth, 1992; Schelosky et al, 1995). Parkinson's patients are often deficient in vitamins, minerals and trace elements (Ames, 2011). Micronutrient sufficiency and quality of the lipid supply may play key roles in brain development. It is because of their diverse and vital roles that nutrient element imbalances are frequently found to be factors in degenerative diseases. Since the body cannot manufacture the elements-and daily losses are unavoidable-the nutrient elements are all "essential" and must regularly be taken in through the diet. Erythrocyte element levels are good indicators of body pools of essential elements such as selenium, zinc, magnesium, potassium, and calcium. Often referred to as minerals, the chemical elements are fundamental to every function in the body. It is because of their diverse and vital roles that nutrient element imbalances are frequently found to be factors in degenerative diseases. Since the body cannot manufacture the elements-and daily losses are unavoidable-the nutrient elements are all "essential" and must regularly be taken in through the diet. But they are easily lost in food processing, so it's easy to see how deficiencies can occur. It has been reported that moderate selenium and vitamin K deficiency show damage accumulates over time as a result of vitamin and mineral loss, leading to age-related diseases (Ames, 2006; McCann & Ames, 2011). Therefore, understanding how best to define and measure optimum nutrition will make the application of new technologies to allow each person to optimize their own nutrition a much more realistic possibility than it is today McCann & Ames, 2011).

4. Oxidative stress and Parkinson's disease

Oxidative stress could play an important role in the degenerative process leading to Parkinson's disease. These considerations provide a rationale for therapeutic strategies to diminish oxidative stress in dopaminergic regions of brain. If oxidative stress is a major factor, the agents that selectively and safely chelate iron may be of value. It was reported that the mitochondrial deficiency (Shoffner et al. 1991; Jenner, 1991; Saggu et al. 1989; Perry & Yong, 1986) in electron transport, enhanced lipid peroxidation, elevated superoxide dismutase, diminished capacity to remove excess hydrogen peroxide (suggested by low glutathione and glutathione peroxidase levels) and the presence of increased iron, which catalyses formation of highly reactive hydroxyl ions from hydrogen peroxide, make attractive the suggestion that oxidative stress could play an important role in the degenerative process leading to Parkinson's disease (Ambani et al. 1975).

5. Selenium and other antioxidants in Parkinson

Deficiency of the minerals and other antioxidants required for life are relatively uncommon, however, modest deficiency is very common and often not taken seriously. Selenium is an essential trace element which is necessary for growth and protein synthesis. Selenium protects cellular elements from oxidative damage and may participate in redox type reactions. Low plasma selenium concentrations are associated with subtle neurological impairments reflected in soft neurological signs (Shahar et al. 2010). A statistically significant increase in plasma Se was identified for PD patients (McIntosh et al. 2012). This has been evidenced by an increased lipid peroxidation and reduced glutathione levels (Delanty and Dichter, 2000) and high concentration of iron and free radical generation via autocatalytic mechanisms within neuromelanin-containing catecholaminergic neurons in the substantia nigra. In addition, the observation that exogenous administration of cysteine, N-acetyl cysteine or glutathione decreased the neurotoxic effects of 6-hydroxydopamine in vitro and in vivo reinforces this hypothesis (Soto-Otero et al. 2000). McCann et al. (2011), tested whether selenium-dependent proteins that are essential from an evolutionary perspective are more resistant to selenium deficiency than those that are less essential. The authors demonstrated a highly sophisticated array of mechanisms at cellular and tissue levels that, when selenium is limited, protect essential selenium-dependent proteins at the expense of those that are nonessential. It was also found that mutations in selenium-dependent proteins that are lost on modest selenium deficiency result in characteristics shared by age-related diseases including cancer, heart disease, and loss of immune or brain function (McCann et al., 2011). It was concluded that taking a multivitamin that contains selenium is a good way to prevent deficiencies that, over time, can cause harm in ways that we are just beginning to understand.

6. Zinc in Parkinson

Zinc is essential as a cofactor for a variety of enzymes and transcription factors and plays a role in various biological processes ranging from gene expression to the immune response. There are two distinct gene families of zinc transporters, 10 ZnT (Slc30a) and 14 Zip (Slc39a) transporter genes (Ohno et al., 1985; Liuzzi & Cousins, 2004). The zinc concentration is ~15 times greater in mature RBC than in plasma (Eide, 2006). More than 90% of RBC zinc functions as a component essential for the activity of zinc metalloenzymes, particularly carbonic anhydrase and Cu2+/Zn2+-superoxide dismutase (Ryu et al. 2008). Abnormal levels of Zn2+plays a role in many diseases, including Alzheimer's and type-2 diabetes. Zn is an essential element for plants and other organisms and is involved in many cellular processes, including activation of enzymes, protein synthesis, and membrane stability (Welch et al., 1982). Zinc is involved in numerous aspects of cellular metabolism (Jiménez-Jiménez et al. 1992; Forsleff et al. 1998; Brewer et al. 2010). Zinc deficiency is characterized by growth retardation. The global extent of zinc deficiency is debated, but diets that are high in whole grains and low in meat could lead to deficiency (Qureshi et al. 2006; MacDiarmid et al. 2013). Low zinc supply has the same effect on human cells as on yeast, zinc deficiency might contribute to human diseases that are associated with a build-up of "junked" proteins, such as Parkinson's and Alzheimer's. A similar protective system to Tsa1 also exists in animals, and the research group plans to move ahead by studying that system in human cell culture (MacDiarmid et al. 2013). The authors demonstrated that cells that are low in zinc also produce proteins that counter the resulting stress, including one called Tsa1. Tsa1 could reduce the level of harmful oxidants in cells that are short of zinc (MacDiarmid et al. 2013).

It has been reported that zinc deficiency may be linked to increased inflammation. Liu et al (2013) studied the activity of zinc to control sepsis, the severe systemic response to infection that can lead to death. Using cell models, the team focused on the role of zinc to prevent the inflammation that leads to sepsis; they found that when a pathogen is recognized, the gene that produces the zinc transporter SLC39A8 (ZIP8) is expressed. This transporter then rapidly moves to cell's walls, where it shuttles zinc from the bloodstream into the cell; after cell entry, zinc is then directed to and bonds to a protein that halts further activity (Liu et al., 2013).

7. Is there a role for trace element in human diseases?

Trace elements are metal ions and non-metal ions (e.g. selenium, arsenic) in human body in low concentrations, less than about 0.05 %. Calcium in the body, about 1.4 % is usually considered a macro element but it should be kept in mind that inside cells calcium is present in low concentration as a trace element and needs carefully control as it is a powerful second messenger. Trace elements like vitamins must be added through food as the body can't synthesize trace elements. Some of them are essential e.g. lack may disturb metabolism, sometime causative a disease, Keshan disease. Some examples of essential trace elements: Si, Fe, F, Zn, Cu, Mn, Se, Mo, Co. Knowledge of trace elements has increased a lot since accurate, sensitive, selective analytical technique was developed around 1980, ICP-MS (inductively coupled plasma mass spectrometry).

Trace elements were originally viewed as nutrients and they excerpt pharmacological actions. Some of these possibly essential elements also are receiving attention because of their toxicological or pharmacological properties that can affect health and wellbeing. However possible relation between trace element status and clinical outcomes are insufficient. Extrapyramidal symptoms reflecting nigrostrial dopaminergic hypofunction are common in patients with neuronal ceroid lipofuscinosis and Parkinson's disease. Inadequacy or imbalance of trace elements supply consequently affects a number of physiological functions. Zinc as an elements that may play a protective anti-atherosclerotic role, decreases. Zn is considered an efficient antioxidant (Prasad, 2008). Zn controls metallothionein expression and is involved in, cellular redox regulation (Maret, 2000). Oxidative stress can be corrected by dietary Zn as demonstrated of hepatic antioxidant enzymes (Tupe et. al. 2010). Zn metabolism may be influenced by low intake, lack of protective factors, e.g. Se. Another possibility may be Cd competition with Zn. Cd has higher binding capacity than Zn, e.g. in metallothionein and may displace Zn from its carrier sites. In a study of Parkinson's disease Mn was implicated (Normandie and Hazell, 2002) and another study demonstrated elevated concentrations of Cd in the erythrocytes (Johansson et.al. 2007). Lack of protective elements e.g. selenium in the metabolism makes it easier for heavy metal ions to enter and interfere the metabolism. As trace elements are active in many parts of the cell metabolism the discussion will be focused on possible effects of imbalance due to heavy metal ions in Parkinson's disease.

8. Elemental profiles as an indicator of metal ion and ligand homeostasis

The cell metabolism is a complex balance of proteins, fatty acids, carbohydrates, metal ions and trace elements regulated by DNA and RNA in nucleus and mitochondria. As the metabolism involve many molecular reactions and species not practical to be monitored a simplified indication of metal ion-ligand status, elemental profile, may be a substitute to monitor effects of important cell reactions. The elemental profile may be looked upon as the integrated results of reactions at the moment the sample was taken. It is important to underline that deviations in the elemental profile may also include effects of compounds with strong association to the examined elements. These deviations may give biochemical and physiological insights to observe early changes in the metabolism. Changes of metabolism of metal ions in e.g. erythrocytes may help to understand early reactions, if it is normal or an indication of an early pathophysiological process.

9. Membrane trafficking and dynamics in presence of heavy metal ions

In a study of 12 patients (9 men and 3 women) with Parkinson's disease (Johansson et.al. 2013) erythrocytes showed significant increased concentration of Pb and Ag. The concentration of Cd (9/12) was also higher than that of controls. The observed increased of concentrations of Pb, Ag and Cd may have effects at different levels, e.g. 1. ATP-metabolism and heavy metal ion metabolism 2. Pb, Ag, Cd interactions with dopamine metabolism 3. Axonal transport and membrane trafficking 4. ROS formation by increased activity of hemeoxidases and displaced iron 5. Preapoptosis signals and possible activation of second messengers 6. Pb and porphyrine synthesis

10. Possible sources of metal ion supply

10.1. ATP-metabolism and heavy metal ion interactions

Pb, Cd and Ag has higher association to binding sites than Mg, Ca. Possible effect is displacement of Mg from enolase enzyme which introduces a double bond in the phosphate group. Mg may also be blocked in the phospho-mutase reaction when phosphoglycerate is transferred from position 3 to position 2. Another effect of cadmium ions is inhibition of Na/K ATPase enzyme by 50% in ABC-transporters (Lijnen et. al. 1991). Examples above indicate possible effects of heavy metal ions in the ATP-metabolism.

10.2. Pb, Ag, Cd interactions with dopamine metabolism

In patients with Parkinon's disease the micoenvironment is full of misfolded alfa-Synuclein (George et.al. 2013) in brain (striatum) which may promote aggregation of cells and cause losses in dopamine synthesis. The synthesis in substantia nigria may be blocked by the increased concentrations of Pb, Ag and Ag. Transport of compounds (dopamine, acetylcholine) by vesicles (Kornberg and McConnell, 1971) in axons may be blocked by reactions with heavy metal ions.

10.3. Axonal transport and membrane trafficking

The axonal transport of mitochondria (Hollenbeck and Saxton, 2006, Gunter et.al 2000) may be disturbed by Pb, Cd and Ag by carry over effects. Mitochondria were transported by kinosin, dynein and myosin motors (Zhang and Zhao, 2007). Interactions with the motor transport in axons may be expected to slow down or stop movements when exposed to Pb, Ag and Cd. The transport of Ca (Perin et.al.1990) may be blocked by Pb, Cd and due to stronger association to binding sites in the mitochondria and ER (endoplasmatic reticulum) resulting in poor nerve signals in the axons.

10.4. ROS formation by increased activity of hemeoxidases and displaced iron

The accumulated heavy metal ions in the erythrocytes may disturb oxygen transport and interact with important brain cells. Cd may be used in heme metabolism, reducing heme concentration when sufficient. In a previous study significantly increased concentration of Cd was observed in the erythrocytes (Johansson et.al. 2007). The gene for hemeoxygenases HO-1, HO-2 is Cd dependent (Koizumi et.al.2007, Alami et.al.2000). HO-1, HO-2 hemeoxygenases are important for cleaning up residues of senescent erythrocytes. Low concentrations of Cd may be involved in cleaning up heme residues, too high concentration of Cd may support formation of reactive oxygen species (ROS), superoxide anion, hydroxy free radicals, and singlet oxygen. In the porphyrine synthesis it is important that introduction of iron (ferrochelatase, frataxin) is not blocked by excess Cd, Pb, Ag (Johansson et.al. 2007). Uncontrolled iron may react with oxygen and produce free radicals, Haber-Weiss reactions.

10.5. Preapoptosis signals and possible activation of second messengers

Cd may enter Ca channels (e.g. Gardos channels) in the erythrocyte membrane and introduce interactions in cells (Verbost et.al.1989). Cd, Pb, Ag may release Ca from calmodulin (superfamily of Ca-carriers) due to weaker binding. Ca Is an important secondary messengers in cells activating e.g. flippases. Liberated Ca may activate translocators, flippases, within the cell (Devaux et.al. 2006). Phosphatidylserine in the inner leaflet may be transferred by trans locators to outer membrane giving an apoptosis marker for the macrophages. Phosphatidylserine is normally situated below leflet (Martin et.al. 1995). Increased Pb, Cd, Ag may start too early apoptosis of important cells e.g. neurons (Sopjani et.al.2009).

10.6. Pb and porphyrine synthesis

Pb is not known to be essential to man. Pb has redox capacity (Pb2+or Pb4+) and usually associated in reduced form to other molecules. As about 99% of Pb is associated to erythrocytes in blood one target will be the metabolism of erythrocytes. Pb is known to interfere with aminolevulinic acid dehydratase in the heme synthesis (Flindt et.al. 1976, Kelada et.al.2001). Pb is also known to interact with Ca channels by allowing increased input of calcium starting too early senescence (Lang et.al. 2010).

10.7. Possible sources of metal ion supply

In the study of 12 Parkinson patients (Johansson et.al.2013) there was no information of food habits for individual patients. In Finland cadmium uptake from food is about 5-10 μg/day, lead 20-66 μg /day, silver was not mentioned. In Sweden cadmium uptake from wheat, rice, potatoes, root-crops is about 10-20 μg /day, lead 15-30 μg /day, silver was not reported. In view of contribution from nutrition of heavy metal ions it is interesting to note that cadmium rich diet in Nigeria decreased Hb and erythrocyte counts in mice (Asagba & Eriyamremu 2007). It cannot be excluded that cadmium, lead in food after long time may accumulate in human erythrocytes and likely decrease erythrocyte counts and hemoglobin synthesis. Smoker may have higher cadmium values in blood but there was no information about smoking habits. Implanters may be a source of metal ion supply. Amalgam is an alloy which is not stable but will release mercury, silver (Johansson E1991, Johansson E et.al.1994, Johansson E and Liljefors T, 1991). Studies indicate that released mercury from amalgam will be found in liver, kidney and brain only minor amounts of mercury will be found in the blood indicating need for looking after other indicators. The effects of silver are often missing but should be included due to effects of silver on important antioxidant compounds containing selenium, sulphur. Some amalgam fillings may have small sticks of guttapercha in the cavity. Some trademarks of Gutta-percha contain cadmium but the released amount is not known for the examined patients (Johansson E and Liljefors T 1991).The observations of problems possibly attributed to implanters should be considered in the early diagnosis.

10.8. The discoid shape of erythrocytes and heavy metal ions

Erythrocytes must be able to shrink and expand during transport (Huang et.al. 2010). If Cd, Pb, Ag, are associated to stabilizing proteins, erythrocytes possess a spectrin-based cytoskeleton they may lose their capacity to shrink and expand (Zhang and Zhao, 2007, Bosman et.al. 2008) in the capillaries.

Author details

Erland Johansson[1], Tuomas Westermarck[2] and Faik Atroshi[3]

1 Selenium consultant Ltd, Sweden

2 Rinnekoti Research Centre, Espoo, Finland

3 Pharmacology & Toxicology, University of Helsinki, Finland

References

[1] Liu MJ, Bao S, Galvez-Peralta M, Pyle CJ, Rudawsky AC, Pavlovicz RE, Killilea DW, Li C, Nebert DW, Wewers MD, Knoell DL. "ZIP8 Regulates Host Defense through Zinc-Mediated Inhibition of NF-[kappa]B." Cell Rep. 2013;3(2):386-400.

[2] Gellein K, Syversen T, Steinnes E, Nilsen TI, Dahl OP, Mitrovic S, Duraj D, Flaten TP Trace elements in serum from patients with Parkinson's disease--a prospective case-control study: the Nord-Trøndelag Health Study (HUNT).Brain research 1219: 2008 Jul 11: 111-5.

[3] Schelosky L, Raffauf C, Jendroska K, Kava and dopamine antagonism (letter). J Neurol Neurosurg Psychiatry 58: 639-40. 1995.

[4] Dan Beth-El. Magic beans? Natural sources of L-Dopa in the treatment of Parkinson's Disease. International J of Comp Med: 11-13. September 1992.

[5] Samii A, Nutt JG, Ransom BR (May 2004). "Parkinson's disease". Lancet 363 (9423): 1783–93.

[6] Poewe W (December 2006). "The natural history of Parkinson's disease". J. Neurol. 253 (Suppl 7): VII2–6.

[7] Davie CA (2008). "A review of Parkinson's disease". Br. Med. Bull. 86 (1): 109–27.

[8] de Lau LM, Breteler MM (June 2006). "Epidemiology of Parkinson's disease". Lancet Neurol. 5 (6): 525–35.

[9] Castagnoli K, Murugesan T (2004 Jan). "Tobacco leaf, smoke and smoking, MAO inhibitors, Parkinson's disease and neuroprotection; are there links?". Neurotoxicology 25 (1–2): 279–91.

[10] Tolosa E, Katzenschlager R (2007). "Pharmacological management of Parkinson's disease". In Tolosa E, Jankovic JJ. Parkinson's disease and movement disorders. Hagerstwon, MD: Lippincott Williams & Wilkins. pp. 110–45.

[11] Hughes AJ, Daniel SE, Ben-Shlomo Y, Lees AJ. The accuracy of diagnosis of parkinsonian syndromes in a specialist movement disorder service. Brain 2002;125:861–870.

[12] Gelb DJ, Oliver E, Gilman S. Diagnostic criteria for Parkinson disease. Arch Neurol 1999;56:33–39.

[13] Sofic E, Lange KW, Jellinger K, Riederer P. Reduced and oxidized glutathione in the substantia nigra of patients with Parkinson's disease. Neurosci Lett. 1992 Aug 17;142(2):128-30

[14] Barichella M, Cereda E, Pezzoli G (October 2009). "Major nutritional issues in the management of Parkinson's disease". Mov. Disord. 24 (13): 1881–92.

[15] Tanner, C. M., Langston, J. F. 1990. Do environmental toxins cause Parkinson's disease? A critical review.Neurology 40(3): 17-31.

[16] de Lau LM, Breteler MM. Epidemiology of Parkinson's disease. Lancet Neurol. 2006 Jun;5(6):525-35.

[17] Noyce AJ, Bestwick JP, Silveira-Moriyama L, Hawkes CH, Giovannoni G, Lees AJ, Schrag A. "Meta-analysis of early nonmotor features and risk factors for Parkinson disease". Annals of Neurology, 2012, 72 (6): 893–901.

[18] Van Maele-Fabry G, Hoet P, Vilain F, Lison D. "Occupational exposure to pesticides and Parkinson's disease: a systematic review and meta-analysis of cohort studies". 2012, Environ Int 46: 30–43.

[19] DeLong MR, Juncos JL. Parkinson's Disease and Other Movement Disorders. In: Kasper DL, Fauci AS, Longo DL, Braunwald E, Hauser SL, Jameson JL, editors. Harrison's Principles of Internal Medicine. 17th ed. New York: McGraw-Hill Medical Publishers; 2008. pp. 2406–17

[20] Di Fabio R, De Filippis S, Cafariello C, Penna L, Marianetti M, Serrao M, Pierelli F. Low doses of rotigotine in patients with antipsychotic-induced parkinsonism. Clin Neuropharmacol. 2013 Sep-Oct;36(5):162-5.

[21] Samii A, Nutt JG, Ransom BR (May 2004). "Parkinson's disease". Lancet 363 (9423): 1783–93.

[22] Poewe W (December 2006). "The natural history of Parkinson's disease". J. Neurol. 253 (Suppl 7): VII2–6.

[23] Davie CA (2008). "A review of Parkinson's disease". Br. Med. Bull. 86 (1): 109–27.

[24] de Lau LM, Breteler MM (June 2006). "Epidemiology of Parkinson's disease". Lancet Neurol. 5 (6): 525–35.

[25] Castagnoli K, Murugesan T (2004 Jan). "Tobacco leaf, smoke and smoking, MAO inhibitors, Parkinson's disease and neuroprotection; are there links?". Neurotoxicology 25 (1–2): 279–91.

[26] Tolosa E, Katzenschlager R (2007). "Pharmacological management of Parkinson's disease". In Tolosa E, Jankovic JJ. Parkinson's disease and movement disorders. Hagerstwon, MD: Lippincott Williams & Wilkins. pp. 110–45.

[27] McCann JC, Ames BN. Adaptive dysfunction of selenoproteins from the perspective of the triage theory: why modest selenium deficiency may increase risk of diseases of aging. The FASEB Journal, 2011; DOI: 10.1096/fj.11-180885

[28] Ames BN. Proc. Low micronutrient intake may accelerate the degenerative diseases of aging through allocation of scarce micronutrients by triage. Natl. Acad. Sci. USA,Vol. 103, pp. 17589-17594, November 2006

[29] Shoffner, J. M . , Watts, R. L. , Juncos,J. L . , Torroni, A . , Wallace, D. C .1991 . Mitochondrial oxidative phosphorylation defects in Parkinson's disease.Ann. Neurol. 30:332-39.

[30] Jenner, P. 1991 . Oxidative stress as a cause of Parkinson's disease. Acta N eurol. Scand. 1 36:6-15 (Supp\.)

[31] Saggu, H., Cooksey, J . , Dexter, D., Wells, F. R . , Lees, A . , et a1. 1989. A selective increase in particulate superoxide dismutase activity in parkinsonian substantia nigra. J. Neurochem.1 53:692-97

[32] Perry, T. L . , Yong, V. W. 1986. Idiopathic Parkinson's disease, progressive supranuclear palsy and glutathione metabolism in the substantia nigra of patients. Neurosci. Lett. 67:269-74.

[33] Ambani, L. M . , Van Woert, M. H . ,Murphy, S . 1975 . Brain peroxidase and catalase in Parkinson's disease.Arch. Neurol. 32: 1 14-1 8.

[34] Shahar A, Patel KV, Semba RD, Bandinelli S, Shahar DR, Ferrucci L, Guralnik JM. Plasma selenium is positively related to performance in neurological tasks assessing coordination and motor speed. Mov Disord. 2010 Sep 15;25(12):1909-15.

[35] McIntosh KG, Cusack MJ, Vershinin A, Chen ZW, Zimmerman EA, Molho ES, Celmins D, Parsons PJ. Evaluation of a prototype point-of-care instrument based on

monochromatic x-ray fluorescence spectrometry: potential for monitoring trace element status of subjects with neurodegenerative disease. J Toxicol Environ Health A. 2012;75(21):1253-68.

[36] Delanty N.; Dichter M. Antioxidant Therapy in Neurologic Disease. Archives of Neurology. 57(9):1265-1270, 2000.

[37] Dworkin RH. Linoleic acid and multiple sclerosis. Lancet 1981; 1153-4.

[38] Soto-Otero R, Mendez-Alvarez E, Hermida-Ameijeiras A, et al. Autoxidation and neurotoxicity of 6-hydroxydopamine in the presence of some antioxidants: potential implication in relation to the pathogenesis of Parkinson's disease. J Neurochem 2000; 74:1605-1612.

[39] McCann JC, Ames BN. Adaptive dysfunction of selenoproteins from the perspective of the triage theory: why modest selenium deficiency may increase risk of diseases of aging. The FASEB Journal, 2011; DOI: 10.1096/fj.11-180885.

[40] Jiménez-Jiménez FJ,; Fernández-Calle, P.; Martínez-Vanaclocha, M.; Herrero, E.; Molina, J.A.; Vázquez, A. and Codoceo, R. Serum levels of zinc and copper in patients with Parkinson's disease. J. Neurol. Sci. 1992, 112(1-2) 30-33.

[41] Forsleff, L.; Schauss, A.G.; Bier, I.D. and Stuart, S. J. Evidence of functional zinc deficiency in Parkinson's disease. Altern. Complement. Med. 1998, 5(1):57-64.

[42] Brewer G.J.; Kanzer, S.H.; Zimmerman, E.A.; Molho, E.S.; Celmins, D.F.; Heckman, S.M. and Dick, R. Subclinical zinc deficiency in Alzheimer's disease and Parkinson's disease. Am. J. Alzheimers Di.s Other Demen. 2010, 25(7):572-575.

[43] MacDiarmid CW, J. Taggart, K. Kerdsomboon, M. Kubisiak, S. Panascharoen, K. Schelble, D. J. Eide. Peroxiredoxin chaperone activity is critical for protein homeostasis in zinc-deficient yeast. Journal of Biological Chemistry, 2013; DOI: 10.1074/jbc.M113.512384.

[44] Qureshi GA, Qureshi AA, Memon SA, Parvez SH.Impact of selenium, iron, copper and zinc in on/off Parkinson's patients on L-dopa therapy. J Neural Transm Suppl. 2006;(71):229-36.

[45] Liuzzi JP, Cousins RJ. Mammalian zinc transporters. Annu Rev Nutr. 2004;24:151–72.

[46] Eide DJ. Zinc transporters and the cellular trafficking of zinc. Biochim Biophys Acta. 2006;1763:711–22.

[47] Ohno H, Doi R, Yamamura K, Yamashita K, Iizuka S, Taniguchi N. A study of zinc distribution in erythrocytes of normal humans. Blut. 1985;50:113–6

[48] Ryu MS, Lichten LA, Liuzzi JP, Cousins RJ. Zinc Transporters ZnT1 (Slc30a1), Zip8 (Slc39a8), and Zip10 (Slc39a10) in Mouse Red Blood Cells Are Differentially Regulated during Erythroid Development and by Dietary Zinc Deficiency.J. Nutr. November 2008 vol. 138 no. 11 2076-2083.

[49] Welch RW, Webb MJ, Loneragan JF (1982) Zinc in membrane function and its role in phosphorus toxicity. In A Scaife, ed, Plant Nutrition 1982, Proceedings of the Ninth International Plant Nutrition Colloquium, Warwick University, UK, August 22–27, 1982. Commonwealth Agricultural Bureaux, Farnham House, Farnham Royal, UK, pp 710–715

[50] Liu MJ, Bao S, Galvez-Peralta M, Pyle CJ, Rudawsky AC, Pavlovicz RE, Killilea DW, Li C, Nebert DW, Wewers MD, Knoell DL. "ZIP8 Regulates Host Defense through Zinc-Mediated Inhibition of NF-[kappa]B." Cell Rep. 2013 Feb 8.

[51] Prasad AS: Clinical, immunological, and antioxidant roles of zinc. Exp.gerontol. 2008.

[52] Maret W: The function of zinc metallothionein, a link between cellular zinc and redox state. J.Nutr.2000,130 (5S Suppl):1455S-8S.

[53] Tupe RS, Tupe SG,Tarwadi KV, Agte VV: Effect of different dietary zinc levels on hepatic antioxidant and micronutrients indices under oxidative stress conditions . Metabolism. 2010. 59(11): 1603-1611.

[54] Normandie I and Hazell AS: Manganese, neurotoxicity: an update of pathophysiological mechanisms. Metab.BrainDis. 2002,17(4), 375-387.

[55] Johansson E, Westermarck T, Hasan MY, Nilsson B, Stephen S, Adem A: Alteration in nickel and cadmium concentrations in erythrocytes and plasma of patients with Parkinson's disease, 2007. Trends in Biomedicine in Finland XXI, vol.2(4), 17-32.

[56] Johansson E, Holmkvist M, Ek P, Westermarck T, Atroshi F: Erythrocytes as biomarkers of changed metal ion homeostais in patients Parkinson's disease. Abstract ISTERH, 2013, Tokyo.

[57] Lijnen P, Staessen J, Fagard R, Amery A :Effect of cadmium on transmembrane Na+ and K+ transport systems in human erythrocytes. 1991. Br.J.Ind.Med.48, 392-398.

[58] George S, Rey NL, Reichenbach N, Steiner JA, Brundin P. • -Synuclein:The long distance runner. 2013. Brain Pathol. 23(3), 350-357.

[59] Kornberg RD and McConnell HM: Inside-outside translocation of phospholipids in vesicle membranes. 1971. Biochemistry 10, 1111-1120.

[60] Hollenbeck PJ and Saxton WM: The axonal transport of mitochondria. 2006. CellScience 118, 5411-5419.

[61] Gunter TE, Buntinas L, Sparagna G, Eliseev R and Gunter K: Mitochondrial calcium transport: mechanisms and functions. 2000. Cell calcium, 288, 285-296.

[62] Zhang Q and Zhao Y: The diverse biofunctions of LIM domain proteins determined by subcellular localization and protein-protein interaction. 2007. Biol.Cell 99, 489-502.

[63] Perin MS, Fried VA, Mignery GA, Jahn R, Südhof TC: Phospholipid binding by a synaptic vesicle protein homologous to the regulatory region of protein kinase C. 1990. Nature 345,260-263.

[64] Koizumi S, Gong PG, Suzuki K and Murata M: Cadmium responsive element of the human heme oxygenase-1 gene mediates heat shock factor 1-17. 2007. J.Biol.Chem. 282, 8715-8723.

[65] Alami J, Wickel C, Syewart D, Gongi P, Touchardi C, Otterbein S, Choi AMK, Burow ME, Ton Jen-sie: Mechanism of heme oxygenase-1, gene activation by cadmium on MCF-7 epithelial cells. 2000, J.Biol.Chem. 275(36), 27694-27702.

[66] Verbost PM, Flik G. Pang PK, Lock RAC and Bonga: SEW: Cadmium inhibition of the erythrocyte Ca2+ pump. 1989. J.Biol.Chem. 264(10), 5613-5616.

[67] Devaux PF, Lopez-Montero I, Bryde S: Proteins involved in lipid translocation in eu-caryotic cells. 2006. Chemistry and physics of lipids, 141, 119-132.

[68] Martin SJ, Reutelingsperger CP, McGahon AJ, Rader JA, van Schie RC, LaFace DM, Green DR: Early redistribution of plasma membrane phosphatidylserine is a general feature of apoptosis regardless of the initiating stimulus: inhibition by overexpression of Bcl-2 and Abl. 1995. J.Exp.Med.182(5), 1545-1556.

[69] Sopjani M, Föller M, Haendeler J, Götz F, Lang F: Silver ion-induced suicidal erythrocyte death. 2009. J.Appl.Toxicol.29(6), 531-536.

[70] Flindt ML, King E, Walsh DB: Blood level and erythrocyte delta-aminolevulinic acid dehydratase levels in Manchester taxi drivers. 1976. Br.J.Ind.Med. 33(2), 79-84.

[71] Kelada SN, Shelton E, Kaufmann RB, Khory MJ: δ-Aminolevulinic acid dehydratase genotype and lead toxicity: a HuGe review. 2001. Am.J.Epidemiol.154(1), 1-13.

[72] Lang F, Gulbins E, Lang FA, Zappulla D and Föller M: Ceramide in suicidal death of erythrocytes Cell Physiol. Biochem. 2010. 26(1), 21-28..

[73] Asagba SO & Eriyamremu GE: Oral cadmium exposure alters haematological and liver function parameters of rats fed a Nigerian-like diet. 2007. J.Nutr.Environ.Med. 16(3-4), 267-274.

[74] Johansson E: Selenium and its protection against the effects of mercury and silver. 1991. J.TraceElem.ElectrolytesHealthDis., 5(4), 273-274.

[75] Johansson E, Liljefors T and Plantin L-O: Comparison ICP-MS estimation of elements using quantitative mode and conditional factors, In Trace Element Analytical Chemistry in Medicine and Biology, Madrid 1994, pp.141-146.

[76] Johansson E and Liljefors T: Heavy elements in root tips from teeth with amalgam fillings, In TEMA-7, Zagreb 1991, pp. 11-18-11-20.

[77] Hollenbeck PJ and Saxton WM: The axonal tranport of mitochondria. 2006. J. Cell Science, 118(23), 5411-5419.

[78] Huang Y-X, Wu Z-J, Mehrishi J, Huang B-T, Chen X-Y, Zheng X-Y, Liu W-J, Liu M: Human red cell aging:correlative changes in surface charge and cell properties. 2010. J.Cell Mol. Med., 15(12), 2634-2642.

[79] Bosman GJ, Werre JM, Willekens FL, Novotny VM: Erythrocyte ageing in vivo and in vitro: structural aspects and implications for transfusion. 2008. Transfus.Med.18(6), 335-347.

11

Trace Elements, Antioxidant Enzymes and Free Carnitine Levels among Epileptic Patients Treated with Valproate Monotherapy

Elżbieta Płonka-Półtorak, Tuomas Westermarck, Pekka Kaipainen, Markus Kaski and Faik Atroshi

1. Introduction

1.1. Epilepsy and oxidative stress

Epilepsy is a common chronic neurological disorder with a prevalence of 0, 4 – 1 % of the general population [1]. The highest incidence rates are in children and elderly. Epilepsy is characterized by recurrent unprovoked seizures, generalized or focal. The epileptic seizure is a clinical manifestation of transient excessive and hyper synchronous activity of neurones in the brain. It may include alterations of consciousness, motor or autonomic components or subjective sensory or psychic phenomena. An epilepsy syndrome is a complexity of signs and symptoms defining a unique condition. One of the most common syndromes is Juvenile myoclonic epilepsy accounting for up to 10% of all epilepsies [2].

Etiology of epilepsy in the majority is not identified [3]. Genetic defect or structural-metabolic disorder of the brain may be the cause of some chronic seizures. The commonest acquired causes of epilepsy include vascular diseases, tumours, trauma, and infections of the central nervous system [2]. However, the mechanisms of epileptogenesis are not well understood.

Experimental and human studies suggested that the homeostasis of trace elements and membrane lipid peroxidation due to increase of free radicals or decreased of antioxidant defence mechanisms have been causally involved in some forms of epilepsies. They were directly or indirectly implicated as taking part in the pathophysiology of neuronal excitability, neuronal excitotoxicity, seizure recurrence and its resistance to treatment with antiepileptic drugs [4].

Oxidative stress is a common pathogenic mechanism in neurodegenerative disorders. The central nervous system is particularly susceptible to reactive oxygen species (ROS) due to high oxygen demands of the brain, low concentration of endogenous antioxidants and concomitant accumulation of reactive iron. Furthermore, the abundance of polyunsaturated fatty acids and excess of predominant neurotransmitter glutamate, favour cell toxicity [5]. ROS can activate a self-accelerating vicious cycle leading to mitochondrial damage and neuronal cell death [6].

In epilepsy, the oxidative/antioxidative balance can have a role in both seizure controls and side effects of often life-long pharmacotherapy.

2. Pharmacotherapy of epilepsy-Valproic acid

There are a large range of antiepileptic drugs with different mechanisms of action, pharmacokinetics, pharmacology, and important side effects. Pharmacotherapy of epilepsy is symptomatic.

Valproic acid (VPA) which is an eight-carbon branched-chain fatty acid, is one of the most widely used effective antiepileptic drugs. The main mechanism of the action includes a blockade of sodium channels, activating calcium dependent potassium conductance and GABAergic effect [7]. VPA is metabolized by microsomal glucuronide conjugation, mitochondrial beta-oxidation and cytochrome P450-dependent omega-, (omega-1)-and (omega-2)-oxidation [8]. Therefore, an involvement of lipid peroxidation seems to be probable during pharmacotherapy with VPA.

Serious side effects are relatively rare but include fatal hepatotoxicity and acute haemorrhagic pancreatitis. They occur mainly in children on polypharmacy and those with organic brain disease. Hyperammonaemic encephalopathy has been reported in patients with urea cycle disorder. Benign elevation of liver enzymes is common during valproate therapy and dose depended. Thrombocytopenia and other haematological abnormalities should be controlled. Other troublesome adverse effects are weight gain, gastrointestinal disturbances, hair loss and tremors. Hormonal disturbances with polycystic ovary syndrome and risk of teratogenicity, including a 1 to 3% risk of neural tube defects, make the use of VPA in some women undesirable [7].

In numerous studies there was found to be an imbalance in oxidative status of the patient with epilepsy treated with VPA [9].

3. Role of trace elements and antioxidant enzymes in epilepsy

3.1. Iron

In several neurodegenerative diseases, iron accumulates in brain tissues. Since post-mortem examinations cannot distinguish whether iron accumulation is a cause or consequence of brain damage, it is necessary to manipulate iron to assess its causal role. In the animal model of epilepsy, iron supplementation increased damage in various brain regions, and a tight relationship between iron and zinc in micro gliosis was found [10]. In general, iron is kept safe by binding itself to protein; transported in form of transferrin-bound iron or stored in form of ferritin. The liberation of free iron can augment generation of active free radicals and it appears to play a crucial role in the posttraumatic epilepsy [11]. Iron deposition results in tissue damage by either directly damaging cells or changing the cellular environment so that it is more susceptible to toxins or other pathologic processes. On the other hand, iron is a cofactor of catalase (CAT), which plays a role in antioxidant defence systems by catalysing the decomposition of hydrogen peroxide. The proper balance of iron without excessive supplementation is very important for oxidant status.

The surrogate markers of iron status may be non-transferrin bound iron (NTBI). There was found an increase in NTBI in patients treated due to epilepsy with VPA [12].

3.2. Selenium, cooper, zinc

The trace elements selenium (Se), cooper (Cu) and zinc (Zn) are important cofactors of antioxidant enzymes such as superoxide dismutase (Cu-SOD, Zn-SOD), glutathione peroxidise (GPX) as well as protein with antioxidant properties, ceruloplasmin (CRL, copper-binding protein). SOD and GPX play a predominant role as free radical scavengers in the brain tissue, whilst CAT is deficient [13]. SOD and GPX are also important for detoxification of xenobiotics, and may be involved in the oxidative injury caused by antiepileptic drugs [14].

Results of various studies on trace elements levels and activities of main antioxidant enzymes during pharmacotherapy of epilepsy are conflicting. A selected bias of patients and different laboratory methods might be responsible, as well as the influence of lifestyle with consumption of natural antioxidants or their supplementation [4, 15, 16].

A decrease in the trace elements selenium and copper was reported in epileptic patients receiving sodium valproate [17]. One of the main selenium status marker is plasma glutathione peroxidise (GPX3). The product of plasma SOD (pSOD) activity, H_2O_2, is the major substrates for GPX3. An involvement of lipid peroxidation seems to be probable and the elevated activity of pSOD in some studies may be explained by this induction. Significant effects of duration of VPA therapy, activity of seizures and gender were found on Zn, pSOD, and erythrocyte SOD (eSOD) levels [4, 9]. Also in prospective studies [18, 19] were reported increased levels of eSOD in epileptic children after implementation of VPA treatment. Some other authors did not find a significant difference in enzyme activity or even a reduced level of pSOD was found in young people with epilepsy treated using valproate [20].

pSOD is a sensitive index of Cu status, while plasma Cu is not a reliable marker of copper status [21]. Zinc supplements can decrease SOD activity, primarily due to the antagonistic relationship between high zinc intakes and copper absorption [22, 23]. A few authors reported lower or normal Zn concentrations in persons with epilepsy [24, 25]

4. Carnitine and cellular energy

L-carnitine is the key factor in mitochondrial beta oxidation of fatty acids for the generation of metabolic energy. Apart from carrying the long-chain fatty acids into the mitochondrial matrix, it takes part in transporting from peroxysomes into mitochondria the products of oxidation of very long-chain fatty acids and in removing from mitochondria medium and short-chain fatty acids, which can be toxic at a high level. As a donor of acetyl group, it participates in the synthesis of neurotransmitter acetylocholine. It also takes part in the reaction of detoxication, including the removal of some drugs, and in chelation of iron [26].

L-carnitine is synthesized in the liver, kidneys and brain from essential amino acids lysine and methionine, with participation of the vitamins C, B_6, PP, and iron. The main source of L-carnitine in the diet is meat and dairy products. When the diet is rich in the aforementioned products and there are no liver and kidney diseases, the risk of carnitine deficiency is low. Bioavailability of carnitine from medical preparations is only ca. 20% [27].

Carnitine deficiency can result from fatty acid oxidation disorders, organic acidemias, renal insufficiency, and treatment with some drugs, as valproic acid. The clinical symptoms of L-carnitine deficiency involve brain with enhanced risk of hypoketonic-hypoglycemic and hepatic encephalopathy, or skeletal and cardiac myopathy. Carnitine deficiency in case of fatty acids oxidative disorders can cause epileptic seizures. The seizures may result from cerebral bioenergetic failure associated with acute episodes of hypoglycemic, hypoketotic encephalopathy, or hypoxic-ischemic encephalopathy due to cardiac arrhythmias and/or cardiomyopathy [28].

In numerous studies, reduced carnitine levels were found during VPA therapy, especially with prolonged use and with high dosage levels [29]. The mechanism of this may include: 1) the formation of valproylcarnitine, 2) the reduction of tubular reabsorption of carnitine in the kidneys, 3) the inhibition of selected enzymes, which take part in biosynthesis of carnitine, 4) the inhibition of the membrane carnitine transporter and 5) the impairment of recycling of carnitine from long-chain acylcarnitines by the VPA-induced decrease of mitochondrial free Co-A level. Deficiency of carnitine is one possible mechanism which explains the VPA induced hepatotoxity. Carnitine depletion can impair the urea cycle (by influence on its enzymes) and cause accumulation of ammonia, what can be found in hepatic failure [30]. The impairment of beta-oxidation can shift the metabolism of VPA toward predominantly peroxisomal gamma-oxidation, resulting in excessive production and accumulation of toxic metabolite 4-en-VPA. It is postulated that carnitine supplementation may increase the beta-oxidation of VPA and limit production of its toxic metabolites. Carnitine inhibits free radicals generation preventing the impairment of fatty acid betaoxidation in mitochondria and protects tissues from damage by repairing oxidized membrane lipids [31].

5. New therapeutic approaches

Some of side effects of therapy with VPA have been suggested by alteration the homeostasis of trace elements and antioxidants. Seriously increase membrane lipid peroxidation at the expense of protective antioxidants; this may lead to an increase in the frequency of seizures and an idiosyncratic drug effect.

Adequate trace elements and antioxidants supply is essential for normal brain functions, and is particularly important for protection against neurological disorders. To elucidate the mechanism of action such substances in the brain should result in new safe therapeutic approaches.

Author details

Elżbieta Płonka-Półtorak[1], Tuomas Westermarck[2], Pekka Kaipainen[2], Markus Kaski[2] and Faik Atroshi[3]

1 Antiepileptic Outpatient Clinic, Provincial Hospital No. 2, Lwowska, Rzeszow, Poland

2 Rinnekoti Research Center, Espoo, Finland

3 Pharmacology & Toxicology, University of Helsinki, Finland

References

[1] http://www.who.int/mediacentre/factsheets/fs999/en/

[2] Shorvon S. Epilepsy. ONL Series. Oxford Neurology Library. Oxford University Press, 2009.

[3] Banerjee PN, Filippi D, Allen Hauser W. The descriptive epidemiology of epilepsy-a review. Epilepsy Res 2009; 85(1):31-45.

[4] Hamed S, Abdullah M. Trace elements and electrolytes homeostasis and their relation to antioxidant enzyme activity in brain hyperexcitability of epileptic patients. J Pharmacol Sci 2004; 96:349-59.

[5] Naziroglu M. (New molecular mechanism on the activation of TRPM2 channels by oxidative stress and ADP-ribose. Neurochem Res 2007; 32:1990-2001.

[6] Patel M. Mitochondrial dysfunction and oxidative stress: cause and consequence of epileptic seizures. Free Radic Biol Med 2004; 37(12):1951–1962.

[7] Panayiotopoulos CP. Pharmacopoeia of prophylactic antiepileptic drugs. In: The epilepsies: seizures, syndromes and management. Bladon Medical Publishing, Oxfordshire (UK) 2005;pp 504-506.

[8] Perucca E. Pharmacological and therapeutic properties of valproate: a summary after 35 years of clinical experience. CNS Drugs 2002; 16:695-714.

[9] Płonka-Półtorak E, Zagrodzki P, Chłopicka J, Bartoń H, Westermarck T, Kaipainen P, Kaski M, Atroshi F. Valproic acid modulates superoxide dismutase, uric acid-independent FRAP and zinc in blood of adult epileptic patients. Biol Trace Elem Res 2011;143(3):1424-34.

[10] Shoham, S, Youdim MBH. Iron involvement in neural damage and microgliosis in models of neurodegenerative diseases. Cell. Mol. Biol 2000; 46: 743–760.

[11] Choi, BH. Oxygen, antioxidants and brain dysfunction. Yonsei Med J 1993; 34(1):1–10.

[12] Ounjaijean S, Westermarck T, Partinen M, Plonka-Poltorak E, Kaipainen P, Kaski M, Fucharoen S, Srichairatanakool S, Atroshi F. Increase in non-transferrin bound iron and the oxidative stress status in epilepsy patients treated using valproic acid monotherapy. Int J Clin Pharmacol Ther 2011; 49(4): 268-7

[13] Halliwell B, Gutteridge JM. Free radicals in biology and medicine. Oxford University Press,1999, Oxford.

[14] Maertens P, Dyken P, Graf W, et al. Free radicals, anticonvulsants, and the neuronal ceroid-lipofuscinoses. Am J Med Genet 1995; 57:225-228.

[15] Sudha K, Rao AV, Rao A. Oxidative stress and antioxidants in epilepsy. Clin Chim Acta 2001; 303:19-24.

[16] Cengiz M, Yüksel A, Seven M. The effects of carbamazepine and valproic acid on the erythrocyte glutathione, glutathione peroxidase, superoxide dismutase and serum lipid peroxidation in epileptic children. Pharmacol Res 2000;41:423-425

[17] Armutcu F, Ozerol E, Gurel A, et al. Effect of long-term therapy with sodium valproate on nail and serum trace element status in epileptic children. Biol Trace Elem Res 2004; 102:1-10.

[18] Yiş U, Seçkin E, Kurul SH, Kuralay F, Dirik E. Effects of epilepsy and valproic acid on oxidant status in children with idiopathic epilepsy. Epilepsy Res 2009; 84:232-237

[19] Yüksel A, Cengiz M, Seen M, Ulutin T Erythrocyte glutathione, glutathione peroxidase, superoxide dismutase and serum lipid peroxidation in epileptic children with valproate and carbamazepine monotherapy.J Basic Clin Physiol Pharmacol 2000; 11:73-81

[20] Solowiej E, Sobaniec W. The effect of antiepilepticdrug therapy on antioxidant enzyme activity and serum lipid peroxidation in young patients with epilepsy. Neurol Neurochir Pol 2003; 37:991-1003

[21] Harvey LJ, McArdle HJ. Biomarkers of copper status: a brief update. Brit J Nutr 2008; 99:S10–S13

[22] Mariani E, Mangialasche F, Feliziani FT, et al. Effects of zinc supplementation on antioxidantenzyme activities in healthy old subjects. Exp Gerontol 2008; 43:445-451

[23] Hughes S, Samman S. The effect of zinc supplementation in humans on plasma lipids, antioxidant status and thrombogenesis. J Am Coll Nutr 2006; 25:285-291

[24] Barbeau A, Donaldson J. Zinc, taurine, and epilepsy. Arch Neurol 1974; 30: 52-58

[25] Higashi A, Ikeda T, Matsukura M, Matsuda I. Serum zinc and vitamin E concentrations in handicapped children treated with anticonvulsants. Dev Pharmacol Ther 1982; 5:109-113

[26] Arrigoni-Martelli E, Caso V. Carnitine protects mitochondria and removes toxic acyls from xenobiotics. Drugs Exp Clin Res 2001; 27: 27–49.

[27] Verrotti A, Greco R, Morgese G, Chiarelli F. Carnitine deficiency and hyperammonemia in children receiving valproic acid with and without other anticonvulsant drugs. Int J Clin Lab Res 1999; 29(1):36-40.

[28] Tein I, Xie ZW. Reversal of valproic acid-associated impairment of carnitine uptake in cultured human skin fibroblasts. Biochem Biophys Res Commun1994; 28, 204(2): 753-8.

[29] Płonka-Półtorak E, Zagrodzki P, Chłopicka J, Bartoń H, Westermarck T, Kaipainen P, Kaski M, Atroshi F. Valproic acid modulates superoxide dismutase, uric acid-independent FRAP and zinc in blood of adult epileptic patients. Biol Trace Elem Res. 2011; 143(3):1424-34

[30] Lheureux PE, Penaloza A, Zahir S, Gris M. Science review: carnitine in the treatment of valproic acid-induced toxicity-what is the evidence? Crit Care 2005; 9(5):431-40

[31] Gulcin I. Antioxidant and antiradical activities of L-carnitine. Life Sci 2006; 78:803-811.

12

Green Tea: Just a Drink or Nutraceutical

Sakaewan Ounjaijean, Suthat Fucharoen and
Somdet Srichairatanakool

1. Introduction

Brewed tea has been the most widely consumed beverage throughout history. Attractively, this is attributed to its present taste, aromatic odor and healthful effects to the human body. Tea (*Camellia sinensis*) is used for the production of green tea, oolong tea and black tea, depending on the fermentation process. Without fermentation, green tea can be made from fresh tea shoots at a high temperature, thereby inactivating the oxidizing enzymes such as polyphenol oxidase (PPO) and leaving the intact polyphenols. Many ingredients persisting in green tea products are flavonols, flavanols, chlorogenic acid, coumarylquinic acid, theogallin (3-galloylquinic acid), vitamin P (flavonoids), alkaloids, caffeine, theophylline, theobromine, theanine, volatile compounds, fluoride, minerals (e.g. aluminium and magnesium), trace elements and other unidentified compounds. During fermentation, these polyphenolic compounds undergo PPO-catalyzed oxidative polymerization giving rise to the formation of theaflavins and thearubigins which are the major antioxidants in black tea [1]. Besides being a world-wide, well-known beverage, green tea has many benefits for health, including anti-oxidative, free radical scavenging, iron-chelating, anti-hyperglycemic and anti-diabetic, weight-lowering, anti-aging, neuro-protective and rescue, thrombosis-inhibitory, anti-inflammatory, exercise-endurating, hepatoprotective, hepatic phase II enzyme activity-inducing, cardioprotective, neoangioprotective, anti-mutagenic, anti-carcinogenic and cancer-preventive, anti-microbial, as well as immunomodulatory activities. Tea products generally provide refreshment and diuretic benefits, as well as contributing to feelings of alertness; however; green tea extraordinarily exhibits such biological and pharmacological properties depending on several specific active phytochemical constituents; particularly catechins. Nowadays, crude extracts, purified catechin fractions and synthetic catechin derivatives of green tea are applicable in alternative and complementary medicines for the prevention, treatment and co-treatment of many diseases and disorders.

2. Sources and compositions of green tea

Tea has traditionally been cultivated across four continents in the manufacturing of a refreshing drink. The tea products that are available are directly related to the process used at the origin, and can be classified as black tea, green tea, yellow tea, red tea, green pressed tea, as well as instant tea and tea dyes [1]. Green tea is manufactured by using conventional and modified methods. One of these methods involves a 2-3-day process of to drying fresh tea leaves and then rolling the dry leaves with a commercial machine. Alternatively, another method involves the very rapid process of baking the tea leaves in a house-hold microwave oven (800 watt, 3 minutes) at a working temperature of 115 °C. This process will shock the persisting PPO enzyme and result in higher catechins content [2]. A typical green tea beverage is normally prepared at a proportion of 1 g dry weight of tea leaves in 100 ml of hot water in a 3-minute brew (an approximate temperature of 80 °C). This brew usually contains 250 – 350 mg tea solids, 30 – 42% catechins (74 mg) and 3–6% caffeine [3]. HPLC analysis shows the green tea extract (GTE) is comprised of at least six major catechins, including (-)-epicatechin (EC), (-)-epicatechin 3-gallate (ECG), (-)-epigallocatechin (EGC), (-)-epigallocatechin 3-gallate (EGCG), (+)-catechin (C) and (-)-gallocatechin (GC), of which EGCG is the major isomer followed by ECG, EGC and EC (Figure 1) [4]. Gallic acid (GA) is derivatized to one of the hydroxyl groups of the catechins, which has been directly attributed to the biological activities of the catechin species.

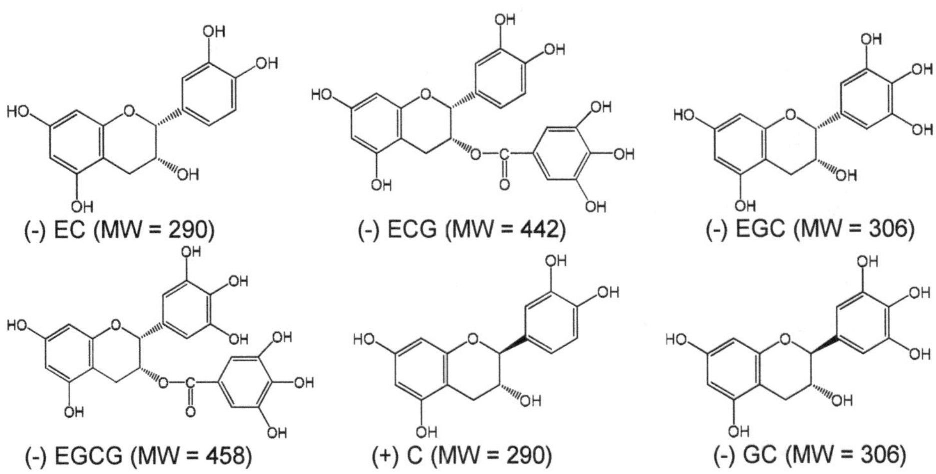

Figure 1. Chemical structures of catechins in green tea (Redrawn from [4])

Moreover, tea products have different amounts and compositions of catechins, which is possibly due to biodiversity, different processing methods, different planting areas and different varieties of tea strains. For instance, Khokhar and colleagues reported that 1 g dry weight of tea product contained 48.4 mg total catechins (9.1 mg EGC, 7.9 mg EC, 22.9 mg EGCG, and 8.5 mg ECG) for Ceylon (NL) black tea; 5.6 mg total catechins (<0.5 mg EGC, 3.1 mg EC,

1.8 mg EGCG, and 0.8 mg ECG) for Yule (India) black tea; 7.5 mg total catechins (<0.5 mg EGC, 4.0 mg EC, 2.6 mg EGCG, and 1.0 mg ECG) for PG tips (UK) black tea;5.15 mg total catechins (16.3 mg EGC, 4.7 mg EC, 26.3 mg EGCG, and 4.4 mg ECG) for Chinese green tea; 84.9 mg total catechins (28.7 mg EGC, 9.4 mg EC, 40.8 mg EGCG, and 5.9 mg ECG) for Japanese green tea; and 21.1 mg total catechins (7.7 mg EGC, 1.7 mg EC, 11.5 mg EGCG, and 0.5 mg ECG) for Chinese oolong tea [5]. EGCG has so far received the most attention because it represents approximately 59% catechin content, EGC at approximately 19%, ECG at approximately 13.6%, and EC at approximately 6.4% of the total catechin content [6]. Green tea also contains other phenolic acids, such as chlorogenic acid and caffeic acid, as well as other flavonols, such as kaempferol, myricetin and quercetin [7].

Green tea catechins have proven to be quite stable in water that is room temperature; however, they can be destroyed at a rate of 20% under brewing at 98 °C for 7 hours and epimerized to other derivatives (e.g. EGCG → GCG) under autoclaving at 120 °C for 20 minutes [8]. Fresh tea leaves are unusually rich in polyphenolic catechins that may constitute up to 30% of the dry leaf weight [9]. As a result of the immediate inactivation of PPO enzyme, the compositions of catechins in green tea are very similar to those of the fresh tea leaves. Various quinines, which are subsequently produced by the enzymatic oxidations, undergo condensation reactions to produce *bis*-flavanols, theaflavins, epitheaflavic acids and thearubigens. These compounds impart the characteristic taste and color properties of black and oolong tea [10].

In our Thai green tea, EGCG was found to be the most abundant catechin (at about 60% of the total catechin content), followed by EGG, ECG, and EC, respectively and the assay yield of the total green tea catechin content was found to be 26-29 g/100 g dry tea leaves (Table 1) [2]. In comparison, Taiwan green tea (1 g dry weight) contained 93.3 mg total catechin content, followed by 43.2 mg EGCG, 33.6 mg ECG, 0.7 mg C, 3.3 mg EC and 2.7 mg ECG [11].

Amounts	EGCG	EGC	ECG	EC	Total catechins
mg/g dry weight	169.4±7.2	60.1±6.2	19.3±2.6	16.3±5.6	279.8±15.2
% (*w/w*)	60.6±2.2	21.5±1.4	6.9±1.0	5.9±2.1	100

Table 1. HPLC analysis of catechin compositions in six green tea extract solutions (2 g%, *w/v*).

3. Nutritional value of green tea

In general, an antioxidant refers to any substance capable of preventing the oxidation catalyzed by reactive oxygen species (ROS)/reactive nitrogen species (RNS). Thus, an antioxidant that protects against iron toxicity is a substance that can: i) chelate iron and prevent the reaction with oxygen or peroxides; ii) chelate iron and maintain it in a redox state that makes iron unable to reduce molecular oxygen; iii) trap already formed radicals, which is a putative action of any substance that can scavenge free radicals in biological systems, regardless of whether they have originated from iron-dependent reactions or not. Not only can natural products chelate iron, but also synthetic compounds are capable of chelating iron *in vivo,* thereby limiting its participation in free radical reactions. Thus, iron chelators also serve as antioxidants by suppressing iron-mediated oxidation in biological systems. Surprisingly, thiol compounds (e.g. glutathione) that are synthesised by mammals can afford significant antioxidant protection. This protection is related to the ability of glutathione to trap radicals, reduce peroxides, as well asits ability to work to maintain the redox state of the cells [12].

The potential of green tea to prevent or ameliorate chronic diseases is currently the subject of considerable scientific investigations. Although a number of mechanisms have been proposed for their beneficial effects, the radical scavenging and antioxidant properties of green tea catechins are frequently cited as important contributors. Emerging evidence has also shown that catechins and their metabolites possessmany additional mechanisms of action [13] by affecting numerous sites, potentiating endogenous antioxidants and eliciting dual actions during oxidative stress. Much of the evidence supporting an antioxidant function for green tea catechins is derived from assays of their antioxidant activity *in vitro.* However, the evidence that green tea catechins are acting either directly or indirectly as antioxidants *in vivo* is limited [14]

4. Anti-oxidative and iron-chelating properties

Green tea catechins stoichiometrically bind ferric ion to form a redox-inactive iron-phenolic complex [15, 16] and potentially protect vital biomolecules from oxidative damage. Incredibly, the catechins could be capable of chelating excessive redox iron in iron overloaded diseases, such as thalassemia, and play important preventive or/and protective roles in this unpleasant condition [2, 17-19]. The phytochemical compounds therefore play a double role in reducing the rate of oxidation because they can participate in: i) iron chelation [19], and ii) trapping radicals [2, 20]. Catechins can protect culture cells from iron-mediated damage [21, 22], ameliorate iron accumulation [17] and inhibit hepatic iron-induced lipid oxidation [23], and also play a dual effect in decreasing labile plasma iron (LPI) in iron-loaded rats [18]. Animal studies offer a unique opportunity to assess the contribution of green tea administration to the physiological effects on different models of oxidative-related diseases. In a combination of free-radical scavenging activity with iron-chelating properties, green tea may have a capacity of chelating excess iron in iron-overloaded conditions and play important preventive and/or protective roles in this unpleasant condition.

Like the deferiprone (DFP) treatment, oral administrations of GTE and EGCG significantly lowered levels of plasma non-transferrin bound iron (NTBI) and LPI in wild-type (WT), heterozygous β-globin gene knockout (BKO) thalassemic and double heterozygous β-globin gene knockout carrying human β^{E} gene (DH) mice (strain C57BL/6J) with iron overload, when compared to the DW group (Table 2) (Sakaewan Ounjaijean and Somdet Srichairatanakool, unpublished data). Elimination of these two toxic irons by green tea extract and EGCG fraction would relieve redox iron-induced oxidative stress and tissue damage in the body. GTE treatment efficiently depleted plasma malondialdehyde (MDA) concentrations in the iron-loaded mice (approximately 50% in WT, 30% in BKO and 40% in DH mice), whereas EGCG treatment caused significantly lower plasma MDA levels (approximately 30% in all the mice), suggesting that GTE and EGCG are strong antioxidants and exert potent anti-plasma lipid peroxidation. Consistently, the GTE and EGCG increased levels of reduced glutathione (GSH) in the plasma of all the mice despite under iron overload. Thus, it can be said that green tea catechins, particularly EGCG, chelate the redox irons and consequently inhibit the iron-catalyzed lipid peroxidation reactions in plasma lipids, as well as membrane phospholipids, resulting in an improvement of a powerful antioxidants as reduced glutathione is reduced in the plasma compartment.

Mice	N diet	Fe diet (0.2% ferrocene, w/w)			
	+DW	+DW	+GTE (90 mg/kg/day)	+EGCG (50 mg/kg/day)	+DFP (50 mg/kg/day)
			Plasma NTBI concentrations (μM)		
WT (n = 24)	-0.27±0.23	11.17±0.26*	6.83±1.49†	6.80±1.75†	6.81±2.23†
BKO (n = 16)	0.34±0.26	19.78±1.36*	10.20±1.92†	10.66±1.60†	11.75±1.21†
DH (n = 10)	-0.07±0.11	13.41±1.84*	7.74±1.38†	7.81±0.71†	7.83±1.41†
			LPI concentrations (μM)		
WT (n = 24)	-2.49±1.00	1.19±0.42*	-2.26±1.98†	-2.47±1.25†	-2.01±2.76†
BKO (n = 16)	0.87±0.22	2.30±1.08*	0.30±2.57†	-0.21±1.37†	0.35±1.05†
DH (n = 10)	-0.15±0.52	0.81±0.26*	0.26±0.61†	0.47±0.63	0.34±0.70
			Plasma MDA concentrations (μM)		
WT (n = 24)	13.39±5.10	39.97±8.67*	23.26±8.30†	28.39±6.66†	32.58±8.73†
BKO (n = 16)	26.80±3.59	54.34±9.88*	37.62±9.23†	41.85±11.8†	52.29±7.51†
DH (n = 10)	18.79±2.31	46.89±4.56*	26.62±5.14†	32.72±2.46†	38.13±5.09†
			Plasma GSH concentrations (μM)		
WT (n = 24)	11.53±2.50	7.73±4.70*	15.15±7.72†	16.04±6.61†	15.89±8.43†
BKO (n = 16)	7.73±4.25	6.24±3.89	15.12±9.76*,†	15.63±7.74*,†	16.50±8.75*,†
DH (n = 10)	10.97±5.00	5.81±1.44*	14.78±5.16†	17.03±7.27†	14.19±4.89†

*p <0.05 compared to N diet; †p <0.05 compared to DW.

Table 2. NTBI, LPI, MDA and GSH concentrations (mean+SD) in the WT, BKO and DH mice fed with a normal (N) diet (iron content 180 mg/kg) and an iron (Fe) diet (iron content 780 mg/kg) and treated with deionized water (DW), 90 mg/kg/day GTE, 50 mg/kg EGCG and 50 mg/kg DFP for 6 months.

5. Fate of green tea catechins in the body

5.1. Gastrointestinal absorption

Among these polyphenolic compounds, the hierarchy of antioxidant activity is ECG > EGCG > EGC > GA > EC ≈ C [24]. With the chelating activity of such prooxidant metals as iron (Fe^{2+}), green tea is able to reduce dietary nonheme iron absorption [25]. The ratio of EGC, EGCG, ECG or EC to the iron was 3:2, 2:1, 2:1 and 3:1, respectively [26]. Unlike most flavonoids, tea catechins existing as aglycone are found in the blood following oral ingestion and subsequently metabolized in the liver by methylation, sulfation and glucoronidation reactions [27]. Structure-activity studies have shown that the presence of the galloyl ring in the 3-position and trihydroxyphenyl B ring are of significant importance in terms of the antioxidant properties of the catechins [26].

After green tea (25 mg/kg) and pure EGCG fractions (10 mg/kg) were intravenously administered into rats, a study of the pharmacokinetic (concentration-time curves) properties of the catechins in the plasma was conducted. Beta-elimination half-lives ($T_{1/2}\beta$) were found to be 212, 45, and 41 minutes; clearances were 2.0, 7.0, and 13.9 ml•minute/kg; and apparent distribution volumes (V_d) were 1.5, 2.1, and 3.6 dl/kg for EGCG, EGC, and EC, respectively. In comparison, EGCG had a shorter $T_{1/2}\beta$ (135 minute), a larger clearance (72.5 ml•minute/kg), and a larger volume (V_d) (22.5 dl/kg) than the other two. When the green tea was intragastrically given (200 mg/kg), around 0.1, 13.7 and 31.2% of EGCG, EGC and EC were detected in the plasma compartment. The EGCG level was found to be the highest in the intestine samples and declined with a $T_{1/2}$ of 173 minute. EGC and EC levels were found to be the highest in the kidneys and declined rapidly with $T_{1/2}$ of 29 and 28 minute, respectively. EGCG, EGC, and EC levels in the liver and lungs were lower than those recorded in the intestine and the kidney [28]. This implies that EGCG is mainly excreted through bile, while EGC and EC are excreted through urine and bile. Inter-individual variations in the bioavailability of green tea catechins can be substantial and may be due, in part, to differences in colonic microflora and genetic polymorphisms among the enzymes involved in polyphenol metabolism [29]. The effect of green tea drinking may also differ by genotype [30].

Following oral administration of green tea catechin solutions (0.6%, *w/v*) to the rats, plasma levels of the catechins measured at 6:00 AM., 9:00 AM., 0:00 PM and 6:00 PM on the same day were found to be 983.9±114.2, 372.89±56.7, 186.89±34.5 and 548.1±221.6 ng/ml EGC; 1,527.3±163.7, 449.2±82.7, 224.6±58.0 and 845.6±374.0 ng/ml ECG; and 105.0±12.6, 85.5±15.8, 95.7±18.3 and 114.8±45.6 ng/ml EGCG, respectively, for which the plasma EGCG concentrations were found to be even lower than those of EGC and EC. There wasa gradual increase in plasma concentrations of EGC, EC and EGCG during Days 1-4. Levels of EGC and EC in the plasma on Day 14 were approximately three times higher than those on Day 1. Plasma levels of these three catechins decreased after Day 14, and by Day 28, plasma levels of the EGC and EC returned to the levels recorded on Day 1. On Days 4, 14 and 28, the catechins were mostly present in glucuronic acid (MW=194)/sulfuric acid (MW=98) conjugated-EGC (91.4, 95.6 and 86.4 ng/ml, respectively) and-EC (92.4, 95.5 and 89.4 ng/ml, respectively), while a much lower proportion of EGCG was found in the conjugated form (21.2, 60.7 and 39.3 ng/ml, respectively). The highest EGC concentration was found in the bladder; the highest EGCG concentration was found in the large intestine; very high concentrations of EGC and EGCG were found in the kidneys, prostate gland and lungs; and low levels of these three catechins were present in the liver, spleen, heart, and thyroid glands [31].

5.2. Organ metabolism

EC was not glucuronidated by uridine diphosphate-glucuronosyltransferases (UGT) and sulfotransferases (SULT) in human liver and small intestinal microsomes. However, the compound was efficiently glucuronidated in rat liver microsomes with the formation of two different glucuronides, and was also sulfated in human liver cytosol, mainly through the SULT1A1 isoform, as well as in the intestine through the SULT1A1 and SULT1A3 isoforms. In comparison, the EC was much less sulfated in the rat liver than in the human liver [32]. EGCG and ECG constituents in green tea drinks (10%, *w/v*) almost completely, competitively inhibited the activities of the SULT1A1 and SULT1A3 enzymes that play an important role in the presystemic inactivation of β_2 agonists in the liver and intestine, respectively [33]. When EGCG was glucuronidated by the liver microsomal UGT enzymes; four EGCG-glucuronides were identified as EGCG-3-glucuronide, EGCG-3′-glucuronide, EGCG-4′-glucuronide and EGCG-7-glucuronide. Under the same conditions, EGC was metabolized into two EGC-glucuronides as EGC-7-glucuronide and EGC-3′-glucuronide [34]. Since rate of the glucuronidation of EGCG and ECG in liver microsomes is rather low (12.2±0.2 and 7.5±0.2%, respectively for 3 hours) due to the galloyl ring, the two potent catechins are therefore recognized to be circulating in the plasma in unconjugated forms [35]. One study claimed that catechins were toxic to rat liver cells in the order of EGCG (LD_{50} 200±19 μM) > ECG (LD_{50} 2,000±214 μM) > GA (LD_{50} 3,000±298 μM), EGC (LD_{50} 3,000±304 μM) > EC (LD_{50} >10,000 μM), and this was likely due to the mitochondrial membrane potential ($\Delta\psi_m$) collapse, and the depletion of GSH and ROS formation. The EGCG and GA dose dependently affected GSH conjugation, methylation, metabolism by NAD(P)H:quinoneoxidoreductase 1 (NQO1) in the hepatic detoxification step (Figure 2), as monitored by a significant increase of plasma alanine aminotransferase (ALT) activity in mice [36].

5.3. Excretion

Most polyphenolic catechins in green tea may not be absorbed in the small intestine. The nonabsorbed catechins will be converted by large bow bacterial flora into simpler phenolic compounds, such as hippuric acid, then absorbed into the blood and excreted in the urine (4.22±0.28 mmol/24 hours), when compared to non-consumption (1.89+0.28 mmol/24 hours) [37].

6. Health benefits

6.1. Health promotion

The potential health effects of green tea catechins depend not only on the amount consumed, but also on their bioavailability, which appears to be substantially varied. Following the oral administration of tea catechins to rats [38] and mice [39], the four principal catechins have been identified in the portal vein, indicating that tea catechins are absorbed intestinally. There appear to be species-related differences in the bioavailability of EGCG compared to other tea

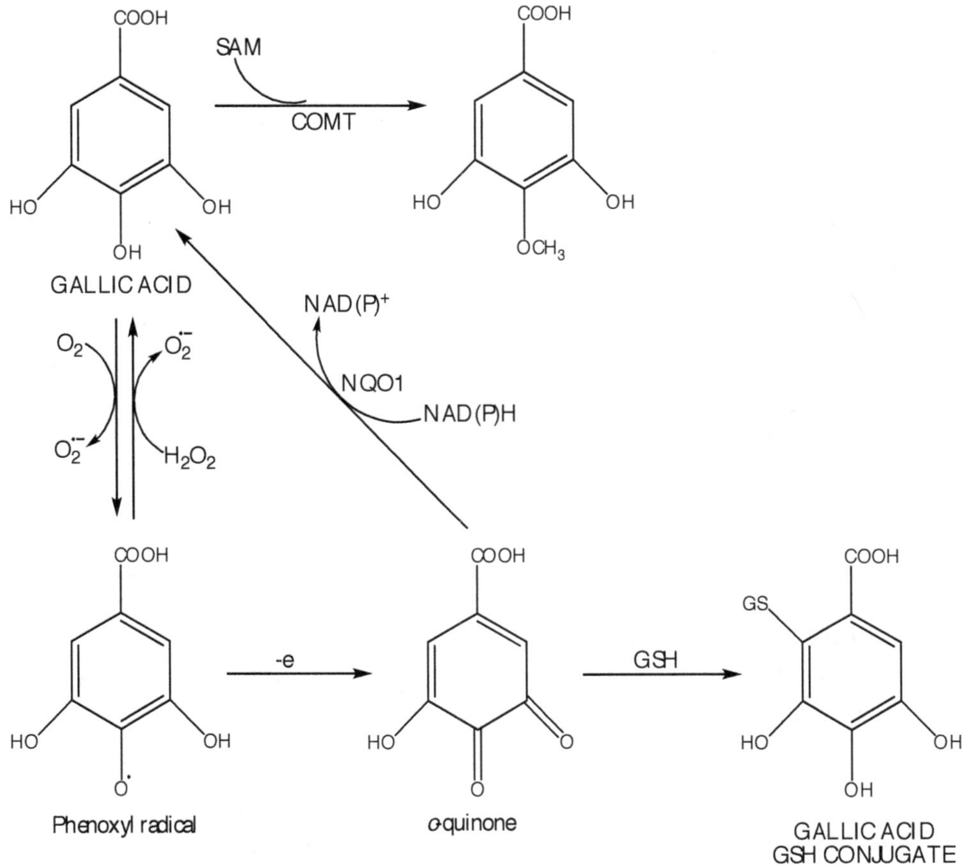

Figure 2. Possible mechanism for the hepaticgalloyl ring metabolism (Redrawn from [36]). Abbreviations: COMT=catechol-*O*-methyltransferase; GSH=reduced glutathione;NAD(P)+=nicotinamide adenine dinucleotide phosphate; NAD(P)H=reduced nicotinamide adenine dinucleotide phosphate; NQO1=NAD(P)H:quinone oxidoreductase-1; SAM=*S*-adenosyl methionine

catechins [7]. The epicatechin isomers purified from green tea were effective agents in protecting human low-density lipoproteins (LDL) and red blood cell (RBC) membranes from oxidative modification [40]. These effects are partly due to their free-radical scavenging abilities [20] and their iron-chelating properties, which are capable of binding any available iron, thus greatly reducing their bioavailability. They also have many pharmacological properties, including anti-hypertensive [41], anti-atheroslcerotic [42], anti-carcinogenic [43-45] and hypocholesterolemic effects [46, 47]. Health benefits of green tea consumption were achieved in the rodents within relatively short periods: three weeks [48], four weeks [49, 50], five weeks [51, 52] and eight weeks [53, 54].

Surprisingly, catechins inhibited xanthine oxidase (XO) activity *in vitro* [55– 58] and the XO inhibition constant (K_i) of EGCG was comparable to that of the common XO inhibitor allopurinol (0.76 versus 0.30 μmol) [56]. GTE consumption was found to decrease levels of serum uric acid concentrations observed in human subjects [59-61]; for instance, by decreasing serum uric acid levels from 4.54 to 4.22 mg/dl ($p<0.05$) within 7 days [59]. Our group has currently found that the consumption of GTE (2, 4 and 6 g/day), of which the 2 g/day dose was found to be the most effective, lowered levels of serum uric acid (3.53%) and also increased serum trolox-equivalent antioxidant capacity (TEAC) values in healthy volunteers (n=11) (unpublished data), suggesting an hypouricemic effect by XO inhibition or an increase of urinary uric acid excretion.

6.2. Hematologic disorders

In consideration of the evidence for its iron chelating properties, strong antioxidant capacity, low toxicity, and orally available administration, green tea has potential to be used as a pharmacological agent in the management of diseasesrelated to iron overload. Hypothetically, the removal of iron could reduce oxidative damage to the cellular biomolecules, including lipids, proteins, carbohydrates and nucleic acids, and this can consequently prevent, as well as improve the vital organ dysfunctions. DFP, known to readily permeate and mobilize nonheme iron from β-thalassemic patient erythrocytes, serves as a benchmark against which orally effective agents; catechins in GTE and purified EGCG products have been compared. Our studies have paid particular attention to the efficacy of GTE and EGCG in terms of the aspects of anti-oxidation and the potential for iron chelation in order to alleviate oxidative stress and iron overload in β-thalassemic mice in the past experiments, and in Thai β-thalassemia patients with regard to the near future.

Though the pathological role of redox iron in the hemosiderosis (such as hereditary hemochromatosis and thalassemia) is well characterized, excessive accumulation of the iron can result in significant organ dysfunction and abnormality. Recognition of the role of iron in conditions beyond transfusion-dependent iron overload may bring significant implications for the management of metabolic, infectious, and degenerative diseases. New findings obtained during the past years, especially in terms of the discovery of mutations in the genes associated with brain iron metabolism, have provided key insights into the mechanisms of brain iron homeostasis and the pathological mechanisms responsible for neurodegenerative diseases. Increased iron in the brain, which is rich in oxygen and fatty acids, provides an ideal environment for oxidative stress and possible irreparable tissue damage. Oxidative stress, resulting from increased brain iron levels, and possibly also from defects in antioxidant defense mechanisms, is widely believed to be associated with neuronal death in brain disorders.

The interaction between iron overload and dietary antioxidants has been well characterized; especially, with respect to vitamins E and C. Vitamin E has been extensively studied with respect to its capacity to protect molecules from the *in vitro* and *in vivo* effects of iron toxicity [62, 63]. Elevated levels of ROS tended to normalize in response to oral therapy with vitamin E, with patients exhibiting improvement in the antioxidant–oxidant balance in plasma and decreased lipid peroxidation in erythrocytes [64]. However, prolonged administration of vitamin E did not result in any significant changes in Hb levels in patients with β-thalassemia intermedia [65]. Therefore, vitamin E by itself is probably insufficient in inducing major changes in the rate of RBC hemolysis and in prolonging their survival, resulting in increased Hb levels.

The interaction of another dietary antioxidant, vitamin C (ascorbic acid) and iron is less clear. Ascorbic acid can reduce 'free iron' (ferric) to a ferrous form, promoting the initiation and propagation of free radical reactions [66, 67]. In people under a risk of iron overload, in which the elevated levels of iron could lead to higher 'free iron' concentrations, an excess of vitamin C could have deleterious effects. Plant flavonoids (including rutin and curcumin) are another group of antioxidants, which may have therapeutic potential in thalassemia. However, despite their apparent salutary effects on erythrocytes, antioxidants have not yet been shown to ameliorate the anemia of the patients [68]. Antioxidants may be more effective if used in combination with an iron chelator. This approach, if successful, could be particularly useful in countries with limited financial resources.

The potential of green tea to prevent or ameliorate chronic disease is currently the subject of considerable scientific investigation. Although a number of mechanisms have been proposed as being responsible for green tea's beneficial effects, the radical scavenging and antioxidant properties of green tea catechins are frequently cited as important contributors. Emerging evidence has shown that catechins and their metabolites have many additional mechanisms of action [69] by affecting numerous sites, potentiating endogenous antioxidants and eliciting dual actions during oxidative stress. Much of the evidence supporting the antioxidant function for green tea catechins has been derived from assays of their antioxidant activity *in vitro*. However, evidence that green tea catechins are acting directly or indirectly as antioxidants *in vivo* is more limited [14]. Interestingly, green tea catechins can play a double role in reducing the rate of oxidation, as they can participate in: i) iron chelation [19]; and ii) trapping radicals [2, 20]. The catechins have been shown to protect culture cells from iron-mediated damage [21, 22]. In animal models of iron overload, they have been reported to ameliorate iron accumulation [17] and inhibit iron-induced lipid oxidation in the liver [23]. They also play a dual effect in decreased labile iron in the plasma and consequently depleting oxidative stress in iron-loaded rats [18]. Animal studies offer a unique opportunity to assess the contribution of the antioxidant properties of the catechins in terms of the physiological effects of tea administration in different models of oxidative-related diseases. Combining free-radical scavenging with iron-chelating properties, green tea catechins may have a capacity of chelating an excess of iron under iron-overloaded conditions and play the important preventive and/or protective roles in this unpleasant condition. None of the treatments over 2 months affected the levels of blood hemoglobin (Hb) in the WT, BKO and DH mice challenged by iron overload, there were fed a high iron-diet. Nonetheless, iron-induced oxidative stress as well as GSH content in the RBC cytoplasm, and lipid-peroxidation in the RBC plasma membrane were reversed by the GTE that was used in the testing, as well as the EGCG, when compared to the DW treatment (Table 3). We also found that these two green tea products increased the survival rate or half-life of the RBC of the WT and BKO mice significantly (Sakaewan Ounjaijen and Somdet Srichairatanakool, unpublished data). Our results suggest that GTE and EGCG treatment might directly increase the erythropoietic rate, either in normal mice or in thalassemic mice, but probably do protect red cells from ROS-induced hemolysis.

Mice	Fe diet (0.2% ferrocene, w/w)								
	+DW			+GTE (90 mg/kg/day)			+EGCG (50 mg/kg/day)		
	Month 0	Month 1	Month 2	Month 0	Month 1	Month 2	Month 0	Month 1	Month 2
Blood Hb concentration (g/dl)									
WT (n = 24)	14.80±1.14	15.19 ±1.11	15.15±1.06	15.22±1.23	15.37±1.23	15.32±1.14	15.29±1.25	15.40±1.13	15.41±1.00
BKO (n = 16)	9.45 ±0.56	9.35 ±0.40	9.28 ±0.31	9.55 ±0.59	9.60 ±0.45	9.54 ±0.48	9.45 ±0.56	9.53 ±0.36	9.56 ±0.39
DH (n = 10)	15.97±1.09	15.80±1.01	15.85±0.88	16.11±0.84	16.25±0.85	16.17±0.77	16.33±0.76	16.41±0.72	16.29±0.71
Erythrocyte ROS (Fluorescent intensity unit)									
WT (n = 10)	38.46±9.17	38.29 ±10.93	42.62±9.63	31.74±9.14	23.29±3.99†	22.45±3.39†	33.07±8.08	26.87±3.72†	23.26±3.02†
BKO (n = 10)	48.29±8.01	53.92 ±9.69	59.81±8.96	35.07±7.68	33.69±7.83†	38.50±6.90†	33.88±7.08	31.47±8.93†	36.67±5.16†
DH (n = 10)	43.08±4.38	44.38 ±3.78	49.60±4.25	31.97±4.23	31.57±4.31	27.88±3.65†	31.51±5.38	31.50±4.38	28.17±4.64†
Erythrocyte MDA (pmol/g Hb)									
WT (n = 8)	ND	ND	48.23±6.15	ND	ND	36.80±3.23†	ND	ND	36.82±2.71†
BKO (n = 8)	ND	ND	60.63±3.28	ND	ND	44.26±2.87†	ND	ND	44.74±2.79†
DH (n = 8)	ND	ND	50.86±1.90	ND	ND	42.00±2.85†	ND	ND	40.36±2.83†
Erythrocyte GSH (μmol/g Hb)									
WT (n = 8)	ND	ND	2.80 ±0.52	ND	ND	3.61 ±0.32†	ND	ND	3.73 ±0.29†
BKO (n = 8)	ND	ND	2.56 ±0.22	ND	ND	3.31 ±0.40†	ND	ND	3.24 ±0.36†
DH (n = 8)	ND	ND	2.76 ±0.18	ND	ND	3.49 ±0.22†	ND	ND	3.46 ±0.19†

$^{\dagger}p$ <0.05 compared to DW.

Table 3. Levels of blood Hb, erythrocyte ROS, GSH and MDA (mean±SD) in WT, BKO and DH mice fed with an Fe diet (iron content 780 mg/kg) and treated with DW, GTE and EGCG for 2 months.$^{\dagger}p$ <0.05 compared to DW treatment. ND=not done.

The inhibition of the growth of blast cells from patients with acute myelocytic leukemic (AML) by EGCG affected hematopoietic growth factors (HGF), granulocyte colony stimulating factor (G-CSF), granulocyte macrophage colony stimulating factor (GM-CSF) or interleukin-3 (IL-3), was useful in terms of the stimulation of leukemic cell proliferation. EGCG dosage and time dependently reduced the survival of NSF60 leukemic cell lines [69, 70]. These factors can lead to an induction of cell apoptosis, including endonuclease activation, p53 induction, caspase 3 protease activation *via* a Bcl-2-insensitive pathway, free-radical production and sphinganine accumulation. Chemopreventive effects in multi-step carcinogenesis by EGCG have also been mentioned [71]. From in vitro studies, green tea and EGCG (dose 9-27 μg/ml) displayed a significant level of inhibition of the peripheral blood T-lymphocytes of adult T-lymphocytes patients, along with a moderate level of inhibition of human T-cell lymphotropic virus type I (HTLV-I)-infected T-cell line, but not of T-lymphocytes in the healthy controls. This was possibly due to a suppression of HTLV-I pX gene expression and induction of cell apoptosis [72].Consistently, Japanese HTLV-1 carriers who had taken green tea extract powder (9 capsules/day equivalent to 10 cups of regular green tea drinking) for 5 months showed a significant decrease in the HTLV-1 provirus load, suggesting that green tea drinking could inhibit the proliferation of HTLV-1-infected lymphocytes [73].

Surprisingly, EGCG diminished the phosphorylation of vascular endothelial growth factor (VEGF) receptors, potent angiogenic cytokines that are essential for the survival of tumor cells in the autocrine pathway, in chronic lymphocytic leukemia B cells that have been isolated from leukemic patients, leading to cell apoptosis [74]. EGCG decreased human telomerase reverse transcriptase (hTERT) promoter methylation and histone H_3 Lys9 acetylation, but increased hTERT repressor E_2F-1 binding at the promoter of MCF-7 breast cancers and HL60 promyelocytic leukemia cell cultures [75]. EGCG treatment induced death-associated protein kinase 2 (DAPK2) in multiple myeloma cells and dose dependently increased levels of the DAPK2 in HL60 and NB4 AML cells, while a combined treatment of EGCG (0 – 40 μM) with all-*trans* retinoic acid (ATRA) (1 μM) cooperatively induced and potentially differentiated the DAPK2 enzyme [76]. After ten patients with stage-0 chronic lymphocytic leukemia (CLL) had been orally given GTE for 6 months; eight patients showed decreases in lymphocytosis and circulating regulatory T cells (T_{reg}) numbers, while one patient revealed stable lymphocytosis with decreased T_{reg} numbers, and one patient showed increased lymphocytosis and T_{reg} numbers [77].

The results of the phase 2 clinical study demonstrated that patients with early stage CLL consumed GTE (Polyphenon E preparation, dose of 2000 mg/day, twice daily) for 6 months showed decreases in the absolute lymphocyte counts and lymphadenopathy [78].

6.3. Cardiovascular diseases

Epigenetics, hypercholesterolemia, diabetes, hypertension, heavy smoking, physical inactivity, stress and obesity are all risk factors for atherosclerosis and cardiovascular diseases (CVD). Green tea catechins have been reported to exert anti-obesity effects, including a reduction of adipocyte differentiation and proliferation; decreases in lipogenesis, fat mass, body weight, fat absorption, plasma levels of triglycerides, free fatty acids, cholesterol, glucose, insulin and leptin; and increases in β-oxidation and thermogenesis.

Yang and Koo reported that the ECG and EGCG that are present in Chinese green tea reduced lipid deposition-caused weight, as well as the cholesterol content of the liver, importantly lowered levels of serum cholesterol levels and the atherogenic index in the rats fed with a cholesterol-enriched diet [54]. Rats fed with the green tea powder (20 g/kg)-enriched diet showed a significant increase in the lag-phase oxidation of plasma with very low density in lipoproteins (VLDL) and LDL by 33% when compared to the control diet [48]. EGCG was proposed to be a competitive inhibitor of β-ketoacyl reductase of the FAS enzyme complex in the liver [79]. EGCG and ECG lowered FAS and malate enzymes in rat liver cytosol, resulting in a significant decrease in visceral fat deposition and hepatic triglyceride content [80]. Nonetheless, experiments showed that GTE lowered serum cholesterol and triglyceride concentrations in the hamsters fed with high fat diet (200 g lard and 1 g cholesterol/kg) in a concentration-dependent manner, for which the mechanism was most likely due to its influence on the absorption of dietary fat and cholesterol, but not on the inhibition of the synthesis of cholesterol or fatty acid [49]. Another study supports the evidence that Chinese green tea lowered plasma cholesterol levels by increasing fecal bile acids and cholesterol excretion, but not by inhibiting activities of three major lipid metabolizing enzymes, including 3-hydroxy-3-methylglutaryl-coenzyme A (HMG-Co A) reductase, cholesterol 7α-hydroxylase and FAS [53]. More importantly, high plasma cholesterol levels, fatty liver, renal dysfunctions and severe atherosclerotic aorta were observed in the LDL knockout mice fed with a normal diet, but not in those fed with a 4% green tea catechins-enriched diet for 35 weeks [81].

GTE, which had greater effects than oolong tea and black tea, decreased high serum triglyceride (195 vs. 119 mg/dl) and cholesterol (104 vs. 73 mg/dl) levels to normal levels, and also decreased hepatic triglyceride content in sucrose-induced hyperlipidemic rats (8.4±1.5 vs. 27.7±7.9 mg/g wet weight (p<0.05); possibly by limiting the intestinal absorption of dietary fat and storage of fat in the liver [52]. EGCG (dose of 0.5 g/kg for 4 weeks) can interfere with the micellar solubilization of dietary cholesterol in the gastrointestinal tract and subsequently reduce cholesterol absorption in the rats fed with a high cholesterol diet [50].

Green tea catechins functioned against membrane phospholipid peroxidation [82], showed a strong synergistic anti-oxidative activity with α-tocopherol in micelles [83],as well as in human LDL levels [84], and had a protective effect of high-density lipoprotein (HDL) on endothelial cell-dependent vasodilatation [85]. They have many pharmacological activities, including anti-hypertensive [41] and anti-atherosclerotic [86, 87] effects. Clearly, green tea catechins; especially EGCG, has a potential hypolipidemic effect, possibly by interfering with the emulsification, digestion, and micellar solubilization of lipids in the critical steps of intestinal absorption of dietary lipids [88]. Bursill and coworkers found that GTE (2% catechins, *w/w*) decreased the levels of total cholesterol (-60%), VLDL-and intermediate density lipoprotein (IDL)-cholesterol (-70%), LDL-cholesterol (-80%) in plasma, total cholesterol (622 versus 800 μmol/g,-10%) and unesterified cholesterol (323 versus 399 μmol/g,-15%) in the liver, and cholesterol (-25%) in the thoracic aorta (0.73 versus 0.98 μmol/g,-25%) and aortic arch fatty streak (1.93 versus 2.35 μmol/g) of the rabbits fed with a high cholesterol (0.25%, *w/w*) diet compared with the placebo group, possibly due to a decrease in cholesterol synthesis and an upregulation of hepatic LDL receptor gene expression [89, 90]. Controversial data has indicated that the consumption of high doses of green tea polyphenols (714 mg/day) for 3 weeks resulted in decreases in the total cholesterol:HDL-cholesterol ratio, but had no effects on the risk biomarkers of CVD [91].

6.4. Neurological diseases

The errors in brain iron metabolism found in neurological disorders are found to be multifactorial, however treatment conditions seem to be particularly important. Epilepsy, an oxidative related disorder of the brain, has served as a model for the investigation in the role of iron, especially NTBI in neurological disorders. The effect of antiepileptic drug treatment on changes of iron status and oxidative stress parameters were determined [92]. Recent genetic and biochemical manipulations of iron overload have placed iron at the centre of research into neurodegenerative diseases. This is supported by the discovery of genetic and non-genetic misregulations of the iron metabolism in these disorders. In many neurodegenerative disorders, abnormally high levels of iron in specific regions of the brain have been reported [93]. Evidence for iron contribution to diseases by augmentation of oxidative stress have led to an examination of the contribution of iron to other diseases, in which oxidative stress may be involved, including epilepsy [94]. It has not been possible to determine whether the accumulated iron is in the labile iron pool (LIP), which can participate in the Fenton reaction to generate the reactive hydroxyl radical. The reduction in GSH during disease progression and in response to neurotoxins, together with increased iron accumulation and ROS generation, might be taken as evidence for the presence of free iron [95].

Oxidative stress, resulting from increased brain iron levels, and possibly also from defects in antioxidant defensive mechanisms, is widely believed to be associated with neuronal death in these disorders [96, 97], along with a reduced availability of GSH and other antioxidant substances in the brain. Changes in the integrity of the blood brain barrier (BBB) due to altered vascularization of the tissue or inflammatory events could be another initial cause. However, neuronal death by any initial cause could lead to large amounts of iron release and increased ROS formation [98]. Therefore, iron and iron-induced oxidative stress could possibly be a common mechanism involved in the development of neurodegeneration [99] (Figure 3). Available data strongly support this hypothesis [100, 101]

Based on this hypothesis, therefore, therapeutic efforts should be devoted to reducing brain iron levels and inhibiting the generation of ROS. A few recent studies have shown that the iron chelator, deferrioxamine, may be a significant factor in an effective therapy for the prevention and treatment of brain disorders [102]. One possible non-toxic approach with natural metal chelators could make use of green tea catechins, especially EGCG. This compound comprising antioxidant, iron chelating and anti-inflammatory activities; has been shown to be neuroprotective in animal models of Parkinson's disease (PD) and Alzheimer's disease (AD), and also regulates the processing of amyloid precursor protein (APP) through a non-amyloidogenic pathway [103, 104]. Understanding the timing of iron mismanagement in relation to the progression of neuronal losses would provide important information on pathogenesis, and

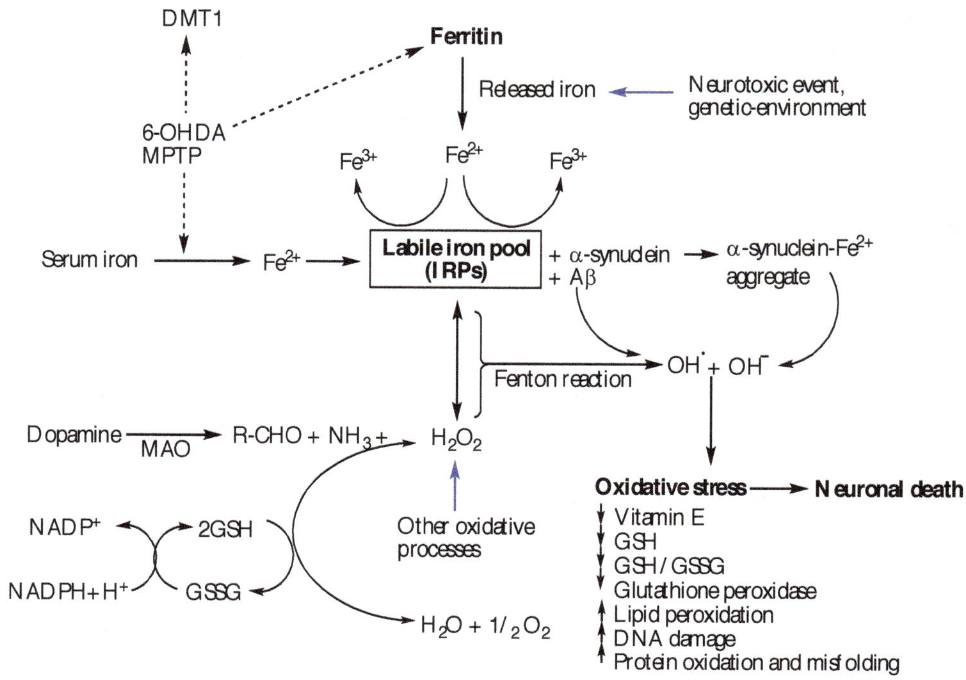

Figure 3. Mechanism of iron-induced neurodegeneration and its prevention [95]. Abbreviations: DMT1=divalent metal ion transporter-1; GSH=reduced glutathione; GSSG=oxidized glutathione; IRPs=iron regulatory proteins; MAO=monoamine oxidase; MPTP=1-methyl-4-phenyl-1,2,3,6-tetrahydropyridine;NADP+=nicotinamide adenine dinucleotide phosphate; NADPH=reduced nicotinamide adenine dinucleotide phosphate; 6-OHDA=6-hydroxydopamine

would raise the possibility of monitoring iron changes as a marker of disease progression, and perhaps even in a pre-clinical diagnosis in conditions where iron misregulation is an early event.

More *in vitro* and *in vivo* studies should be done to investigate how iron misregulation/accumulation synergizes with common endogenous and environmental toxins. Iron misregulation/accumulation alone can kill neurons only in genetic disorders where iron imbalance occurs rapidly and is extensive. However, in most cases, the amount of iron build-up is relatively low and the neurotoxic mechanism might involve a combination of iron and other toxins. Future investigations of iron in the brain, including how to best monitor iron deposition *in vivo*, the clinical relevance of excessive iron deposition, and the mechanistic relationship between iron deposition and disease pathophysiology, hold the promise of advancements in the field of neurotherapeutics.

6.5. Mutagenicity and cancinogenesis

Topical applications of green tea polyphenol fractions (such as EGCG, EGC and ECG) inhibitedbenz[a]-pyrene (BP)-and 7,12-dimethylbenz[a]-anthracene (DMBA)-initiated and 12-*O*-tetradecanoylphorbol-13-acetate (TPA)-promoted tumorigenesis of mouse skin, possibly by inhibiting ROS production, inflammation and hyperplasia [105]. Green tea catechins can counteract against tumorigenesis and DNA damage [106]. Mu and colleagues have identified an association between tea consumption and decreased cancer risk [107]. Surprisingly, EGCG in green tea exerted inhibitory effects on skin cancer, hepatocellular carcinoma and duodenal cancer, on metastasis of the melanoma cell line in lung cancer in mice, possibly by blocking the interaction of their tumor promoters with their own membrane receptors called sealing effects. Green tea significantly prevented growth of Namalwa, RAP1-EIO and HS-Sultan tumors transplanted intraperitoneally in the NOD/SCID mice; possibly by impairment of tumor invasion, anti-angiogenesis and by cell apoptosis induction [108]. EGCG decreased ornithine decarboxylase (ODC) and Ras and Jun oncogene levels, and also inhibited tyrosine kinase (TK) as well as mitogen-activated protein kinase (MAPK) activities in the transformed NIH-pATMras fibroblasts [109].

7. Conclusions

Green tea has long been considered a refreshing beverage that is prepared from tea (*Camellia sinensis*) shoots. It exerts many beneficial health effects, including anti-oxidant, anti-diabetic, hypolipidemic, anti-aging, anti-gout, neuroprotective, cardioprotective, hepatoprotective, anti-inflammatory, anti-carcinogenesis properties, among others. Variations of strain, source, geographic area, altitude, climate, cultivation, duration of fermentation and the preparation process can give rise to differences in the amounts of catechins derivatives, nutritional values, biological activities and the pharmacological properties of green tea products. EGCG is the most abundant type of catechin found in green tea and also the most relevant phytochemical displaying an influencing in several diseases and disorders. Some green tea catechins are not absorbed, while some catechins are absorbed from the intestine into the blood, and then are biologically transformed in liver microsomes by glucuronidation, sulfation and methylation reactions and ultimately excreted through the bile and urine. In this article, we have focused on the efficacy of green tea crude extract and catechins fractions, particularly EGCG in 1) depleting free radicals in normal cells, 2) removing chelatable iron from vital organs with iron overload, 3) lowering the levels of the risk factors of cardiovascular diseases, 4) inhibiting growth and proliferation of leukemic cells and solid malignant tumors, and 5) scavenging ROS and a repletion in the reducing power in neuronal tissues. The recognized benefits of green tea are that it is 1) potent in antioxidation, 2) effective in iron chelation, 3) beneficial in the inhibition of fat digestion, absorption and synthesis, 4) apoptotic induction, and 5) neuroprotection, respectively. Green tea has played a prominent role in the lives of many over time as a beverage, as a component of the diet, and now a substance that can be applied in drugs. The benefits of which have now been evidently documented.

Abbreviations

AD=Alzheimer's disease

ALT=alanine aminotransferase

AML=acute myelocytic leukemia

APP=amyloid precursor protein

ATRA=all-*trans* retinoic acid

BBB=blood brain barrier

BKO=β-globin gene knockout

BP=benz[a]-pyrene

C=catechin

CLL=chronic lymphocytic leukemia

COMT=catechol-*O*-methyltransferase

CVD=cardiovascular diseases

DAPK2=death-associated protein kinase 2

DFP=deferiprone

DH=double heterozygous β-globin gene knockout carrying human β^E gene

DMBA=7,12-dimethylbenz[a]-anthracene

DMT1=divalent metal ion transporter-1

DW=deionized water

EC=epicatechin

ECG=epicatechin 3-gallate

EGC=epigallocatechin

EGCG=epigallocatechin 3-gallate

FAS=fatty acid synthase

GA=gallic acid

GC=gallocatechin

G-CSF=granulocyte colony stimulating factor

GM-CSF=granulocyte macrophage colony stimulating factor

GSH=reduced glutathione

GSSG=oxidized glutathione

GTE=green tea extract

Hb=hemoglobin

HDL=high-density lipoprotein

HGF=hematopoietic growth factors

HMG-Co A=3-hydroxy-3-methylglutaryl-coenzyme A

hTERT=human telomerase reverse transcriptase

HTLV-I=human T-cell lymphotropic virus type I

IDL=intermediate density lipoprotein

IL-3=interleukin-3

IRPs=iron regulatory proteins

K_i=inhibition constant

LD_{50}=lethal dose at 50%

LDL=low-density lipoprotein

LIP=labile iron pool

LPI=labile plasma iron

MAO=monoamine oxidase

MAPK=mitogen-activated protein kinase

MDA=malondialdehyde

MPTP=1-methyl-4-phenyl-1,2,3,6-tetrahydropyridine

MW=molecular weight

$NAD(P)^+$=nicotinamide adenine dinucleotide phosphate

NAD(P)H=reduced nicotinamide adenine dinucleotide phosphate

ND=not determined

NQO1=NAD(P)H:quinoneoxidoreductase 1

NTBI=non-transferrin bound iron

ODC=ornithine decarboxylase

6-OHDA=6-hydroxydopamine

PD=Parkinson's disease

PPO=polyphenol oxidase

RBC=red blood cell

RNS=reactive nitrogen species

ROS=reactive oxygen species

SAM=*S*-adenosyl methionine

SULT=sulfotransferases

$T_{1/2}\beta$=beta-elimination half-lives

TEAC=trolox-equivalent antioxidant capacity

TK=tyrosine kinase

TPA=12-*O*-tetradecanoylphorbol-13-acetate

T_{reg}=regulatory T cells

UGT=uridine diphosphate-glucuronosyltransferase

V_d=distribution volume

VEGF=vascular endothelial growth factor

WT=wild-type

XO=xanthine oxidase

Acknowledgements

This work was partially supported by the Office of Higher Education Commission and Mahidol University under the National Research University Initiative, Thailand Research Fund through Professor Suthat Fucharoen, MD. and by a Research Chair Grant from the National Science and Technology Development Agency (NSTDA) and Mahidol University through Professor Suthat Fucharoen, MD.

Author details

Sakaewan Ounjaijean[1], Suthat Fucharoen[2] and Somdet Srichairatanakool[3*]

*Address all correspondence to: ssrichai@med.cmu.ac.th

1 Research Institute for Health Sciences, Chiang Mai University, Chiang Mai, Thailand

2 Thalassemia Research Center, Institute of Bioscience, Mahidol University, NakornPathom, Thailand

3 Department of Biochemistry, Faculty of Medicine, Chiang Mai University, Chiang Mai, Thailand

References

[1] Bokuchava MA, Skobeleva NI. The Biochemistry and Technology of Tea Manufacture. Critical Reviews in Food Science and Nutrition 1980;12(4) 303-70.

[2] Srichairatanakool S, Ounjaijean S, Thephinlap C, Khansuwan U, Phisalpong C, Fucharoen S. Iron-chelating and Free-radical Scavenging Activities of Microwave-processed Green Tea in Iron Overload. Hemoglobin 2006;30(2) 311-27.

[3] Balentine DA, Wiseman SA, Bouwens LC. The Chemistry of Tea Flavonoids. Critical Reviews in Food Science and Nutrition 1997;37(8) 693-704.

[4] Zuo Y, Chen H, Deng Y. Simultaneous Determination of Catechins, Caffeine and Gallic Acids in Green, Oolong, Black and Pu-erh Teas Using HPLC With a Photodiode Array Detector. Talanta 2002;57(4) 307-16.

[5] Khokhar S, Venema D, Hollman PC, Dekker M, Jongen W. A RP-HPLC Method for the Determination of Tea Catechins. Cancer Letters 1997;114(1-2) 171-2.

[6] McKay DL, Blumberg JB. The Role of Tea in Human Health: an Update. Journal of the American College of Nutrition 2002;21(1) 1-13.

[7] Cabrera C, Artacho R, Gimenez R. Beneficial Effects of Green Tea--a Review. Journal of the American College of Nutrition 2006;25(2) 79-99.

[8] Chen Z, Zhu QY, Tsang D, Huang Y. Degradation of Green Tea Catechins in Tea Drinks. Journal of Agricultural and Food Chemistry 2001;49(1) 477-82.

[9] Rababah TM, Hettiarachchy NS, Horax R. Total Phenolics and Antioxidant Activities of Fenugreek, Green Tea, Black Tea, Grape Seed, Ginger, Rosemary, Gotu Kola, and Ginkgo Extracts, Vitamin E, and Tert-butylhydroquinone. Journal of Agricultural and Food Chemistry 2004;52(16) 5183-6.

[10] Graham HN. Green Tea Composition, Consumption, and Polyphenol Chemistry. Preventive Medicine 1992;21(3) 334-50.

[11] Kuo YC, Yu CL, Liu CY, Wang SF, Pan PC, Wu MT, et al. A Population-based, Case control Study of Green Tea Consumption and Leukemia Risk in Southwestern Taiwan. Cancer Causes and Control 2009;20(1) 57-65.

[12] Milchak LM, Douglas Bricker J. The Effects of Glutathione and Vitamin E on Iron Toxicity in Isolated Rat Hepatocytes. Toxicology Letters 2002;126(3) 169-77.

[13] Sutherland BA, Rahman RM, Appleton I. Mechanisms of Action of Green Tea Catechins, With a Focus on Ischemia-induced Neurodegeneration. Journal of Nutritional Biochemistry 2006;17(5) 291-306.

[14] Frei B, Higdon JV. Antioxidant Activity of Tea Polyphenols in Vivo: Evidence From Animal Studies. Journal of Nutrition 2003;133(10) 3275S-84S.

[15] Grinberg LN, Newmark H, Kitrossky N, Rahamim E, Chevion M, Rachmilewitz EA. Protective Effects of Tea Polyphenols Against Oxidative Damage to Red Blood Cells. Biochemical Pharmacology 1997;54(9) 973-8.

[16] Morel I, Lescoat G, Cillard P, Cillard J. Role of Flavonoids and Iron Chelation in Antioxidant Action. Methods in Enzymology 1994;234 437-43.

[17] Saewong T, Ounjaijean S, Mundee Y, Pattanapanyasat K, Fucharoen S, Porter JB, et al. Effects of Green Tea on Iron Accumulation and Oxidative Stress in Livers of Iron challenged Thalassemic Mice. Medicinal Chemistry 2010;6(2) 57-64.

[18] Ounjaijean S, Thephinlap C, Khansuwan U, Phisalapong C, Fucharoen S, Porter JB, et al. Effect of Green Tea on Iron Status and Oxidative Stress in Iron-loaded Rats. Medicinal Chemistry 2008;4(4) 365-70.

[19] Thephinlap C, Ounjaijean S, Khansuwan U, Fucharoen S, Porter JB, Srichairatanakool S. Epigallocatechin-3-gallate and Epicatechin-3-gallate From Green Tea Decrease Plasma Non-transferrin Bound Iron and Erythrocyte Oxidative Stress. Medicinal Chemistry 2007;3(3) 289-96.

[20] van Acker SA, van Balen GP, van den Berg DJ, Bast A, van der Vijgh WJ. Influence of Iron Chelation on the Antioxidant Activity of Flavonoids. Biochemical Pharmacology 1998;56(8) 935-43.

[21] Kostyuk VA, Potapovich AI, Vladykovskaya EN, Korkina LG, Afanas'ev IB. Influence of Metal Ions on Flavonoid Protection Against Asbestos-induced Cell Injury. Archives of Biochemistry and Biophysics 2001;385(1) 129-37.

[22] Raza H, John A. In Vitro Protection of Reactive Oxygen Species-induced Degradation of Lipids, Proteins and 2-Deoxyribose by Tea Catechins. Food and Chemical Toxicology 2007;45(10) 1814-20.

[23] Higuchi A, Yonemitsu K, Koreeda A, Tsunenari S. Inhibitory Activity of Epigallocatechin Gallate (EGCg) in Paraquat-induced Microsomal Lipid Peroxidation--a Mechanism of Protective Effects of EGCg against Paraquat Toxicity. Toxicology 2003;183(1-3) 143-9.

[24] Salah N, Miller NJ, Paganga G, Tijburg L, Bolwell GP, Rice-Evans C. Polyphenolic flavanols as Scavengers of Aqueous Phase Radicals and As Chain-breaking Antioxidants. Archives of Biochemistry and Biophysics 1995;322(2) 339-46.

[25] Samman S, Sandstrom B, Toft MB, Bukhave K, Jensen M, Sorensen SS, et al. Green Tea or Rosemary Extract Added to Foods Reduces Nonheme-iron Absorption. American Journal of Clinical Nutrition 2001;73(3) 607-12.

[26] Guo Q, Zhao B, Li M, Shen S, Xin W. Studies on Protective Mechanisms of Four Components of Green Tea Polyphenols Against Lipid Peroxidation in Synaptosomes. Biochimica et Biophysica Acta 1996;1304(3) 210-22.

[27] Valcic S, Burr JA, Timmermann BN, Liebler DC. Antioxidant Chemistry of Green Tea Catechins. New Oxidation Products of (-)-Epigallocatechin Gallate and (-)-Epigallocatechin From Their Reactions With Peroxyl Radicals. Chemical Research in Toxicology 2000;13(9) 801-10.

[28] Chen L, Lee MJ, Li H, Yang CS. Absorption, Distribution, Elimination of Tea Polyphenols in Rats. Drug Metabolism and Disposition 1997 Sep;25(9) 1045-50.

[29] Scalbert A, Williamson G. Dietary Intake and Bioavailability of Polyphenols. Journal of Nutrition 2000;130(8S Suppl) 2073S-85S.

[30] Loktionov A, Bingham SA, Vorster H, Jerling JC, Runswick SA, Cummings JH. Apolipoprotein E Genotype Modulates the Effect of Black Tea Drinking on Blood Lipids and Blood Coagulation Factors: a Pilot Study. British Journal of Nutrition 1998;79(2) 133-9.

[31] Kim S, Lee MJ, Hong J, Li C, Smith TJ, Yang GY, et al. Plasma and Tissue Levels of Tea Catechins in Rats and Mice During Chronic Consumption of Green Tea Polyphenols. Nutrition and Cancer 2000;37(1) 41-8.

[32] Vaidyanathan JB, Walle T. Glucuronidation and Sulfation of the Tea Flavonoid (-)-Epicatechin by the Human and Rat Enzymes. Drug Metabolism and Disposition 2002;30(8) 897-903.

[33] Nishimuta H, Ohtani H, Tsujimoto M, Ogura K, Hiratsuka A, Sawada Y. Inhibitory Effects of Various Beverages on Human Recombinant Sulfotransferase Isoforms SULT1A1 and SULT1A3. Biopharmaceutics & Drug Disposition 2007;28(9) 491-500.

[34] Lu H, Meng X, Li C, Sang S, Patten C, Sheng S, et al. Glucuronides of Tea Catechins: Enzymology of Biosynthesis and Biological Activities. Drug Metabolism and Disposition 2003;31(4) 452-61.

[35] Crespy V, Nancoz N, Oliveira M, Hau J, Courtet-Compondu MC, Williamson G. Glucuronidation of the Green Tea Catechins, (-)-Epigallocatechin-3-gallate and (-)-Epicatechin-3-gallate, by Rat Hepatic and Intestinal Microsomes. Free Radical Research 2004;38(9) 1025-31.

[36] Galati G, Lin A, Sultan AM, O'Brien PJ. Cellular and in Vivo Hepatotoxicity Caused by Green Tea Phenolic Acids and Catechins. Free Radical Biology and Medicine 2006;40(4) 570-80.

[37] Mulder TP, Rietveld AG, van Amelsvoort JM. Consumption of Both Black Tea and Green Tea Results in an Increase in the Excretion of Hippuric Acid into Urine. American Journal of Clinical Nutrition 2005;81(1 Suppl) 256S-60S.

[38] Okushio K, Matsumoto N, Kohri T, Suzuki M, Nanjo F, Hara Y. Absorption of Tea Catechins into Rat Portal Vein. Biological and Pharmaceutical Bulletin 1996;19(2) 326-9.

[39] Lambert JD, Lee MJ, Lu H, Meng X, Hong JJ, Seril DN, et al. Epigallocatechin-3-gallate is Absorbed but Extensively Glucuronidated Following Oral Administration to Mice. Journal of Nutrition 2003;133(12) 4172-7.

[40] Zhang A, Zhu QY, Luk YS, Ho KY, Fung KP, Chen ZY. Inhibitory Effects of Jasmine Green Tea Epicatechin Isomers on Free Radical-induced Lysis of Red Blood Cells. Life Sciences 1997;61(4) 383-94.

[41] Henry JP, Stephens-Larson P. Reduction of Chronic Psychosocial Hypertension in Mice by Decaffeinated Tea. Hypertension. 1984;6(3) 437-44.

[42] Hertog MG, Feskens EJ, Hollman PC, Katan MB, Kromhout D. Dietary Antioxidant Flavonoids and Risk of Coronary Heart Disease: the Zutphen Elderly Study. Lancet 1993;342(8878) 1007-11.

[43] Cutter H, Wu LY, Kim C, Morre DJ, Morre DM. Is The Cancer Protective Effect Correlated with Growth Inhibitions by Green tea (-)-Epigallocatechin Gallate Mediated Through an Antioxidant Mechanism? Cancer Letters 2001;162(2) 149-54.

[44] Shi ST, Wang ZY, Smith TJ, Hong JY, Chen WF, Ho CT, et al. Effects of Green Tea and Black Tea on 4-(Methylnitrosamino)-1-(3-pyridyl)-1-butanone Bioactivation, DNA Methylation, and Lung Tumorigenesis in A/J mice. Cancer Research 1994;54(17) 4641-7.

[45] Wang ZY, Huang MT, Lou YR, Xie JG, Reuhl KR, Newmark HL, et al. Inhibitory Effects of Black Tea, Green Tea, Decaffeinated Black Tea, and Decaffeinated Green Tea on Ultraviolet B Light-induced Skin Carcinogenesis in 7,12-Dimethylbenz[a]anthracene-initiated SKH-1 Mice. Cancer Research 1994;54(13) 3428-35.

[46] Imai K, Nakachi K. Cross Sectional Study of Effects of Drinking Green Tea on Cardiovascular and Liver Diseases. British Medical Journal 1995;310(6981) 693-6.

[47] Kono S, Shinchi K, Ikeda N, Yanai F, Imanishi K. Green Tea Consumption and Serum Lipid Profiles: a Cross-sectional Study in Northern Kyushu, Japan. Preventive Medicine 1992;21(4) 526-31.

[48] Anderson JW, Diwadkar VA, Bridges SR. Selective Effects of Different Antioxidants on Oxidation of Lipoproteins from Rats. Proceedings of the Society for Experimental Biology and Medicine 1998;218(4) 376-81.

[49] Chan PT, Fong WP, Cheung YL, Huang Y, Ho WK, Chen ZY. Jasmine Green Tea Epicatechins are Hypolipidemic in Hamsters (Mesocricetus auratus) Fed a High Fat Diet. Journal of Nutrition 1999;129(6) 1094-101.

[50] Raederstorff DG, Schlachter MF, Elste V, Weber P. Effect of EGCG on Lipid Absorption and Plasma Lipid Levels in Rats. Journal of Nutritional Biochemistry 2003;14(6) 326-32.

[51] Skrzydlewska E, Ostrowska J, Farbiszewski R, Michalak K. Protective Effect of Green Tea Against Lipid Peroxidation in the Rat Liver, Blood Serum and the Brain. Phytomedicine 2002;9(3) 232-8.

[52] Yang M, Wang C, Chen H. Green, Oolong and Black Tea Extracts Modulate Lipid Metabolism in Hyperlipidemia Rats Fed High-sucrose Diet. Journal of Nutritional Biochemistry 2001;12(1) 14-20.

[53] Yang TT, Koo MW. Chinese Green Tea Lowers Cholesterol Level Through an Increase in Fecal Lipid Excretion. Life Science 2000;66(5) 411-23.

[54] Yang TT, Koo MW. Hypocholesterolemic Effects of Chinese Tea. Pharmacological Research 1997;35(6) 505-12.

[55] Lam le H, Sakaguchi K, Ukeda H, Sawamura M. Flow Injection Determination of Xanthine Oxidase Inhibitory Activity and Its Application to Food Samples. Analytical Sciences 2006;22(1) 105-9.

[56] Aucamp J, Gaspar A, Hara Y, Apostolides Z. Inhibition of Xanthine Oxidase by Catechins From Tea (Camellia sinensis). Anticancer Research 1997;17(6D) 4381-5.

[57] Ozyurek M, Bektasoglu B, Guclu K, Apak R. Measurement of Xanthine Oxidase Inhibition Activity of Phenolics and Flavonoids With a Modified Cupric Reducing Antioxidant Capacity (CUPRAC) Method. Analytica Chimica Acta 2009;636(1) 42-50.

[58] Lin JK, Chen PC, Ho CT, Lin-Shiau SY. Inhibition of Xanthine Oxidase and Suppression of Intracellular Reactive Oxygen Species in HL-60 Cells by Theaflavin-3,3'-digallate, (-)-Epigallocatechin-3-gallate, and Propyl Gallate. Journal of Agricultural and Food Chemistry 2000;48(7) 2736-43.

[59] Kimura M, Umegaki K, Kasuya Y, Sugisawa A, Higuchi M. The Relation Between Single/double or Repeated Tea Catechin Ingestions and Plasma Antioxidant Activity in Humans. European Journal of Clinical Nutrition 2002;56(12) 1186-93.

[60] Gomikawa S, Ishikawa Y, Hayase W, Haratake Y, Hirano N, Matuura H, et al. Effect of Ground Green Tea Drinking for 2 Weeks on the Susceptibility of Plasma and LDL to the Oxidation ex Vivo in Healthy Volunteers. Kobe journal of medical sciences 2008;54(1) E62-72.

[61] Sone T, Kuriyama S, Nakaya N, Hozawa A, Shimazu T, Nomura K, et al. Randomized Controlled Trial For an Fffect of Catechin-enriched Green Tea Consumption on Adiponectin and Cardiovascular Disease Risk Factors. Food and Nutrition Research 2011;55. doi: 10.3402/fnr.v55i0.8326.

[62] Fraga CG, Oteiza PI. Iron Toxicity and Antioxidant Nutrients. Toxicology 2002;180(1)23-32.

[63] Galleano M, Puntarulo S. Dietary Alpha-tocopherol Supplementation on Antioxidant Defenses After in Vivo Iron Overload in Rats. Toxicology 1997;124(1) 73-81.

[64] Tesoriere L, D'Arpa D, Butera D, Allegra M, Renda D, Maggio A, et al. Oral Supplements of Vitamin E Improve Measures of Oxidative Stress in Plasma and Reduce Oxidative Damage to LDL and Erythrocytes in Beta-thalassemia Intermedia Patients. Free Radical Research 2001;34(5) 529-40.

[65] Rachmilewitz EA, Weizer-Stern O, Adamsky K, Amariglio N, Rechavi G, Breda L, et al. Role of Iron in Inducing Oxidative Stress in Thalassemia: Can It Be Prevented by Inhibition of Absorption and by Antioxidants? Annals of the New York Academy of Sciences 2005;1054 118-23.

[66] Buettner GR, Jurkiewicz BA. Catalytic Metals, Ascorbate and Free Radicals: Combinations to Avoid. Radiation Research 1996;145(5) 532-41.

[67] Herbert V, Shaw S, Jayatilleke E. Vitamin C-driven Free Radical Generation from Iron. Journal of Nutrition 1996;126(4 Suppl) 1213S-20S.

[68] Rund D, Rachmilewitz E. Beta-thalassemia. The New England Journal of Medicine 2005;353(11) 1135-46.

[69] Otsuka T, Ogo T, Eto T, Asano Y, Suganuma M, Niho Y. Growth Inhibition of Leukemic Cells by (-)-Epigallocatechin Gallate, the Main Constituent of Green Tea. Life Sciences 1998;63(16) 1397-403.

[70] Asano Y, Okamura S, Ogo T, Eto T, Otsuka T, Niho Y. Effect of (-)-Epigallocatechin Gallate on Leukemic Blast Cells from Patients With Acute Myeloblastic Leukemia. Life Sciences 1997;60(2) 135-42.

[71] Surh Y. Molecular Mechanisms of Chemopreventive Effects of Selected Dietary and Medicinal Phenolic Substances. Mutation Research 1999;428(1-2) 305-27.

[72] Li HC, Yashiki S, Sonoda J, Lou H, Ghosh SK, Byrnes JJ, et al. Green Tea Polyphenols Induce Apoptosis in Vitro in Peripheral Blood T Lymphocytes of Adult T-Cell Leukemia Patients. Japanese Journal of Cancer Research 2000;91(1) 34-40.

[73] Sonoda J, Koriyama C, Yamamoto S, Kozako T, Li HC, Lema C, et al. HTLV-1 Provirus Load in Peripheral Blood Lymphocytes of HTLV-1 Carriers is Diminished by Green Tea Drinking. Cancer Science 2004;95(7) 596-601.

[74] Beliveau R, Gingras D. Green tea: Prevention and Treatment of Cancer by Nutraceuticals. Lancet 2004;364(9439) 1021-2.

[75] Berletch JB, Liu C, Love WK, Andrews LG, Katiyar SK, Tollefsbol TO. Epigenetic and Genetic Mechanisms Contribute to Telomerase Inhibition by EGCG. Journal of Cellular Biochemistry 2008;103(2) 509-19.

[76] Britschgi A, Simon HU, Tobler A, Fey MF, Tschan MP. Epigallocatechin-3-gallate Induces Cell Death in Acute Myeloid Leukaemia Cells and Supports All-trans Retinoic Acid-induced Neutrophil Differentiation via Death-associated Protein Kinase 2. British Journal of Haematology 2010;149(1) 55-64.

[77] D'Arena G, Simeon V, De Martino L, Statuto T, D'Auria F, Volpe S, et al. Regulatory T-cell Modulation by Green Tea in Chronic Lymphocytic Leukemia. International Journal of Immunopathology and Pharmacology 2013;26(1) 117-25.

[78] Shanafelt TD, Call TG, Zent CS, Leis JF, LaPlant B, Bowen DA, et al. Phase 2 Trial of Daily, Oral Polyphenon E in Patients With Asymptomatic, Rai Stage 0 to II Chronic Lymphocytic Leukemia. Cancer 2012;119(2) 363-70.

[79] Wang X, Tian W. Green Tea Epigallocatechin Gallate: a Natural Inhibitor of Fatty acid Synthase. Biochemical and Biophysical Research Communications 2001;288(5) 1200-6.

[80] Ikeda I, Hamamoto R, Uzu K, Imaizumi K, Nagao K, Yanagita T, et al. Dietary Gallate Esters of Tea Catechins Reduce Deposition of Visceral Fat, Hepatic Triacylglycerol, and Activities of Hepatic Enzymes Related to Fatty Acid Synthesis in Rats. Bioscience, Biotechnology, and Biochemistry 2005;69(5) 1049-53.

[81] Suzuki J, Ogawa M, Izawa A, Sagesaka YM, Isobe M. Dietary Consumption of Green Tea Catechins Attenuate Hyperlipidaemia-induced Atherosclerosis and Systemic Organ Damage in Mice. Acta Cardiologica 2005;60(3) 271-6.

[82] Kondo K, Kurihara M, Miyata N, Suzuki T, Toyoda M. Scavenging Mechanisms of (-)-Epigallocatechin Gallate and (-)-Epicatechin Gallate on Peroxyl Radicals and Formation of Superoxide During the Inhibitory Action. Free Radical Biology and Medicine 1999;27(7-8) 855-63.

[83] Zhou B, Wu LM, Yang L, Liu ZL. Evidence for Alpha-tocopherol Regeneration Reaction of Green Tea Polyphenols in SDS Micelles. Free Radical Biology and Medicine 2005;38(1) 78-84.

[84] Liu Z, Ma LP, Zhou B, Yang L, Liu ZL. Antioxidative Effects of Green Tea Polyphenols on Free Radical Initiated and Photosensitized Peroxidation of Human Low Density Lipoprotein. Chemistry and Physics of Lipids;106(1) 53-63.

[85] Li XP, Zhao SP, Zhang XY, Liu L, Gao M, Zhou QC. Protective Effect of High Density Lipoprotein on Endothelium-dependent Vasodilatation. International Journal of Cardiology 2000;73(3) 231-6.

[86] Geleijnse JM, Launer LJ, Hofman A, Pols HA, Witteman JC. Tea Flavonoids May Protect Against Atherosclerosis: the Rotterdam Study. Archives of Internal Medicine 1999;159(18) 2170-4.

[87] Vinson JA, Teufel K, Wu N. Green and Black Teas Inhibit Atherosclerosis by Lipid, Antioxidant, and Fibrinolytic Mechanisms. Journal of Agricultural and Food Chemistry 2004;52(11) 3661-5.

[88] Koo SI, Noh SK. Green Tea as Inhibitor of the Intestinal Absorption of Lipids: Potential Mechanism for Its Lipid-lowering Effect. Journal of Nutritional Biochemistry 2007;18(3) 179-83.

[89] Bursill CA, Abbey M, Roach PD. A Green Tea Extract Lowers Plasma Cholesterol by Inhibiting Cholesterol Synthesis and Upregulating the LDL Receptor in the Cholesterol-fed Rabbit. Atherosclerosis 2007;193(1) 86-93.

[90] Bursill CA, Roach PD. A Green Tea Catechin Extract Upregulates the Hepatic Low-Density Lipoprotein Receptor in Rats. Lipids 2007;42(7) 621-7.

[91] Frank J, George TW, Lodge JK, Rodriguez-Mateos AM, Spencer JP, Minihane AM, et al. Daily Consumption of an Aqueous Green Tea Extract Supplement Does Not Impair Liver Function or Alter Cardiovascular Disease Risk Biomarkers in Healthy Men. Journal of Nutrition 2009;139(1) 58-62.

[92] Ounjaijean S, Westermarck T, Partinen M, Plonka-Poltorak E, Kaipainen P, Kaski M, et al. Increase in Non-transferrin Bound Iron and the Oxidative Stress Status in Epilepsy Patients Treated Using Valproic Acid Monotherapy. International Journal of Clinical Pharmacology and Therapeutics 2011;49(4) 268-76.

[93] Snyder AM, Connor JR. Iron, the Substantia Nigra and Related Neurological Disorders. Biochimica et Biophysica Acta. 2009;1790(7) 606-14.

[94] Thompson KJ, Shoham S, Connor JR. Iron and Neurodegenerative Disorders. Brain Research Bulletin 2001;55(2) 155-64.

[95] Zecca L, Youdim MB, Riederer P, Connor JR, Crichton RR. Iron, Brain Ageing and Neurodegenerative Disorders. Nature Reviews Neuroscience 2004;5(11) 863-73.

[96] Andrews NC. Iron Homeostasis: Insights from Genetics and Animal Models. Nature Reviews Genetics 2000;1(3) 208-17.

[97] Halliwell B. Role of Free Radicals in the Neurodegenerative Diseases: Therapeutic Implications for Antioxidant Treatment. Drugs and Aging 2001;18(9) 685-716.

[98] Andersen JK. Oxidative Stress in Neurodegeneration: Cause or Consequence? Nature Medicine 2004;10 Suppl S18-25.

[99] Ke Y, Qian ZM. Brain Iron Metabolism: Neurobiology and Neurochemistry. Progress in Neurobiology 2007;83(3) 149-73.

[100] Youdim MB, Stephenson G, Ben Shachar D. Ironing Iron Out in Parkinson's Disease and Other Neurodegenerative Diseases With Iron Chelators: a Lesson From 6-Hydroxydopamine and Iron Chelators, Desferal and VK-28. Annals of the New York Academy of Sciences 2004;1012 306-25.

[101] Richardson DR. Novel Chelators for Central Nervous System Disorders That Involve Alterations in the Metabolism of Iron and Other Metal Ions. Annals of the New York Academy of Sciences 2004;1012 326-41.

[102] Liu G, Men P, Perry G, Smith MA. Nanoparticle and Iron Chelators As a Potential Novel Alzheimer Therapy. Methods in Molecular Biology 2010;610 123-44.

[103] Mandel SA, Amit T, Weinreb O, Reznichenko L, Youdim MB. Simultaneous Manipulation of Multiple Brain Targets by Green Tea Catechins: a Potential Neuroprotective Strategy for Alzheimer and Parkinson Diseases. CNS Neuroscience and Therapeutics 2008;14(4) 352-65.

[104] Mandel S, Amit T, Reznichenko L, Weinreb O, Youdim MB. Green Tea Catechins as Brain-permeable, Natural Iron Chelators-antioxidants For the Treatment of Neurodegenerative Disorders. Molecular Nutrtion and Food Research 2006;50(2) 229-34.

[105] Huang MT, Ho CT, Wang ZY, Ferraro T, Finnegan-Olive T, Lou YR, et al. Inhibitory Effect of Topical Application of a Green Tea Polyphenol Fraction on Tumor Initiation and Promotion in Mouse Skin. Carcinogenesis 1992;13(6) 947-54.

[106] Anderson RF, Fisher LJ, Hara Y, Harris T, Mak WB, Melton LD, et al. Green Tea Catechins Partially Protect DNA From (.)OH Radical-induced Strand Breaks and Base Damage Through Fast Chemical Repair of DNA Radicals. Carcinogenesis 2001;22(8) 1189-93.

[107] Mu LN, Zhou XF, Ding BG, Wang RH, Zhang ZF, Chen CW, et al. [A Case-control Study on Drinking Green Tea and Decreasing Risk of Cancers in the Alimentary Canal Among Cigarette Smokers and Alcohol Drinkers]. Zhonghua Liu Xing Bing Xue Za Zhi 2003;24(3) 192-5.

[108] Bertolini F, Fusetti L, Rabascio C, Cinieri S, Martinelli G, Pruneri G. Inhibition of Angiogenesis and Induction of Endothelial and Tumor Cell Apoptosis by Green Tea in Animal Models of Human High-grade Non-Hodgkin's Lymphoma. Leukemia 2000;14(8) 1477-82.

[109] Wang YC, Bachrach U. The Specific Anti-cancer Activity of Green Tea (-)-Epigallocatechin-3-gallate (EGCG). Amino Acids 2002;22(2) 131-43.

13

Impact of CoQ_{10}, L-Carnitine and Cocktail Antioxidants on Oxidative Stress Markers in HIV Patients

M Sauka, G Selga, A Skesters, A Silova, T Westermarck, A Latvus and F Atroshi

1. Introduction

Nutritional deficiencies have long been recognized as an important problem among HIV-1-seropositive individuals. They have a great demand for nutrients because of the stress placed on their immune systems. Moreover, poor nutrition may also affect drug effectiveness or increased toxicity [34-37]. It has been shown that micronutrient deficiencies are associated with more rapid HIV-disease progression and higher HIV-1 related mortality [38-40]. Supplementation of micronutrient has delayed time to AIDS and improved survival, suggesting that supplementation could offer a simple and relatively inexpensive strategy to slow HIV-1 progression [41, 42].

HIV infected patients present changes in components of the antioxidant defense system, which may be the result of excessive production of oxygen-derived species during the development of the disease (Pace and Leaf, 1995) and that cells infected with HIV can enhance production of $O_2^{\bullet-}$ [43]. This phenomenon combined with a deficiency in key antioxidant enzymes superoxide dismutase and catalase, and a decreased concentrations of the antioxidant vitamins [44] may lead to severe oxidative stress in HIV-infected patients. Humans infected with human immunodeficiency virus (HIV) have been shown to be under chronic oxidative stress [44-46], which is the result of imbalance between free radical (or pro-oxidant) production and antioxidant action. In HIV infection, oxidative stress may be caused by both overproduction of reactive oxygen species (ROS) and a simultaneous deficiency of antioxidant defenses [47, 48]. Oxidative stress induced by ROS play a critical role in the stimulation of HIV replication and the development of immunodeficiency [49, 50].

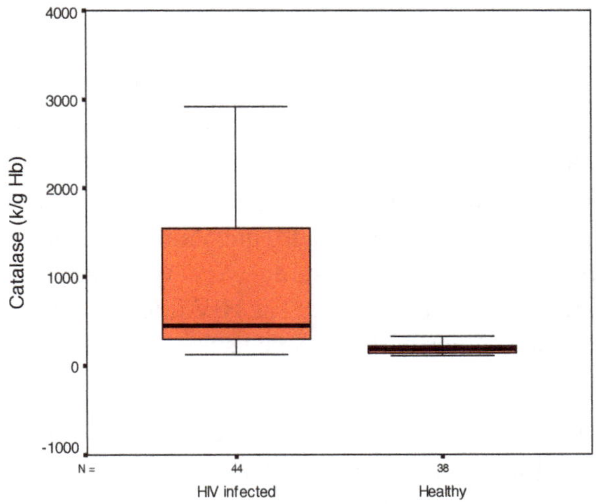

Figure 1. Catalase level of HIV infected individuals and healthy subjects (k/g Hb)Catalase level of

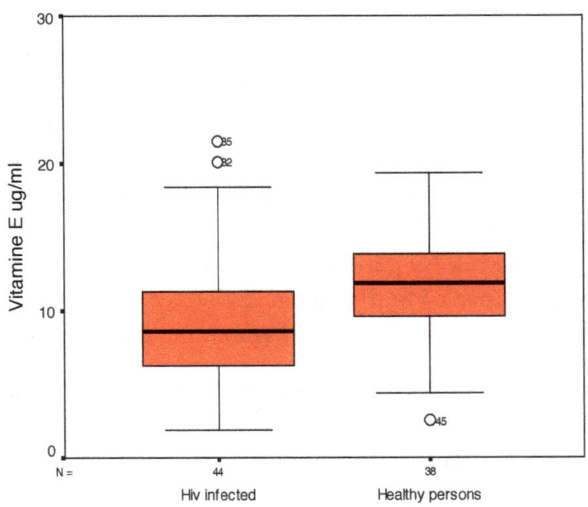

Figure 2. Vitamin E level of HIV infected individuals and healthy subjects (μg /ml)

Many studies have focused on the role of nutritional supplements to attenuate signs and symptoms of HIV. Of these, some have reported favorable results, while many others have reported no benefit of the selected nutrient. Despite these mixed findings, recommendations for the use of nutritional supplements for the purposes of attenuating HIV are rampant. Based on this background, we have assessed the antioxidant status among HIV-infected patients on oxidative stress after antioxidant supplementation.

2. Subjects and methods

2.1. Subjects

Open clinical trial study was implemented to access antioxidant status among HIV-infected male volunteers in Latvia. Twenty six HIV-positive males (age 35.3 ± 2.5) whose serostatus are known were studied. They were recruited among two non-governmental HIV infected patients' support organizations by "snow-ball" methodology using gatekeepers as contact persons. All participants in the research study were volunteers and their agreement to participate was get through their gatekeepers. The HIV-infected subjects represented a broad range of disease progression. None of the screened subjects had (CD4) T cell counts less than $200x10^9/L$.

Exclusion criteria for the study groups were as follows: they were over 18 years old, have not used antioxidants as food supplement two months before the study, had no active opportunistic infections or malignancies, had readily mobile, and were no drug users. Any information of partner identifications was not used in the written information

For the control group 10 uninfected males were selected among uninfected friends and relatives of HIV-infected individuals. Control subjects had no acute or chronic illness and were not taking any medications or nutritional supplements.

HIV-infected individuals used food supplements– antioxidant cocktail for 6 month, including 250 mg L-carnitine (Bio-Carnitine$^{TM)}$, 800 µg vitamin A, 15 mg vitamin E, 90 mg vitamin C, 2 mg vitamin B_6, 15 mg Zn, 100 mg CoQ_{10} and 75 µg selenium (organic) (Bio-Selenium^{TM+}Zn) a day. All subjects underwent an initial screening and after 6 months that included an anthropometric (weight and height) and biochemical (complete blood count, bilirubin, albumin, from liver panel-alanine aminotranferase (ALT) and alkaline aminotranferase (), from lipid profile total holesterol and triglicerides. All patients were evaluated with regard to the blood antioxidant system, specifically superoxide dismutase (SOD), catalase (CAT) selenium-dependent glutathione peroxidase (GSH-Px, trace element selenium, and α-tocopherol).

Participants will be involved in the study only after obtaining informed consent. The study protocol was approved by the ethics committee of the Latvian Institute of Cardiology for Clinical and Physiological Research, Drug and Pharmaceutics Product Clinical Investigation.

2.2. Laboratory analysis

After overnight fasting, venous blood samples were collected from all study subjects. Biochemical determinations were done at the hospital laboratory. CD4+and CD8+cell count was estimated by FACSscan flowcytometry (BD Becton Dickimon). Alanine aminotranferase (ALT) and alkaline aminotranferase were estimated by kinetic reaction (Hitachi 917, Roche Diagnostics), bilirubin, albumin and total protein by two point colour reaction (Hitachi 917, Roche Diagnostics). From lipid profile total holesterol and triglycerides were estimated by using fermentative colour reaction (Hitachi 917, Roche Diagnostics). Blood antioxidant system was evaluated at Riga Stradinš University laboratory. Selenium and α-Tocophrol concentrations in plasma were measured using fluorometric method. Other measurements were also included such as catalase and GSHPX.

2.3. Statistical analyses

Using the SPSS 14.0 for Windows software standard version, statistical analyses were performed. All group data are expressed as means ± SEMs. The HIV-positive group was compared with the seronegative control subjects by using one way ANOVA. The minimal level of significance was identified at $P < 0.05$. All patients were evaluated with regard to the blood antioxidant system, specifically superoxide dismutase (SOD) and glutathione peroxidase.

3. Results

Subject characteristics, including CD4+cell count, CD8+cell count, and CD4/CD8 ratio, weight, body mass index (BMI, in kg/m^2), are shown in Table 1. At initial screening HIV-infected subjects were significantly lower weight and BMI compared to healthy subjects. There were insignificant changes between initial screening and after 6 months. The range of CD4+cell counts was broad, from 282 to 1830 x 10^6 cells/L at the initial screening and from 323 to 1687 after 6 months CD4/CD6 ratio was from 0.1 to 1.7 at the initial screening and from 0.1 to 3.4 after 6 months of using food supplements, CD8+cell counts was from 272 to 4525 at the initial screening and from 222 to 4851 after 6 months.

		Baseline		After 6 months	
		n	Mean±SE	n	Mean±SE
Weight	HIV-infected	26	73.1±2.1	13	74.7±2.8
	healthy uninfected	10	82.4±2.6	9	83.3±2.7
			p<0.05		p<0.05
BMI	HIV-infected	26	22.5±0.6	13	23.0±0.8
	Healthy	10	24.7±0.7	9	25.1±0.7
			p<0.05		NS
CD4+	HIV-infected	25	698.4±74.3	21	743.6±87.4
CD8+	HIV-infected	25	1641.9±188.1	21	1341.0±216.1
CD4+/CD8	HIV-infected	25	0.6±0.1	21	0.9±0.2

Table 1. Effect of antioxidant supplementation on body weight, body mass index and immune function in HIV patients.

Antioxidant status is shown in Table 2. At the baseline HIV-positive patients had significantly lower GSHPX and CAT concentrations compare to healthy subjects (p<0.05), but did not differ after 6 months using food supplements. There were insignificant differences in SOD and MDA measurements and α-Tocopherol concentration at the initial screening, but differed significantly after 6 months compare to HIV-infected and healthy individuals. Changes of biochemical measurements (alanine aminotranferase, alkaline aminotranferase, bilirubin, albumin and total protein, total holesterol and triglicerides) were not significant between groups of HIV-infected and healthy individuals as well as at the initial screening and after 6 months after use of food supplements. Additionally, two HIV-infected individuals from 26 involved in the study reported that after the use of antioxidant cocktail, gingival bleeding was stopped. One reported this symptom for two years before the study and one reports half a year this problem before study.

Measuremetns	groups	Baseline		After 6 months		
		n	Mean±SE	n	Mean±SE	p
GSHPX	infected	25	46.5±1.1	19	45.6±1.3	NS
	healthy	10	50.9±1.6	9	49.5±0.7	NS
	p		0.036		NS	
CAT	infected	26	1023.5±164.1	19	350.3±22.3	0.01
	healthy	10	317.4±34.6	9	377.7±13.1	NS
			0.013		NS	
SOD	infected	25	1074±68.3	19	1419.3±56.6	0.001
	healthy	10	1293.7±36.6	9	1172.8±30.4	0.023
			NS		0.008	
TAS	infected	24	1.0±0.0	17	1.5±0.0	0.001
	healthy	10	1.4±0.0	9	1.4±0.0	NS
			NS		NS	
VITE	infected	26	10.8±0.8	19	13.2±1.2	NS
	healthy	10	9.2±1.0	9	7.4±0.1	NS
			NS		0.003	
SE	infected	25	47.4	21	64.0±3.7	0.000
	healthy	10	51±3.0	9	53.9±3.1	NS
			NS		NS	
MDA	infected	24	3.5±0.1	17	5.1±0.3	0.000
	healthy	10	3.4±0.2	9	3.4±0.2	NS
			NS		0.000	

Table 2. Effect of antioxidants supplementation on antioxidant enzymes, selenium, vitamin E and lipid peroxidation in HIV patients.

4. Discussion

There has been increasing interest in the application of antioxidants to many diseases as information is constantly gathered linking the development of HIV to oxidative stress [51]. Antioxidants are believed to function interactively and synergistically to neutralize reactive oxygen species (ROS). Reactive oxygen species include molecules like hydrogen peroxide; ions like the hypochlorite ion; radicals like the hydroxyl radical; and the superoxide anion, which are an ion and a radical.

All subjects from the current study are at low serum selenium level (which is about 80 – 120 μg /L in Europe), and stayed as that even after use of antioxidants supplements, including selenium. Similar trend was also notice in the selenoenzyme glutathione peroxidase (GSHPx) level among HIV patients. Low serum selenium was defined as a serum level ≤ 85 μg/l [52]. Selenium deficiency, more than any other nutrient, has been documented to correlate with progression and mortality of HIV [53]. Selenium is needed for the proper functioning of the immune system, and appears to be a key nutrient in counteracting the development of virulence and inhibiting HIV progression to AIDS [54]. When taken as a supplement, selenium modulates the cellular response to oxidative stress, inducing a faster restoration of the endogenous antioxidative defence system against the production of reactive oxygen species [55]. Glutathion peroxidase controls the interacellular level of hydrogen peroxide, reducing the formation of reactive oxygen species that can induce lipid peroxidations with consequent damage to the cellular membranes [56].

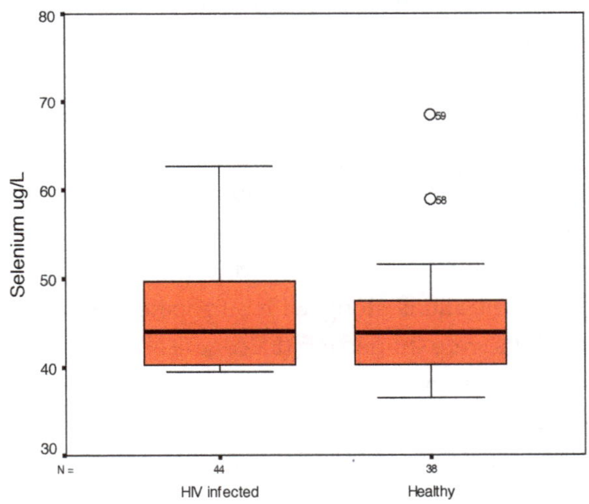

Figure 3. Selenium level of HIV infected individuals and healthy subjects (μ/g Hb)

The loss of CD4 T lymphocytes is a central factor in the progression of HIV infection to AIDS. The key role of these cells in regulating and amplifying the immune response means that any decline in their number results in deficits in both humoral and cell-mediated immunity [57]. Both the CD4 percentage and the CD4:CD8 ratio are also affected by changes in the number of CD8 cells, which tends to rise through the course of HIV infection [58].This study demonstrates that after supplementation, there is an increase in CD4 T cells in HIV patients. Several research studies have indicated that the apoptosis of CD4 cells contributing to HIV progression does not result solely from HIV infection, but largely from antioxidant imbalances in the host [43, 59, 60]. Activation of latent HIV state can be stimulated in the presence of reactive oxygen species (ROS) through the stimulation of oxygen-responsive transcription factors, specifically NF-kB, which induces HIV replication in the infected T-lymphocyte.

The mean serum malondialdehyde (MDA) concentrations in this study were significantly elevated in HIV infected patients. Serum concentration of total serum antioxidant status (TAS) was increased after supplementation. Our data indicate that severe oxidative stress occurs in the serum of HIV patients in comparison with controls ones and the inclusion of antioxidants in the therapeutic approach in managing HIV patients may prevent the additional free radicals damage. It has been shown that cells infected with the HIV undergo a significant amplification of O_2^- generation. This phenomenon combined with a deficiency in key antioxidant enzymes (SOD and CAT) and a decreased concentration of the antioxidant vitamins, may lead to severe oxidative stress in HIV-infected patients. Consequently these conditions may in turn be responsible for the DNA base modifications observed in this study [43]. Serum MDA adducts also tended to correlate inversely with expression of CD127 on T cells was shown [61]. Study in placenta, umbilical cord blood and infant blood in HIV/ART-exposed infants compared with uninfected controls [62] showed that placental mitochondria malondialdehyde (MDA) concentrations and mtDNA content in placenta and cord blood were similar between groups. Supplementation with antioxidant vitamins prevents oxidative modification of DNA in lymphocytes of HIV-infected patients [44]. Furthermore, as an antioxidant, vitamin E [63]and atherosclerotic lesions contain oxidized lipids [64], therefore, supplementation with vitamin E would decrease heart disease risk. It has been reported that α-tocopherol concentrations in serum are regulated by the α-tocopherol transfer protein and are dependent on serum lipid concentrations because α-tocopherol is non-specifically transported by lipoproteins [63]. Serum micronutrient concentrations along with surrogate markers of atherosclerosis in a cohort of HIV infected adults were studied [65](Falcone et al. 2010), the highest tertile of serum vitamin E concentration was associated with higher common and internal carotid intima-media thickness (c-IMT) and coronary artery calcium (CAC) scores [65]. The authors concluded that elevated serum vitamin E values may increase the risk of cardiovascular complications in HIV-infected adults [65].

There appears to be a possible role for antioxidants supplements. However, these supplements cannot effectively eliminate HIV signs and symptoms and the optimal dosage of these nutrients is (whether used alone or in combination) has to defined

Author details

M Sauka[1], G Selga[1], A Skesters[1], A Silova[1], T Westermarck[2], A Latvus[3] and F Atroshi[4]

1 Rīga Stradiņš University, Rīga, LV, Latvia

2 Rinnekoti Research Center, Espoo-Finalnd, Finland

3 Hankintatukku Oy, Museokatu, Helsinki, Finland

4 Pharmacology &Toxicology, University of Helsinki, Finland

References

[1] WHO. HIV/AIDS.Global situation and trends, 2013.

[2] Sicotte M, Langlois EV, Aho J, Ziegler D, Zunzunegui MV. Association between nutritional status and the immune response in HIV + patients under HAART: protocol for a systematic review. Syst Rev. 2014 Feb 10;3(1):9. [Epub ahead of print]

[3] Kaio DJ, Rondó PH, Souza JM, Firmino AV, Luzia LA, Segurado AA. Vitamin A and Beta-Carotene Concentrations in Adults with HIV/AIDS on Highly Active Antiretroviral Therapy. J Nutr Sci Vitaminol (Tokyo). 2013;59(6):496-502.

[4] Fawzi, W. Micronutrients and human immunodeficiency virus type 1 disease progression among adults and children. Clin. Infect. Dis., 2003, 37 Suppl 2, S 112 – 6.

[5] Nkengfack GN, Torimiro JN, Englert H. Effects of antioxidants on CD4 and viral load in HIV-infected women in sub-Saharan Africa - dietary supplements vs. local diet. nt J Vitam Nutr Res. 2012 Feb;82(1):63-72.

[6] van Lettow M, Harries AD, Kumwenda JJ, Zijlstra EE, Clark TD, Taha TE, Semba RD. Micronutrient malnutrition and wasting in adults with pulmonary tuberculosis with pulmonary tuberculosis with and without HIV co-infection in Malawi. BMC Infect Dis 2004;4:61.

[7] Stone CA, Kawai K, Kupka R, Fawzi WW. Role of selenium in HIV infection. Nutr Rev 2010; 68:671–81.

[8] Campa A, Baum MK. Micronutrients and HIV infection. HIV Ther 2010;4:437–69.

[9] Rayman MP. Selenium and human health. Lancet 2012;379:1256–68.

[10] Odeh M. The role of zinc in acquired immunodeficiency syndrome. J Intern Med. 1992 May;231(5):463-9.

[11] Baum MK, Shor-Posner G, Lu Y, Rosner B, Sauberlich HE, Fletcher MA, Szapocznik J, Eisdorfer C, Buring JE, Hennekens CH. Micronutrients and HIV-1 disease progression. AIDS. 1995 Sep;9(9):1051-6.

[12] Graham NM, Sorensen D, Odaka N, Brookmeyer R, Chan D, Willett WC, Morris JS, Saah AJ. Relationship of serum copper and zinc levels to HIV-1 seropositivity and progression to AIDS. J Acquir Immune Defic Syndr. 1991;4(10):976-80.

[13] Tang AM, Graham NM, Saah AJ. Effects of micronutrient intake on survival in human immunodeficiency virus type 1 infection. Am J Epidemiol. 1996 Jun 15;143(12): 1244-56.

[14] Miyamoto H, Araya Y, Ito M, Isobe H, Dosaka H, Shimizu T, Kishi F, Yamamoto I, Honma H, Kawakami Y. Serum selenium and vitamin E concentrations in families of lung cancer patients. Cancer. 1987 Sep 1;60(5):1159-62.

[15] Delmas-Beauvieux MC, Peuchant E, Couchouron A, Constans J, Sergeant C, Simonoff M, Pellegrin JL, Leng B, Conri C, Clerc M. The enzymatic antioxidant system in blood and glutathione status in human immunodeficiency virus (HIV)-infected patients: effects of supplementation with selenium or beta-carotene. Am J Clin Nutr. 1996 Jul;64(1):101-7. Erratum in: Am J Clin Nutr 1996 Dec;64(6):971.

[16] Flax VL, Bentley ME, Combs GF Jr, Chasela CS, Kayira D, Tegha G, Kamwendo D, Daza EJ, Fokar A, Kourtis AP, Jamieson DJ, van der Horst CM, Adair LS. Plasma and breast-milk selenium in HIV-infected Malawian mothers are positively associated with infant selenium status but are not associated with maternal supplementation: results of the Breastfeeding, Antiretrovirals, and Nutrition study. Am J Clin Nutr. 2014 Feb 5. [Epub ahead of print].

[17] Mburu S, Marnewick JL, Abayomi A, Ipp H. Modulation of LPS-induced CD4+ T-cell activation and apoptosis by antioxidants in untreated asymptomatic HIV infected participants: an in vitro study. Clin Dev Immunol. 2013;2013:631063. doi: 10.1155/2013/631063. Epub 2013 Nov 21.

[18] Hillesheim E, Lima LR, Silva RC, Trindade EB. Dietary intake and nutritional status of HIV-1-infected children and adolescents in Florianopolis, Brazil. Int J STD AIDS. 2013 Dec 18. [Epub ahead of print].

[19] Kaiser JD, Campa AM, Ondercin JP, Leoung GS, Pless RF, Baum MK. Micronutrient supplementation increases CD4 count in HIV-infected individuals on highly active antiretroviral therapy: a prospective, double-blinded, placebo-controlled trial. J Acquir Immune Defic Syndr. 2006 Aug 15;42(5):523-8

[20] Baeten JM, McClelland RS, Richardson BA, Bankson DD, Lavreys L, Wener MH, Overbaugh J, Mandaliya K, Ndinya-Achola JO, Bwayo JJ, Kreiss JK. Vitamin A deficiency and the acute phase response among HIV-1-infected and -uninfected women in Kenya. J Acquir Immune Defic Syndr. 2002 Oct 1;31(2):243-9.

[21] Guo Y, Pino-Lagos K, Ahonen CA, Bennett KA, Wang J, Napoli JL, Blomhoff R, Sockanathan S, Chandraratna RA, Dmitrovsky E, Turk MJ, Noelle RJ. A retinoic acid--rich tumor microenvironment provides clonal survival cues for tumor-specific CD8(+) T cells. Cancer Res. 2012 Oct 15;72(20):5230-9.

[22] Irlam JH, Visser MM, Rollins NN, Siegfried N. Micronutrient supplementation in children and adults with HIV infection. Cochrane Database Syst Rev. 2010 Dec 8; (12):CD003650. doi: 10.1002/14651858.CD003650.

[23] Thorne-Lyman AL, Fawzi WW. Vitamin A and carotenoids during pregnancy and maternal, neonatal and infant health outcomes: a systematic review and meta-analysis. Paediatr Perinat Epidemiol. 2012 Jul;26 Suppl 1:36-54. doi: 10.1111/j. 1365-3016.2012.01284.

[24] Forrester JE, Wang XD, Knox TA, Borek CG, Tang AM, Johnson EJ. Factors associated with serum retinol, alpha-tocopherol, carotenoids, and selenium in Hispanics with problems of HIV, chronic hepatitis C, and drug use. J Public Health Policy. 2009 Sep;30(3):285-99.

[25] Monteiro JP, Freimanis-Hance L, Faria LB, Mussi-Pinhata MM, Korelitz J, Vannucchi H, Queiroz W, Succi RC, Hazra R. Both human immunodeficiency virus-infected and human immunodeficiency virus-exposed, uninfected children living in Brazil, Argentina, and Mexico have similar rates of low concentrations of retinol, beta-carotene, and vitamin E. Nutr Res. 2009 Oct;29(10):716-22.

[26] Villamor E, Koulinska IN, Aboud S, Murrin C, Bosch RJ, Manji KP, Fawzi WW. Effect of vitamin supplements on HIV shedding in breast milk. Am J Clin Nutr. 2010 Oct; 92(4):881-6.

[27] Dror DK, Allen LH. Vitamin E deficiency in developing countries. Food Nutr Bull. 2011 Jun;32(2):124-43.

[28] Isanaka S, Mugusi F, Fawzi WW. Standard-dose vs high-dose multivitamin supplements for HIV--reply. JAMA. 2013 Feb 13;309(6):546. doi: 10.1001/jama.2012.216995.

[29] Sudfeld CR, Isanaka S, Mugusi FM, Aboud S, Wang M, Chalamilla GE, Giovannucci EL, Fawzi WW. Weight change at 1 mo of antiretroviral therapy and its association with subsequent mortality, morbidity, and CD4 T cell reconstitution in a Tanzanian HIV-infected adult cohort. Am J Clin Nutr. 2013 Jun;97(6):1278-87.

[30] Abrams B, Duncan D, Hertz-Picciotto I. A prospective study of dietary intake and acquired immune deficiency syndrome in HIV-seropositive homosexual men. J Acquir Immune Defic Syndr. 1993 Aug;6(8):949-58.

[31] Folkers K, Langsjoen P, Nara Y, Muratsu K, Komorowski J, Richardson PC, Smith TH. Biochemical deficiencies of coenzyme Q10 in HIV-infection and exploratory treatment. Biochem Biophys Res Commun. 1988 Jun 16;153(2):888-96.

[32] Cherry CL, Mobarok M, Wesselingh SL, Fain R, Weinstock S, Tachedjian G, Srivastava S, Tyssen DP, Glass JD, Hooker DJ. Ubisol-Aqua: coenzyme Q10 prevents antiretroviral toxic neuropathy in an in vitro model. Curr HIV Res. 2010 Apr;8(3):232-9.

[33] Xue SY, Hebert VY, Hayes DM, Robinson CN, Glover M, Dugas TR. Nucleoside reverse transcriptase inhibitors induce a mitophagy-associated endothelial cytotoxicity that is reversed by coenzyme Q10 cotreatment. Toxicol Sci. 2013 Aug;134(2):323-34.

[34] Hickey, M. S. Nutritional support of patients with AIDS. Surg.Clin.North Am. 71:645-664, June 1991.

[35] Karter DL, Karter AJ, Yarrish R, Patterson C, Kass PH, Nord J, Kislak JW. Vitamin A deficiency in non-vitamin-supplemented patients with AIDS: a cross-sectional study. J Acquir Immune Defic Syndr Hum Retrovirol. 1995 Feb 1;8(2):199-203.

[36] Timbo BB, Tollefson L. Nutrition: a cofactor in HIV disease. J Am Diet Assoc. 1994 Sep;94(9):1018-22.

[37] Augustus LJ. Nutritional care for patients with HIV. Am J Nurs. 1997 Oct;97(10):62-5.

[38] Beach RS, Mantero-Atienza E, Shor-Posner G, Javier JJ, Szapocznik J, Morgan R, Sauberlich HE, Cornwell PE, Eisdorfer C, Baum MK: Specific nutrient abnormalities in asymptomatic HIV-1 infection. AIDS 1992, 6:701-708.

[39] Semba RD, Graham NM, Caiaffa WT, Margolick JB, Clement L, Vlahov D: Increased mortality associated with vitamin A deficiency during human immunodeficiency virus type 1 infection. Arch Intern Med 1993, 153:2149-2154.

[40] Tang AM, Graham NM, Semba RD, Saah AJ: Association between serum vitamin A and E levels and HIV-1 disease progression. AIDS 1997, 11:613-620.

[41] Jiamton S, Pepin J, Suttent R, Filteau S, Mahakkanukrauh B, Hanshaoworakul W, Chaisilwattana P, Suthipinittharm P, Shetty P, Jaffar S: A randomized trial of the impact of multiple micronutrient supplementation on mortality among HIV-infected individuals living in Bangkok. AIDS 2003, 17:2461-2469.

[42] Fawzi WW, Msamanga GI, Spiegelman D, Wei R, Kapiga S, Villamor E, Mwakagile D, Mugusi F, Hertzmark E, Essex M, Hunter DJ: A randomized trial of multivitamin supplements and HIV disease progression and mortality. N Engl J Med 2004, 351:23-32.

[43] Kameoka M, Kimura T, Ikuta K. Superoxide enhances the spread of HIV-1 infection by cell-to-cell transmission. FEBS Lett. 1993 Sep 27;331(1-2):182-6.

[44] Jaruga P, Jaruga B, Gackowski D, Olczak A, Halota W, Pawlowska M, Olinski R. Supplementation with antioxidant vitamins prevents oxidative modification of DNA in lymphocytes of HIV-infected patients. Free Radic Biol Med. 2002, 32(5):414-20.

[45] Peterhans E. Oxidants and antioxidants in viral diseases: disease mechanisms and metabolic regulation.J Nutr. 1997 May;127(5 Suppl):962S-965S.

[46] Pace GW, Leaf CD. The role of oxidative stress in HIV disease. Free Radic Biol Med. 1995 Oct;19(4):523-8.

[47] Smit E, Tang A. Nutritional assessment in intravenous drug users with HIV/AIDS. J Acquir Immune Defic Syndr. 2000 Oct 1;25 Suppl 1:S62-9.

[48] Tang AM, Smit E, Semba RD, Shah N, Lyles CM, Li D, Vlahov D. Improved antioxidant status among HIV-infected injecting drug users on potent antiretroviral therapy.J Acquir Immune Defic Syndr. 2000 Apr 1;23(4):321-6.

[49] Wong GHW, McHugh T, Weber R, Goeddel DV. Tumor necrosis factor alpha selectively sensitizes human immunodeficiency virus infected cells to heat and radiation. Proc Natl Acad Sci U S A 1991;88:4372–6.

[50] Kotler DP. Nutritional management of patients with AIDS-related anorexia. Semin Gastrointest Dis. 1998 Oct;9(4):189-99.

[51] Kupka R, Msamanga GI, Spiegelman D, Morris S, Mugusi F, Hunter DJ, Fawzi WW: Selenium status is associated with accelerated HIV disease progression among HIV-1-infected pregnant women in Tanzania. J Nutr 2004, 134:2556-2560.

[52] Hardy G, Hardy I. Selenium: the Se-XY nutraceutical. Nutrition. 2004 Jun;20(6):590-3.

[53] Baum MK, Shor-Posner G, Lai S, et al. High risk of HIV-related mortality is associated with selenium deficiency. J Acquir Immune Defic Syndr Hum Retrovirol 1997;15:370–4.

[54] Rayman M.P. (2000).The importance of selenium to human health. Lancet. 15;356(9225):233-41.

[55] Jozanov-Stankov O, Demajo M, Djujić I, Mandić M. Selenium intake as a modulator of responsiveness to oxidative stress. J Environ Pathol Toxicol Oncol. 1998;17(3-4): 251-7.

[56] Levander OA, Beck MA. Selenium and viral virulence. Br Med Bull. 1999;55(3): 528-33.

[57] Grossman Z, Meier-Schellersheim M, Sousa AE, Victorino RM, Paul WE. CD4+ T-cell depletion in HIV infection: are we closer to understanding the cause? Nat Med 2002; 8:319–323.

[58] Highleyman, L. (2003). Monitoring tests for people with HIV. Bulletin of Experimental Treatments for AIDS: Retrieved July 2003 from Hogg, R. et. al. (2001). Rates of disease progression based on CD4 cell count and viral load after initiating drug therapy. Journal of the American Medical Association, 286(20). 2568-2577.

[59] Sandstrom PA, Murray J, Folks TM, Diamond AM. Antioxidant defenses influence HIV-1 replication and associated cytopathic effects. Free Radic Biol Med 1998;24:1485-1491.

[60] Droge W, Eck HP, Gmunder H, Mihm S. Requirement for prooxidant and antioxidant states in T cell mediated immune responses. Relevance for the pathogenic mechanisms of AIDS? Klin Wochenschr 1991;69:118-122.

[61] Kalinowska M, Bazdar DA, Lederman MM, Funderburg N, Sieg SF. Decreased IL-7 responsiveness is related to oxidative stress in HIV disease. PLoS One. 2013;8(3):e58764. doi: 10.1371/journal.pone.0058764. Epub 2013 Mar 7.

[62] Ross AC, Leong T, Avery A, Castillo-Duran M, Bonilla H, Lebrecht D, Walker UA, Storer N, Labbato D, Khaitan A, Tomanova-Soltys I, McComsey GA. Effects of in utero antiretroviral exposure on mitochondrial DNA levels, mitochondrial function and oxidative stress. HIV Med. 2012 Feb;13(2):98-106.

[63] Traber MG. Vitamin E regulatory mechanisms. Annu Rev Nutr 2007;27:347–62.

[64] Diaz MN, Frei B, Vita JA, Keaney JFJ. Antioxidants and atherosclerotic heart disease. N Engl J Med 1997;337:408–16.

[65] Falcone EL, Mangili A, Tang AM, et al. Micronutrient concentrations and subclinical atherosclerosis in adults with HIV. Am J Clin Nutr , 2010;91:1213–9

14

Antioxidant-Rich Natural Products and Diabetes Mellitus

Ayodeji B. Oyenihi, Nicole L. Brooks,
Oluwafemi O. Oguntibeju and Guillaume Aboua

1. Introduction

Diabetes mellitus (DM) is one of the most common metabolic disorders worldwide with an estimated 143 million people suffering from the disease [1]. This number may double by 2030 [2]. Although understanding of the pathophysiological processes involved in DM has increased, with great feats achieved in the management of DM, yet serious diabetic complications still confront patients and physicians [3]. Diabetes mellitus is characterized by chronic hyperglycemia (very high blood glucose levels) and disturbances of carbohydrate, fat and protein metabolism associated with absolute or relative deficiency in insulin secretion or insulin action [4-5]. On the basis of aetiology and clinical presentation, DM is classified into two; type 1 diabetes mellitus also called insulin-dependent diabetes mellitus (IDDM) and type 2 which is the non-insulin dependent diabetes mellitus (NIDDM). The effects of DM include long term damage, dysfunction and failure of various organs, especially the eyes, kidneys, livers, hearts, and blood vessels [6].

In the treatment of diabetes, many oral hypoglycemic agents like sulfonylureas, meglitinides, thiazolidines, D-phenylalanine and α-glucosidase inhibitors are used in addition to insulin treatment action along with appropriate diet and exercise [5]. However, none can be termed as an ideal one, due to their toxic side effects and sometimes diminution in response after prolonged use [7]. The limitations and side effects associated with existing synthetic oral hypoglycemic agents had necessitated the search for newer drugs. As a result, natural agents from plants and plant products have been the alternative target to source for new antioxidant and antidiabetic agents based on their traditional use.

2. Hyperglycemia and oxidative stress

A relationship has been established between hyperglycemia, oxidative stress and numerous pathways which can lead to the development of diabetic complications. Four of these pathways are very important: activation of protein kinase C isoforms, increased hexosamine pathway flux, increased advanced glycation end-product (AGE) formation [8-9], and increased aldose-reductase pathway flux [10]. Oxidative stress has been implicated to play a central role in these pathways. Oxidative stress occurs as a result of excessive formation of reactive oxygen species (ROS) and reactive nitrogen species (RNS) collectively described as free radicals. Free radicals are highly unstable and have the ability to attract electrons from macromolecules such as carbohydrates, protein, lipid and DNA [11]. Excessive ROS can cause structural deterioration and instability of the macromolecules, consequently affecting proper cellular signaling pathways, gene regulation and function [12]. Although, the human system has check-in mechanisms to deal with oxidative damage and free radical formation through endogenous and exogenous antioxidants, however, when the rate of formation of ROS overwhelms the detoxifying ability of the antioxidants, oxidative stress can occur [11, 13-14].

The increase in oxidative stress in diabetes mellitus could be attributed to elevated blood glucose levels, which upon auto-oxidation generates free radicals and damages the cell membrane through peroxidation of membrane lipids [15] and protein glycation [16]. Chronic hyperglycemia results in oxidative stress via auto-oxidation of glucose in the presence of transition metals [17]; decreased activities of antioxidant enzymes such as superoxide dismutase (SOD) and glutathione peroxidase [18]; increased oxidative phosphorylation [19], glycosylation of proteins [17]; and activation of the hexosamine pathway [20]. Hyperglycemia-induced oxidative stress has been demonstrated to result in beta cell dysfunction and death [21-22], as well as in fibrosis of pancreatic islets [23-24]. It has also been established that hyperglycemia increases mitochondrial ROS production, which could represent a key event in the development of diabetic complications [19, 25].

Hyperglycemia has been reported to induce oxidative insult and apoptosis in diabetic liver and renal tubular cells [26-27]. Hyperglycemia leads to increased levels of ROS and D-glucose which has been shown to be capable of inducing apoptosis through the activation of Bax-caspase pathway [28]. Caspases are a family of cysteine proteases known to be the effectors of apoptosis. Upon activation of Bax by free radicals, caspases are activated, which alter mitochondrial function by reducing the electrochemical gradient across the mitochondrial membrane leading to the release of mitochondrial cytochrome C into cytoplasm [28-29]. Studies had shown that movement of Bax into the mitochondrial membrane is accompanied by a significant increase in the activities of caspase-3 and caspase-9 [30-32].

3. Levels of antioxidant action

The antioxidants acting in the defense systems act at different levels such as preventive, radical scavenging, repair and de novo, and the fourth line of defense, i.e., the adaptation.

According to Lobo *et al.* [33], the first line of defense is the preventive antioxidants, which suppress the formation of free radicals. Although the precise mechanism and site of radical formation in vivo are not well elucidated yet, the metal-induced decompositions of hydroperoxides and hydrogen peroxide must be one of the important sources. To suppress such reactions, some antioxidants reduce hydroperoxides and hydrogen peroxide beforehand to alcohols and water, respectively, without generation of free radicals and some proteins sequester metal ions. Glutathione peroxidase, glutathione-s-transferase, phospholipid hydroperoxide glutathione peroxidase (PHGPX), and peroxidase are known to decompose lipid hydroperoxides to corresponding alcohols. PHGPX is unique in that it can reduce hydroperoxides of phospholipids integrated into biomembranes. Glutathione peroxidase and catalase reduce hydrogen peroxide to water.

The second line of defense is the antioxidants that scavenge the active radicals to suppress chain initiation and/or break the chain propagation reactions. Various endogenous radical-scavenging antioxidants are known: some are hydrophilic and others are lipophilic. Vitamin C, uric acid, bilirubin, albumin, and thiols are hydrophilic, radical-scavenging antioxidants, while vitamin E and ubiquinol are lipophilic radical-scavenging antioxidants. Vitamin E is accepted as the most potent radical-scavenging lipophilic antioxidant.

The third line of defense is the repair and de novo antioxidants. The proteolytic enzymes, proteinases, proteases, and peptidases, present in the cytosol and in the mitochondria of mammalian cells, recognize, degrade, and remove oxidatively modified proteins and prevent the accumulation of oxidized proteins.

The DNA repair systems also play an important role in the total defense system against oxidative damage. Various kinds of enzymes such as glycosylases and nucleases, which repair the damaged DNA, are known [33].

There is another important function called adaptation where the signal for the production and reactions of free radicals induces formation and transport of the appropriate antioxidant to the right site [34].

4. Antioxidants and diabetes mellitus treatment

The human system employs the use of endogenous enzymatic and non-enzymatic antioxidant defense systems against the onslaught of free radicals and oxidative stress [35-36]. Enzymatic antioxidants include superoxide dismutase, catalase, glutathione peroxidase, glutathione reductase. Non-enzymatic antioxidants include vitamins A, C, and E, glutathione, alpha-lipoic acid, carotenoids, and coenzyme Q. Other antioxidants include biflavonoids, minerals (copper, zinc, manganese, and selenium), and cofactors (folic acid, vitamins B1, B2, B6 and B12). These antioxidants work synergistically with each other using different mechanisms against different free radicals and stages of oxidative stress [37]. Hyperglycemia has been reported to impair the endogenous antioxidant defense systems in many ways during diabetes in addition to generating free radicals [18, 38]. The involvement of hyperglycemia-mediated oxidative damage in diabetes mellitus has led to the hypothesis that drugs that improve glycemic index and/or oxidative stress will be beneficial in the treatment of diabetes mellitus and its complications.

Majority of the drugs currently used in the treatment of diabetes mellitus have antioxidant activities in addition to their primary pharmacological activity. For example, aminoguanidine has been shown to exhibit free radical scavenging properties and inhibit lipid peroxidation [39-43] although clinical trials were discontinued in Europe and in the United States due to its long term toxicity. Troglitazone lowered hydroperoxides and decreased SOD activity in type 2 diabetic rats [44]. Glibenclamide, a sulphonylureas in addition to its glucose lowering effect possesses antioxidant properties due to its ability to restore liver catalase and superoxide dismutase in diabetic rats [45]. Also, repaglinide used in the treatment of type 2 diabetes mellitus exhibited antioxidant properties and inhibited protein peroxidation by upregulating glutathione reductase and glutathione levels in diabetic rabbits in addition to its insulin releasing effects [46].

Several *in vivo* studies have been carried out to ascertain the effects of antioxidants on experimental diabetic models [47-53]. Most of these studies reported the beneficial role of antioxidants against specific biomarkers of oxidative stress and provided the foundation for clinical trials embarked on later [54-60]. Majority of the studies were not designed specifically to assess the effects of antioxidant use in diabetic patients and none has been carried out yet on antioxidant-rich plant products despite the large evidence supporting its use. Medicinal plants and antioxidant-rich plant products definitely hold promise in this area in the near future.

5. Role of flavonoids in diabetes mellitus

The presence of polyphenolic compounds such as flavonoids, phenols, flavonols, and proanthocyanidins in plants is associated with the antioxidant and antidiabetic potentials [61]. A number of studies have reported on the beneficial effect of flavonoids in diabetes mellitus [62-63]. Examples of flavonoids include quercetin, rutin, diosmin, luteolin, lycopene, catechins and cinnamic acids.

5.1. Quercetin

Quercetin (3,3',4',5-7-penta- hydroxyflavone), belongs to the class flavonol, a member of the flavonoid family and is widely distributed in plants. Quercetin and rutin are the flavonoids most abundantly consumed in foods [64]. Sources of quercetin include brassica green vegetables, carrots, berries, onions, apple, legumes, green tea, citrus fruits, red wines etc [65]. Quercetin has been shown to prevent oxidative stress [66] by different mechanisms, including scavenging free radicals [67], inhibiting xanthine oxidase [68], lipid peroxidation, and chelating metal ions [69]. Quercetin is a powerful antioxidant, proven by *in vitro* [70] and *in vivo* studies [71]. Quercetin ameliorated the damage caused by oxidative stress in pancreatic tissues in rats, by directly quenching lipid peroxides and indirectly enhancing the production of endogenous antioxidants [72].

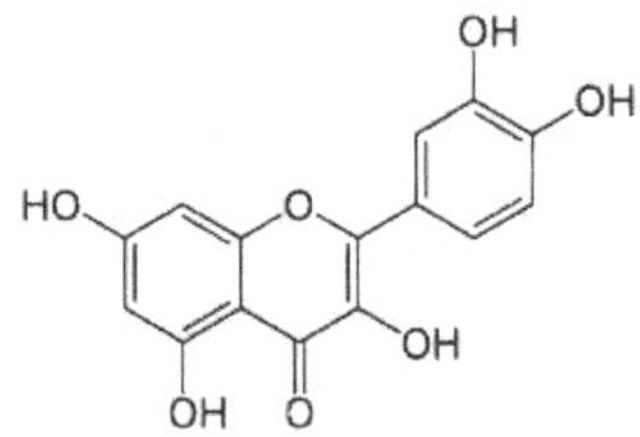

Figure 1. The chemical structure of quercetin.

Quercetin reduces intestinal glucose absorption by inhibiting GLUT 2 in CaCo-2 intestinal cells [73-74]. Quercetin has been extensively investigated in diabetic rat models in recent times. It decreases the fasting blood glucose and improves glucose tolerance [75]; protects against oxidative damage and preserves pancreatic beta cell integrity [76]. Kobori *et al.* [77] reported that quercetin alleviated diabetic symptoms and liver injury in diabetic patients. Quercetin blocks tyrosine kinase thereby interfering with insulin signaling and the propagation of the biological actions of the hormone [78-79]. Quercetin elevated insulin secretion in insulin-secreting cell line induced by glucose and glibenclamide [80] by mediating ERK1/2 pathway [81]. Insulin resistance was improved in genetically obese Zucker rats upon administration of quercetin [82]. Quercetin also reduced maltose-induced postprandial hyperglycemia in type 2 diabetic patients by inhibiting intestinal alpha glucosidase activity [83]. Several mechanisms of action of quercetin in diabetes have been postulated and those included: decreases lipid peroxidation, increases antioxidant enzymes activity like superoxide dismutase (SOD), glutathione peroxidase (GPX), and catalase [76]. Other mechanisms are inhibition of insulin-dependent activation of phosphoinositol-3 kinase (PI-3K) [84], increase adiponectin levels [85], and decrease the intestinal maltose activity [27].

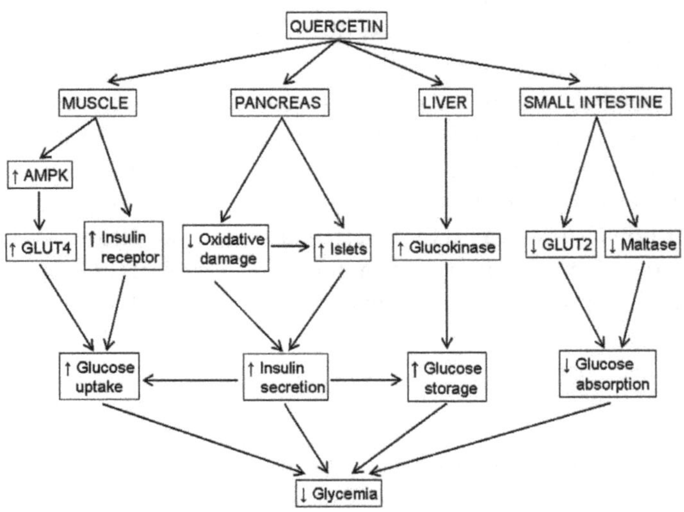

Figure 2. Proposed mechanisms for anti-diabetic effects of Quercetin. Reproduced from Portillo *et al.*, (2011).

5.2. Rutin

Rutin {2-(3,4-dihydroxyphenyl)-5,7-dihydroxy-3-[α-Lrhamnopyranosyl-(1→6)-β-D-gluco pyranosyloxy]-4*H*chromen-4-one} is abundantly present in onions, apples, tea and red wine [86]. The name rutin originated from the plant *Ruta graveolens*. Rutin exhibits multiple pharmacological activities including antibacterial, antitumour, antidiabetic, antiinflammatory, antidiarrhoeal, antiulcer, antimutagenic, myocardial protecting, vasodilator, immunomodulator and hepatoprotective activities [87]. It is a potent antioxidant and anti-inflammatory agent that has the potential to provide a lot of health benefits [88].

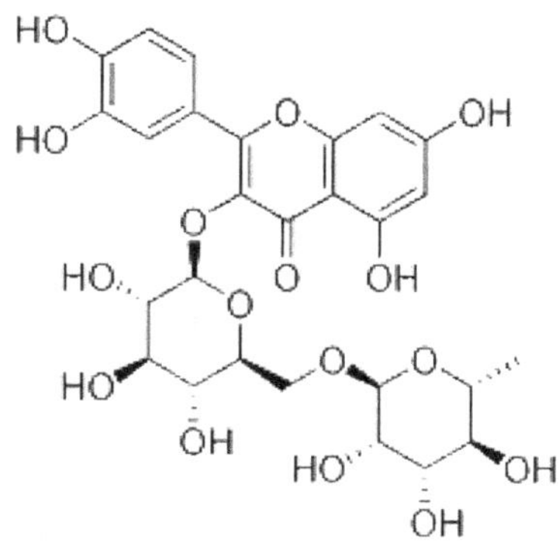

Figure 3. The chemical structure of rutin.

Rutin by its ability to scavenge free radicals and to inhibit lipid peroxidation, prevents streptozotocin-induced oxidative stress and protects pancreatic beta cells resulting in increased insulin secretion and decreased blood glucose levels. Rutin effectively reduced the increased levels of thiobarbituric acid reactive substances and hydroperoxides in the diabetic state *in vivo* [89] and *in vitro* [90]. Rutin reduces hyperglycemia and dyslipidemia while inhibiting the progression of liver and heart dysfunction in diabetic rats [91]. It also significantly decreases elevated reactive oxygen species while increasing endogenous antioxidant enzymes in kidney of diabetic rats and may consequently control or prevent the development of diabetic nephropathy [92]. When Rutin supplementation tablets (500mg) was administered simultaneously with their regular medication for 60 days to patients with type 2 diabetes mellitus, the hypertension, total cholesterol and low-density lipoproteins (LDL) were markedly attenuated. Rutin also decreased the levels of fasting blood glucose, systolic and diastolic blood pressure and improved lipid profiles in the diabetic subjects [93]. Rutin found in *Morus alba* leaves, possesses significant, dose-dependent antidiabetic activity in a type 2 diabetic rat model [94].

5.3. Diosmin

Diosmin (3′,5,7-trihydroxy-4′-methoxyflavone 7-rutinoside) is a naturally occurring flavonoid glycoside that can be isolated from various plant sources or derived by dehydrogenation of the corresponding flavanone glycoside Hesperidin, that is abundant in the pericarp of various citrus fruits [95]. Diosmin was first isolated in 1925 from *Scrophularia nodosa*. Diosmin is considered to be a vascular-protecting agent used to treat chronic venous insufficiency, hemorrhoids, lymphedema, and varicose veins. Diosmin exhibits anti-inflammatory, antioxidant, and anti-mutagenic properties [95-97]. Clinical studies have demonstrated that diosmin can be used to treat venous leg ulcers and hemorrhoids [98]. Also, its anti-inflammatory and anti-apoptotic activity has been demonstrated in neuronal cells [99].

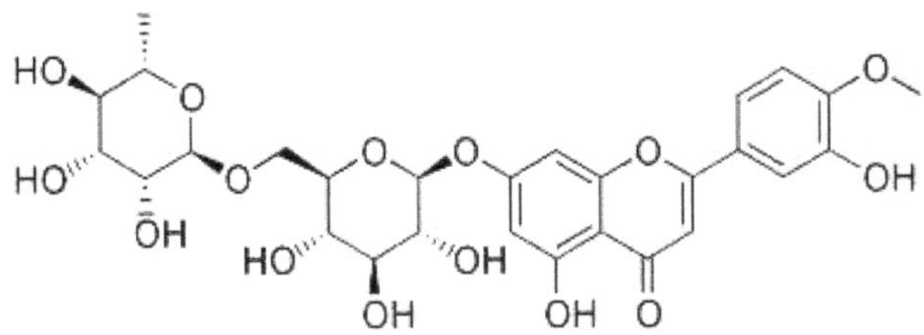

Figure 4. The chemical structure of diosmin.

Diosmin was found to be capable of normalizing capillary filtration rate and prevent ischemia in diabetics [100-101]. Diosmin has been shown to improve factors associated with diabetic complications. A decrease in hemoglobin A1c as well as an increase in glutathione peroxidase was observed in type 1 diabetic patients after an intervention with a diosmin-containing flavonoid mixture [102]. Diosmin and hesperidin are known to lower hepatotoxicity induced by carbon tetrachloride (CCl4) and lipopolysaccharides (LPS), minimize oxidation stress caused by nicotine, reduce blood sugar and cholesterol, and inhibit carcinogenesis of the bladder and colon [31, 103-106]. Administration of diosmin for 45 days significantly lowered plasma glucose level, increased the activities of hepatic key enzymes such as hexokinase and glucose-6-phosphate dehydrogenase in addition to decreasing glucose-6-phosphatase and fructose-1,6-bisphosphatase concentrations in streptozotocin-nicotinamide treated rats exhibiting its antihypeglycemic properties [107]. Diosmin lowered plasma glucose and increased plasma insulin levels in diabetic rats by ameliorating the oxidative stress induced by streptozotocin and nicotinamide. Activities of antioxidant enzymes (superoxide dismutase, catalase, glutathione peroxidase, and glutathione s-transferase), vitamin C, vitamin E and reduced glutathione were increased while lipid peroxidation was reduced in liver and kidney of diabetic rats upon treatment with diosmin. Diosmin was also recently reported to possess antihypertensive property by increasing the activities of antioxidant enzymes,, reducing reactive oxygen species and normalizing marker enzymes in serum and tissues (liver, kidney, heart, aorta) when rats were made hypertensive by deoxycorticosterone acetate (DOCA) salt [108].

5.4. Luteolin

Luteolin (3′,4′,5,7-tetrahydroxyflavone) is a flavonoid widely distributed in the plant kingdom including several such as *Reseda luteola L., Achillea millefolium L, Chamomillae requtita, Cynara scolymus, Thymus vulgaris, Limonium sinuatum* [109]. Luteolin has a variety of pharmacological activities, including anti-mutagenic, anti-tumorigenic [110], anti-inflammatory [111], anti-hypertensive [112], and anti-oxidative [113] properties. It is thought to play an important role in the human body as an antioxidant, a free radical scavenger, an agent in the prevention of inflammation, a promoter of carbohydrate metabolism, and an immune system modulator [114]. The antioxidant activity of luteolin and its glycosides has been associated with their capacity to scavenge reactive oxygen and nitrogen species [115-116], to chelate transition metals that may induce oxidative damage through the Fenton reaction [117] to inhibit prooxidant enzymes [118] and to induce antioxidant enzymes [119-120]. The antioxidant activity of luteolin has been investigated *in vitro* and *in vivo* [121-122].

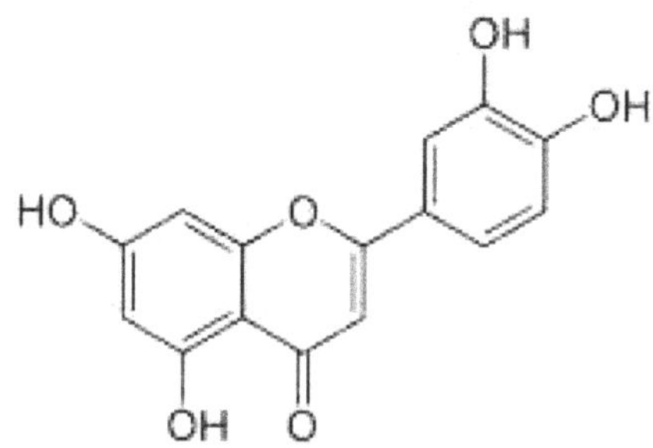

Figure 5. The chemical structure of luteolin.

The antidiabetic property of luteolin was reported by Zarzuelo *et al* [123] where a significant decrease in glycemia levels (> 50%), a 2.5-fold increase in insulin blood levels, elevated pancreatic insulin and DNA content were observed. Luteolin is reported to inhibit alpha-glucosidase and alpha-amylase suggesting that it can suppress postprandial hyperglycemia in patients with non-insulin dependent diabetes mellitus [124]. Recently, luteolin was found to influence insulin action and production of adipokines/cytokines in adipocytes by activating the PPARγ pathway suggesting its role in preventing insulin resistance and type 2 diabetes mellitus [125].

5.5. Lycopene

Lycopene is a carotenoid present in tomatoes (*Lycoperisicon esculentum*). It can be found in many fruits and vegetables like water melon, pawpaw and pink grape fruit. Lycopene is a potent antioxidant according to *in vitro* and human studies, inactivating hydrogen peroxide and nitrogen dioxide [126] and reducing the susceptibility of lymphocyte DNA to oxidative damage [127]. The presence of many conjugated double bonds in lycopene may account for its antioxidant properties [128]. Lycopene quenches singlet oxygen and traps peroxyl radicals [129]. The singlet quenching ability has been reported to be twice as high as that of beta carotene and 10 times higher than that of alpha tocopherol and butylated hydroxyl toluene (BHT) [130-132]. Lycopene is also a potent neuroprotective [133], anti-proliferative, anti-cancer [134], anti-inflammatory [135] and hypocholesterolemic agent [136]. The mechanisms of action against reactive species for lycopene has been proposed to be by adduct formation, electron transfer to radicals and allylic hydrogen attraction [137-141].

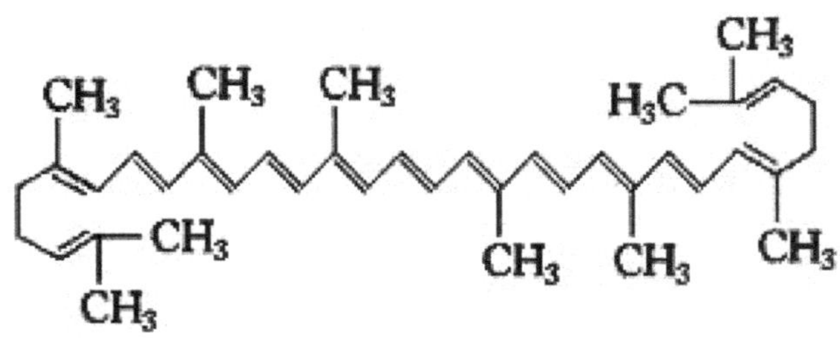

Figure 6. The chemical structure of lycopene.

Lycopene values in serum were found to be significantly lower in patients suffering from type-2 diabetes and impaired glucose metabolism [142-143]. Also, according to data from phase I of the Third National Health and Nutrition Examination Survey (1988-1991), lycopene was found to be inversely related to fasting serum insulin suggesting a possible role for lycopene in the pathogenesis of insulin resistance and diabetes [144]. Lycopene was also found to be useful in the management of neuropathy, a complication of diabetes mellitus, by attenuating cold allodynia and thermal hyperalgesia in streptozotocin induced diabetic rats [145].

5.6. Catechins

Tea (*Camellia sinensis* L) is the most widely consumed beverage in the world, next to water [146-147]. Tea contains catechins, polyphenolic compounds belonging to the flavonoid family. The most important catechins in green tea are: epigallocatechin gallate (EGCG), epigallocatechin (EGC), epicatechin gallate (ECG) and epicatechin (EC) [148]. The antioxidant properties of catechins have been well documented [149-155]. The mechanisms of action of catechins may include free radical scavenging [149-150, 152-153], chelating metal ions to form inactive complexes [150, 152, 156-157], transferring electrons rapidly to ROS induced radical sites on DNA [158] and forming stable semi-quinone free radicals [150]. Catechins also increase the body's endogenous antioxidants to reduce oxidative damage and decrease lipid peroxidation biomarkers in several tissues in rats [158]. Apart from their antioxidant properties, catechins are also anti-carcinogenic, anti-tumorigenic, anti-mutagenic, anti-proliferative, anti-inflammatory, anti-allergic, anti-hypertensive and chemopreventative [159].

In diabetes mellitus, the effects of catechins *in vitro* and *in vivo* studies were investigated [160-163]. In rat models of diabetes, catechins have been demonstrated to have ameliorative effects on biomarkers of oxidative stress on diabetic erythrocytes [164] and on erythrocyte Na/H antiport [165].

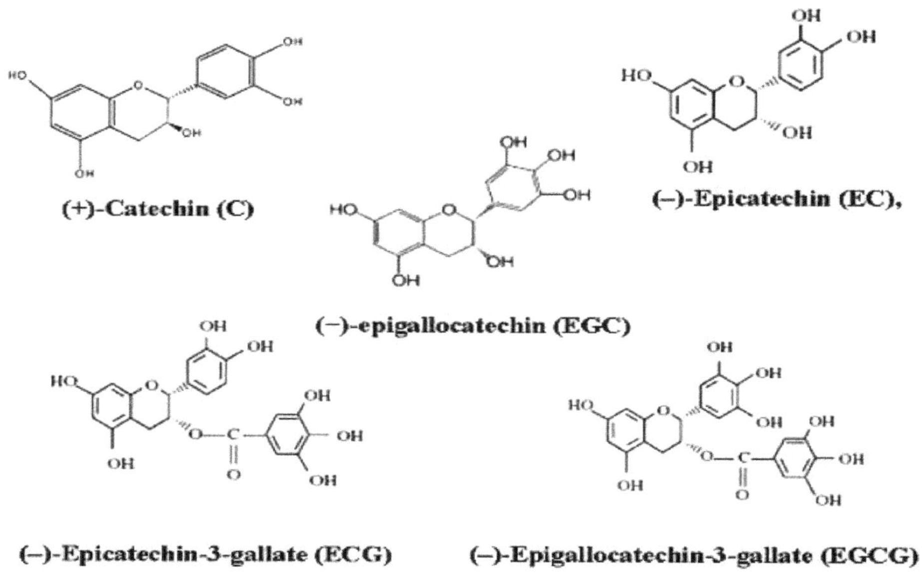

Figure 7. The chemical structure of catechins

5.7. Cinnamic acids

Cinnamon, used extensively since ancient times in food as a herb or spice, has been shown to ameliorate the symptoms of metabolic syndromes, such as insulin resistance and elevated levels of glucose and lipids [166]. Cinnamon bark contains cinnamic acid, cinnamaldehyde and cinnamic alcohol [167]. Cinnamic acid has been reported to exhibit several pharmacological properties including hepatoprotective [168], antioxidant [169] and anti-diabetic properties [170].

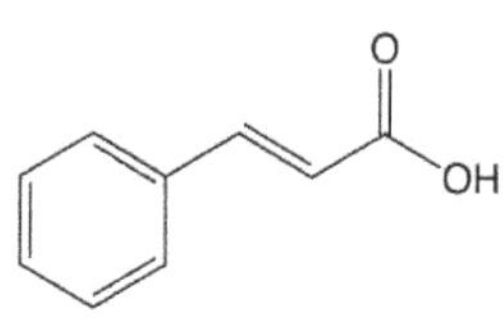

Figure 8. The chemical structure of cinnamic acid.

Cinnamic acid was recently reported to be capable of preventing advanced glucated end-products (AGEs)-mediated diabetic complications. It inhibited the formation of AGEs in a bovine serum albumin (BSA)/fructose system, as well as reduced the levels of fructosamine, the formation of N-(carboxymethyl) lysine (CML) and the level of amyloid cross beta-structure [167]. Sinapic acid is a 4-hydroxy-3, 5-dimethoxy cinnamic acid derivative. It is widely distributed in edible plants such as cereals, nuts, oil seeds and berries [171]. Sinapic acid is a potent antioxidant [172]. Sinapic acid possesses potential anti-hyperglycemic effects, through an increase in insulin production associated with a subsequent increase in the activity of glcolytic enzyme, hexokinase and decrease in the activity of gluconegoenic enzymes, glucose-6-phosphatase and fructose-1, 6-bisphosphatase [173].

6. Selected antioxidant-rich natural plants with antidiabetic potentials

6.1. *Sclerocarya birrea*

Sclerocarya birrea (Family : Anacardiaceae) is a medium-size-to-large deciduous tree widely used for the treatment of proctitis, dysentery, and diarrhea in South Africa and Africa at large and its antimicrobial and antiparasitic properties has been documented [174-175]. *Sclerocarya birrea* is widely used as traditional remedy against diabetes in Africa [176] and has a significant hypoglycemic effect [177]. The methanolic extracts of different parts of the tree such as the leaves, fruit juice, roots and stem-bark has antioxidant properties [61] due to high contents of flavonoids and polyphenolic compounds.

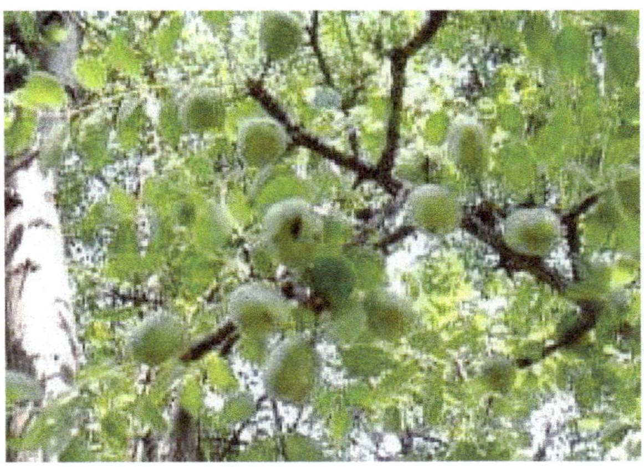

Figure 9. *Sclerocarya birrea* plant

6.2. *Prosopis glandulosa*

Prosopis glandulosa (Family: Fabaceae) commonly known as Honey mesquite is a small to medium height tree or shrub that is thorny and branching near the ground found mostly in southern parts of India. The bark and leaves are used by the tribes and native medical practitioners to treat various ailments such as leprosy, dysentery, bronchitis, asthma, leucoderma, piles, and tremors of the muscles, tumors, eye diseases and rheumatism [178]. It is commonly found in the dry, arid regions of the northern and north-western Cape of South Africa. Literature studies have indicated that the plant contains flavan-3-ol dimer, mesquitol [179-180] and catechin [181]. Phytochemical screening of leaves from *Prosopis glandulosa* indicates the presence of alkaloids, glycosides, flavonoids, phenolic compounds, steroids and terpenoids [182].

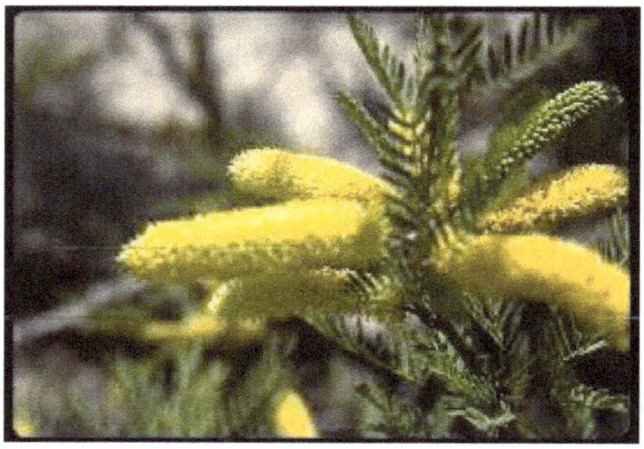

Figure 10. *Prosopis glandulosa* plant

6.3. *Tamarindus indica*

Tamarindus indica Linn (Family: caesalpiniaceae) is a plant that grows naturally in tropical and subtropical regions and has become an important plant for food, herbs in many parts of the world [183]. Literature studies reported *Tamarindus indica* as a traditional medicine for the management of diabetes mellitus in human and experimental animals [184-185]. Siddhuraju [183] reported the potential antioxidant activity of *Tamarindus indica* seeds isolating the antioxidant components 2-hydroxy-30,40-dihydroxyacetophenone, methyl 3,4- ihydroxybenzoate, 3,4-dihydroxyphenylacetate and oligomeric proanthocyanidins. Phenolic compounds such as procyanidin B2, epicatechin, procyanidin trimer, procyanidin tetramer, procyanidin pentamer, procyanidin hexamer, polymeric tannins, polymeric tannins are also present in the seeds of *Tamarindus indica* [186]. It has been postulated that the antidiabetic property of *Tamarindus indica* observed in experimental animals may be due to the presence of the antioxidant-rich compounds [187].

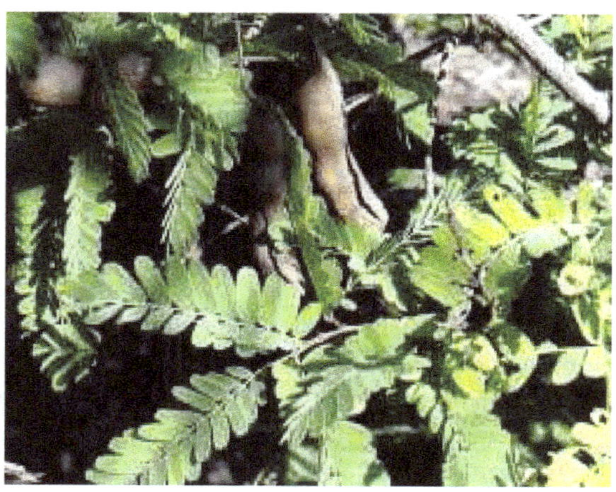

Figure 11. Tamarindus indica plant

7. Conclusion

The pathophysiology of most of the diseases affecting mankind today (*diabetes mellitus* inclusive) seems to have a common denominator, namely oxidative stress. Although, it is a wide topic with several theories, mechanisms, sites and targets of action, reactive oxygen species (ROS) have been implicated in the management of many diseases. As a result, antioxidants have received overwhelming attention in recent years with many outstanding achievements. Most therapeutic agents and drugs are either antioxidants or act primarily to prevent the formation of excess ROS. Therefore it is not surprising to note that natural products with antioxidant properties from plant origin are again gaining prominence in research circles all over the world.

Currently, a lot of therapeutic agents with different modes of action have been designed to combat hyperglycemia; the efficacy and effectiveness of these agents are limited due to several reasons. Individual agent with particular mechanism of action can only act on part of the pathogenic process and only to a partial extent [188-189]. Also, several defects in the pathophysiology of diabetes remain unresolved, and therefore, result in the inability to single out a drug target to focus on as human systems are too interwoven and complex to be fully understood through conventional experimental protocols [190]. However, combination of natural products and phytomedicines from different plants present in most traditional medicines appears to take a different, more holistic approach. These medicinal preparations contain a variety of natural products that act synergistically on a variety of targets through different mechanisms fighting the disease in a more efficient manner. Consequently, the conventional, unidirectional therapeutic method in the management of diabetes seems to be gradually replaced by a more holistic, multidimensional approach

Author details

Ayodeji B. Oyenihi[1], Nicole L. Brooks[2], Oluwafemi O. Oguntibeju[3] and Guillaume Aboua[4]

1 Department of Biochemistry, School of Life Sciences, University of KwaZulu-Natal, Durban, South Africa

2 Department of Wellness Sciences, Faculty of Health & Wellness Sciences, Cape Peninsula University of Technology, Bellville, South Africa

3 Oxidative Stress Research Centre, Departments of Biomedical Sciences, Faculty of Health and Wellness Sciences, Cape Peninsula University of Technology, Bellville, South Africa

4 Department of Biomedical Sciences, Faculty of Health and Wellness Sciences, Cape Peninsula University of Technology, Bellville, South Africa

References

[1] King H, Aubert R.E, and Herman W.H. Global burden of diabetes, 1995-2025: prevalence, numerical estimates, and projections. Diabetes Care. 1998;21(9):1414-1431.

[2] Harris M.I, Flegal K.M, Cowie C.C, Eberhardt M.S, Goldstein D.E, Little R.R, Wiedmeyer H.M, and Byrd-Holt D.D. Prevalence of diabetes, impaired fasting glucose, and impaired glucose tolerance in U.S. adults. The Third National Health and Nutrition Examination Survey, 1988-1994. Diabetes Care. 1998;21:518-524.

[3] Tiwari A.K., and Rao J.M. Diabetes mellitus and multiple therapeutic approaches of phytochemicals: Present status and future prospects. Current Science. 2002;83(1): 30-37.

[4] Jayakar B. and Suresh B. Antihyperglycemic and hypoglycemic effect of Aporosa lindleyana in normal and alloxan induced diabetic rats. Journal of Ethnopharmacology. 2003;84: 247-249.

[5] Bastaki S. Diabetes mellitus and its treatment. International Journal of Diabetes and Metabolism 2005;13:111-134.

[6] Bennett P.H and Knowler W.C. Definition, diagnosis and classification of Diabetes Mellitus and glucose homeostasis: Joslin's Diabetes Mellitus. In: Kahn CR, WEIR GC, KING GL, JACOBSON AM, MOSES AC, SMITH RJ editors. Lippincott, Williams and Wilkins 2005: 331-339.

[7] Chattopadhyay R.R. A comparative evaluation of some blood sugar lowering agents of plant origin. Journal of Ethnopharmacology. 1999;67:367–372.

[8] Vlassara H and Palace M.R. Diabetes and advanced glycation endproducts. Journal of Internal Medicine. 2002;251:87-101.

[9] Peppa M, Uribarri J, and Vlassara H. The role of advanced glycation end products in the development of atherosclerosis. Current Diabetes Reports. 2004;4: 31-36

[10] Rolo A.P and Palmeira C.M. Diabetes and mitochondrial function: role of hyperglycemia and oxidative stress. Toxicology and Applied Pharmacology. 2006;212:167-178.

[11] Valko M., Leibfritz D., Moncola J., Cronin M.T.D., Mazura M., and Telser J. Free radicals and antioxidants in normal physiological functions and human disease. The International Journal of Biochemistry and Cell Biology. 2007;39:44–84.

[12] Pop-Busui R, Sima A, Stevens M. Diabetic neuropathy and oxidative stress. Diabetes/ Metabolism Research and Reviews. 2006;22:257-273.

[13] Ridnour L.A., Thomas D.D., Mancardi D., Espey M.G., Miranda K.M., Paolocci N., Feelisch M., Fukuto J., and Wink D. A. The chemistry of nitrosative stress induced by nitric oxide and reactive nitrogen oxide species. Biological Chemistry. 2004;385:1-10

[14] Halliwell B. Free radicals and antioxidants - quo vadis? Trends in Pharmacological Sciences. 2011;32:125-130.

[15] Baynes J.W and Thorne S. Role of oxidative stress diabetic complications: a new perspective on an old paradigm. Diabetes, 1999;48: 1-9.

[16] Baynes W. Chemical modification of protein by lipids in diabetes. Clinical Chemistry and Laboratory Medicine 2003;41: 1159-1165.

[17] Wolff S.P., Bascal Z.A. and Hunt J.V. "Autoxidative glycosylation": free radicals and glycation theory. Progress in Clinical and Biological Research. 1989;304:259-75.

[18] Blakytny, R. and Harding, J. J. Glycation (non-enzymic glycosylation) inactivates glutathione reductase. Biochemical Journal, 1992;288:303-7.

[19] Nishikawa T., Edelstein D., Du X. L, Yamagishi S., Matsumura T., Kaneda Y., Yorek M.A, Beebe D., Oates P.J., Hammes H.P., Giardino I. and Brownlee M. Normalizing mitochondrial superoxide production blocks three pathways of hyperglycaemic damage. Nature. 2000;404:787-90.

[20] Kaneto H., Xu G., Song K., Suzuma K., Bonner-Weier S., Sharma A. and Weier G. C. Activation of the hexosamine pathway leads to deterioration of pancreas b-cells function through the induction of oxidative stress. Journal of Biological Chemistry. 2001;276:31099-31104.

[21] Donath M. Y.; Gross D. J.; Cerasi E. and Kaiser N. Hyperglycemia-induced b-cell apoptosis in pancreatic islets of Psammomys obesus during development of diabetes Diabetes. 1999;48:738-44.

[22] Robertson R.P, Harmon J, Tran P.O, Tanaka Y, and Takahashi H. Glucose toxicity in beta cells: type 2 diabetes, good radicals gone bad, and the glutathione connection. Diabetes. 2003;52:581–587.

[23] Hayden M.R. Islet amyloid and fibrosis in the cardiometabolic syndrome and type 2 diabetes mellitus. Journal of the Cardio-metabolic Syndrome. 2007;2:70-5.

[24] Hong O., Lee S., Rhee M., Ko S., Cho J., Choi Y., Song K., Son H. and Yoon K. Hyperglycemia and hyperinsulinemia have additive effects on activation and proliferation of pancreatic stellate cells: possible explanation of islet-specific fibrosis in type 2 diabetes mellitus. Journal of Cell Biochemistry. 2007;101:665-75.

[25] Kiritoshi S, Nishikawa T, Sonoda K, Kukidome D, Senokuchi T, Matsuo T, Matsumura T, Tokunaga H, Brownlee M and Araki E. Reactive oxygen species from mitochondria induce cyclooxygenase-2 gene expression in human mesangial cells: potential role in diabetic nephropathy. Diabetes. 2003;52 :2570–2577.

[26] Stitt-Cavanagh E., MacLeod L, and Kennedy C.R.J. The Podocyte in Diabetic Kidney Disease. The ScientificWorld JOURNAL. 2009;9:1127–1139.

[27] Kim Y.J, Kim Y.A, Yokozawa T.. Pycnogenol modulates apoptosis by suppressing oxidative stress and inflammation in high glucose-treated renal tubular cells. Food and Chemical Toxicology. 2011;49:2196–2201.

[28] Green D.R and Reed J.C. Mitochondria and apoptosis. Science 1998;281:1309–1312.

[29] Liu X, Kim CN, Yang J, Jemmerson R and Wang X. Induction of apoptotic program in cell-free extracts: requirement for dATP and cytochrome C. Cell. 1996;86:147–157.

[30] Fraser A. and Evans G. A. license to kill. Cell. 1996;85:781–784.

[31] Yang J, Liu X, Bhalla K, Kim C.N, Ibrado A.M, Cai J, Peng T.I, Jones D.P and Wang X. Prevention of apoptosis by Bcl-2: release of cytochrome c from mitochondria blocked. Science. 1997;275:1129–1132.

[32] Nakagami H, Morishita R, Yamamoto K, Taniyama Y, Aoki M, Yamasaki K, Matsumoto K, Nakamura T, Kaneda Y and Ogihara T. Hepatocyte growth factor prevents endothelial cell death through inhibition of bax translocation from cytosol to mitochondrial membrane. Diabetes. 2002;51:2604–2611.

[33] Lobo V. Patil A. Phatak A. and Chandra N. Free radicals, antioxidants and functional foods: Impact on human health. Pharmacognosy Reviews. 2010;4:118–126.

[34] Niki E. Antioxidant defenses in eukaryotic cells. In: Poli G, Albano E, Dianzani MU, editors. Free radicals: From basic science to medicine. Basel, Switzerland: Birkhauser Verlag;. 1993;365–73

[35] Harris, E.D. Regulation of antioxidant enzymes. Journal of Nutrition. 1992;122:625-626.

[36] Jacob R.A. The integrated antioxidant system. Nutrition Research. 1995;15:755-766.

[37] Maritim A, Sanders R, Watkins J.I. Effects of alpha-lipoic acid on biomarkers of oxidative stress in streptozotic-induced diabetic rats. Journal of Nutrition and Biochemistry. 2003;14(5):288-294.

[38] Saxena A.K, Saxena P, Kale R.K and Baquer N.Z. Impaired antioxidant status in diabetic rat liver: Effect of vanadate. Biochemical Pharmacology. 1993;45:539–542.

[39] Biegelsen E.S and Vita J.A. Human studies of antioxidants and vascular function. In: Keaney Jr. JF, editor. Oxidative stress and vascular disease. Dordrecht: Kluwer Academic Publishers: 1999;213-243.

[40] Gaziano J.M. Antioxidants and cardiovascular disease. In: Keaney Jr. JF, editor. Oxidative stress and vascular disease. Dordrecht: Kluwer Academic Publishers: 1999;245-258.

[41] Kern T.S, Tang J, Mizutani M, Kowluru R.A, Nagaraj R.H, Romeo G., Podesta F., and Lorenzi M. Response of capillary cell death to aminoguanidine predicts the develop-

ment of retinopathy: comparison of diabetes and galactosemia. Investigative Ophthalmology and Visual Science. 2000;41: 3972-3978.

[42] Dobsak P., Courderot-Masuyer C., Siegelova J, Svacinova H., Jancik J.,Vergely-Vanriessen C., Rochette. Antioxidant properties of aminoguanidine: a paramagnetic resonance test Scripta Medica (BRNO). 2001;74 (1): 45–50.

[43] El-Shazly A.M, Mahmoud A.M, and Darwish N.S. Potential prophylactic role of aminoguanidine in diabetic retinopathy and nephropathy in experimental animals. Acta Pharmaceutica. 2009;59: 67–73.

[44] Fukui T, Noma T, Mizushige K, Aki Y, Kimura S, and Abe Y. Dietary troglitazone decreases oxidative stress in early stage type II diabetic rats. Life Sciences. 2000;66:2043–2049.

[45] Elmali E, Altan N, and Bukan N. Effect of the Sulphonylurea glibenclamide on liver and kidney antioxidant enzymes in streptozocin-induced diabetic rats. Drugs. 2004;5:203–8

[46] Gumieniczek A, Hopka H, Rolinski J, Bojarska-Junak A. Antioxidative and anti-inflammatory effects of repaglinide in plasma of diabetic animals. Pharmacology Research 2005;

[47] Mekinova D, Chorvathova V, Volkovova K, Staruchova M, Grancicova E, Klvanoca J, and Ondreicka R. Effect of intake of exogenous vitamins C, E and beta-carotene on the antioxidative status in kidneys of rats with streptozotocin-induced diabetes. Nahrung. 1995;39(4):257-261.

[48] Kocak G, Aktan F, Canbolat O, Ozogul C, Elberg S, Yildizoglu-Ari N, and Karasu C. Alpha-lipoic acid treatment ameliorates metabolic parameters, blood pressure, vascular reavtivity and morphology of vessels already damaged by streptozotocin-diabetes. Nutrition and Metabolism. 2000;13:308-318.

[49] Obrosova I, Fathallah L, and Greene D. Early changes in lipid peroxidation and antioxidative defense in rat retina. European Journal of Pharmacology. 2000;398:139-146.

[50] Cinar M, Ulker S, Alper G, and Evinc A. Effect of dietary vitamin E supplementation on vascular reactivity of thoracic aorta in streptozotocin-diabetic rats. Pharmacology. 2001;62(1):56-64.

[51] Maritim A, Sanders R, Watkins J.I. Effects of alpha-lipoic acid on biomarkers of oxidative stress in streptozotic-induced diabetic rats. Journal of Nutrition and Biochemistry. 2003;14(5):288-294.

[52] Rauscher F, Sanders R, and Watkins J.I. Effects of coenzyme Q10 treatment on antioxidant pathways in normal and streptozotocin- induced diabetic rats. Journal of Biochemistry and Molecular Toxicology. 2001;15:41-46.

[53] Kedziora-kornatowska K, Szram S, Kornatowski T, Szadujkis-Szadurski L, Kedziora J, and Bartosz G. Effect of vitamin E and vitamin C supplementation of antioxidative

state and renal glomerular basement membrane thickness in diabetic kidney. Experimental Nephrology. 2003;95:134-143.

[54] Ziegler D, Hanefeld M, Ruhnau K..J, Meissner H.P, Lobisch M, Schutte K, and Gries F.A Treatment of symptomatic diabetic peripheral neuropathy with the anti-oxidant alpha-lipoic acid. A 3-week multicentre randomized controlled trial (ALADIN Study). Diabetologia. 1995;38(12):1425-1433.

[55] Reljanovic M, Reichel G, Rett K, Lobisch M, Schuette K, Moller W, Tritschler H.J, and Mehnert H. Treatment of diabetic polyneuropathy with the antioxidant thioctic acid (alpha-lipoic acid): a two year multicenter randomized double-blind placebo-controlled trial (ALADIN II). Alpha Lipoic Acid in Diabetic Neuropathy. Free Radical Research. 1999;31(3):171-179.

[56] Ziegler D, Hanefeld M, Ruhnau K, Hasche H, Lobisch M, Schutte K, Kerum G, and Malessa R. Treatment of symptomatic diabetic polyneuropathy with the antioxidant alpha-lipoic acid: a 7- month multicenter randomized controlled trial (ALADIN III Study). ALADIN III Study Group. Alpha-Lipoic Acid in Diabetic Neuropathy. Diabetes Care. 1999;22(8):1296-1301.

[57] Skyrme-Jones R.A, O'Brien R.C, Berry K.L, and Meredith I.T. Vitamin E supplementation improves endothelial function in type I diabetes mellitus: a randomized, placebo-controlled study. Journal of the American College of Cardiology. 2000;36(1): 94-102.

[58] Gaede P, Poulsen H.E, Parving H.H, and Pedersen O. Double-blind, randomized study of the effect of combined treatment with vitamin C and E on albuminuria in Type 2 diabetic patients. Diabetes and Medicine. 2001;18(9):756-760.

[59] Lonn E.M, Yusuf S, Dzavik V, Doris C.I, Yi Q, Smith S, Moore-Cox A, Bosch J, Riley W.A, Teo K.K. Effects of ramipril and vitamin E on atherosclerosis : The study to evaluate carotid ultrasound changes in patients treated with ramipril and vitamin E (SECURE). Circulation. 2001;103(7):919-925.

[60] Beckman J.A, Goldfine A.B, Gordon M.B, Garrett L.A, Keaney J.F Jr, and Creager M.A. Oral antioxidant therapy improves endothelial function in Type 1 but not Type 2 diabetes mellitus. American Journal of Physiology. 2003;285(6):2392-2398.

[61] Mariod A.A., Matthaus B., and Hussein I. H. "Antioxidant properties of methanolic extracts from different parts of Sclerocarya birrea," International Journal of Food Science and Technology. 2008;43:921–926,

[62] Adaramoye O.A. and Adeyemi E.O. Hypoglycaemic and hypolipidaemic effects of fractions from Kolaviron, a biflavonoid complex from Garcinia kola in streptozotocin- induced diabetes mellitus rats. Journal of Pharmacy and Pharmacology. 2006;58:121-128.

[63] Rauter A.P., Martins A., Borges C., Mota-Filipe H., Pinto R., Sepodes B. and Justino J. Antihyperglycaemic and protective effects of flavonoids on streptozotocin-induced diabetic rats. Phytotherapy Research. 2010;24(2): S133-S138.

[64] Nakamura T, Kaneda Y and Ogihara T. Hepatocyte growth factor prevents endothelial cell death through inhibition of bax translocation from cytosol to mitochondrial membrane. Diabetes. 2002;51: 2604–2611.

[65] Hakkinen S.H., Karenlampi S.O., Heinonen I.M., and Mykkanen H. Content of the flavonols quercetin, myricetin, and kaempferol in 25 edible berries. Journal of Agriculture and Food Chemistry. 1999;47:2274-2279.

[66] Larocca L.M., Teofili, L., Sica, S., Pierelli L., and Menichella G. Quercetin inhibits the growth of leukemic progenitors and induces the expression of transforming growth factor-B1 in these cells. Blood. 1995;85:3654-3661

[67] Cox D., Whichelow M.J, and Prevost T.A. Antioxidant effects of flavonoids. Public Health Nutrition. 2000;3:19-29.

[68] Chang W.S, Lee, Y.J, Lu, F.J. and Chiang, H.C. Inhibitory effects of flavonoids on xanthine oxidase. Anticancer Research. 1993;13:2165-2170.

[69] Chen Y.T, Zheng R.L., Jia Z.J. and Ju Y. Flavonoids as superoxide scavengers and antioxidants. Free Radical Biology and Medicine. 1990;9:19-20.

[70] Fiorani M., Guidarelli A., Blasa M., Azzolini C., Candiracci M., Piatti E., and Cantoni O. Mitochondria accumulate large amounts of quercetin: prevention of mitochondrial damage and release upon oxidation of the extra-mitochondrial fraction of the flavonoid. Journal of Nutrition and Biochemistry. 2010;21:397-404.

[71] Meyers K.J., Rudolf J.L. and Mitchell A.E. Influence of dietary quercetin on glutathione redox status in mice. Journal of Agriculture and Food Chemistry. 2008;56:830-836.

[72] Abd El-Baky A.E. Quercetin protective action on oxidative stress, sorbitol, insulin resistance and beta cells function in experimental diabetic rats. International Journal of Pharmaceutical Studies and Research 2011;2(2)11-18.

[73] Kwon O, Eck P, Chen S, Corpe C.P, Lee J.H, Kruhlak M, and Levine M. Inhibition of the intestinal glucose transporter GLUT2 by flavonoids. Federation of American Societies for Experimental Biology Journal. 21: 2007;366-77.

[74] Manzano S and Williamson G. Polyphenols and phenolic acids from strawberry and apple decrease glucose uptake and transport by human intestinal Caco-2 cells. Molecular Nutrition and Food Research. 2010;54:1773-80.

[75] Vessal M, Hemmati M, and Vasei M. Antidiabetic effects of quercetin in streptozocin-induced diabetic rats. Comparative Biochemistry and Physiology Part C: Toxicology. 2003;135:357-64.

[76] Coskun O, Kanter M, Korkmaz A, and Oter S. Quercetin, a flavonoid antioxidant, prevents and protects streptozotocin-induced oxidative stress and β-cell damage in rat páncreas. Pharmacology Research. 2005;51: 117-23.

[77] Kobori M, Masumoto S, Akimoto Y, and Takahashi Y. Dietary quercetin alleviates diabetic symptoms and reduces streptozotocininduced disturbance of hepatic gene expression in mice. Molecular Nutrition and Food Research. 2009;53: 859-68.

[78] Elberg G, Jinping L, Leibovitch A, and Shechter Y. Non-receptor cytosolic protein tyrosine kinases from various rat tissues. Biochimica et Biophysica Acta. 1995;1269:299-306.

[79] Portillo M.P., Aguirre L, Arias N, Macarulla M. T, and Gracia A. Beneficial Effects of Quercetin on Obesity and Diabetes. The Open Nutraceuticals Journal. 2011;4: 189-198.

[80] Youl E, Bardy G, Magous R, Cros G, Sejalon F, Virsolvy A, Richard S, Quignard J.F, Gross R, Petit P, Bataille D, and Oiry C. Quercetin potentiates insulin secretion and protects INS-1 pancreatic b-cells against oxidative damage via the ERK1/2 pathway. British Journal of Pharmacology. 2010;161(4):799-814.

[81] Longuet C, Broca C, Costes S, Hani E.H, Bataille D, and Dalle S. Extracellularly regulated kinases (p44/42 mitogen-activated protein kinases) phosphorylate synapsin I and regulate insulin secretion in the MIN6 beta-cell line and islets of Langerhans. Endocrinology. 2005;146: 643-54.

[82] Rivera L, Morón R, Sánchez M, Zarzuelo A, and Galisteo M. Quercetin ameliorates metabolic syndrome and improves the inflammatory status in obese zucker rats. Obesity. 2008;16:2081-7.

[83] Hussain S.A, Ahmed Z.A., Mahwi T.O., and Aziz T.A. Quercetin Dampens Postprandial Hyperglycemia in Type 2 Diabetic Patients Challenged with Carbohydrates Load International Journal of Diabetes Research. 2012;1(3): 32-35.

[84] Steward L.K, Wang Z, Ribnicky D, Soileau J.L, Cefalu W.T, and Gettys T.W. Failure of dietary quercetin to alter the temporal progression of insulin resistance among tissues of C57BL/6J mice during the development of diet-induced obesity. Diabetologia. 2009;52: 514-23.

[85] Wein S, Behm N, Petersen R.K, Kristiansen K, Wolffram S. Quercetin enhances adiponectin secretion by a PPARℵ independent mechanism. European Journal of Pharmaceutical Sciences. 2010;41:16-22.

[86] Hertog M.G., Hollman P.C., Katan M. B. and Kromhout D. Intake of potentially anticarcinogenic flavonoids and their determinants in adults in The Netherlands. Nutrition and Cancer. 1993;20:21–29.

[87] Janbaz K.H., Saeed S.A. and Gilani A.H Protective effect of rutin on paracetamol- and CCl4-induced hepatotoxicity in rodents. Fitoterapia. 2002;73: 557–563.

[88] Navarro-Núñez L., Lozano M.L, Palomo M, Martínez C, Vicente V, and Castillo J, "Inhibits Platelet Adhesion and Thrombus Formation and Synergizes with Aspirin in the Suppression of the Arachidonic Acid Pathway", Journal of Agriculture and Food Chemistry. 2008;56(9): 2970–6.

[89] Kamalakkannan N and Prince P.S.M. Antihyperglycaemic and Antioxidant Effect of Rutin, a Polyphenolic Flavonoid, in Streptozotocin-Induced Diabetic Wistar Rats. Basic, Clinical Pharmacology and Toxicology. 2006;98: 97–103.

[90] Kozlov A.V., Ostrachovitch E.A. and Afanas'ev I.B. Mechanism of inhibitory effects of chelating drugs on lipid peroxidation in rat brain homogenates. Biochemical Pharmacology. 1994;47:795–799.

[91] Fernandes H., Angélica A., Lourenzi E., Novelli B., Okoshi K., Okoshi M.P, Di Muzio B.P., Guimarães J.F.C, Fernandes A Jnr. Influence of rutin treatment on biochemical alterations in experimental diabetes. Biomedicine and pharmacotherapy. 2010;64(3): 214-219.

[92] Alsaif M.A. Beneficial Effects of Rutin and Vitamin C Coadministration in a Streptozotocin-Induced Diabetes Rat Model of Kidney Nephrotoxicity. Pakistan Journal of Nutrition. 2009;8 (6):745-754.

[93] Sattanathan K., Dhanapal C.K.,and Manavalan R. LDL lowering properties of rutin in diabetic patients. International Journal of Pharma and Bio sciences. 2010;1(4): 0975-6299.

[94] Hunyadi A, Martins A, Hsieh T.J, Seres A, Zupko′ I. Chlorogenic Acid and Rutin Play a Major Role in the In Vivo Anti-Diabetic Activity of Morus alba Leaf Extract on Type II Diabetic Rats. PLoS ONE 2012;7(11): e50619. doi:10.1371/journal.pone.0050619.

[95] Carmada L., Distefano V., DelBosco S.F., and Schillaci D. Antoproliferative activity of citrus juices and HPLC evaluation of their flavonoid composition. Fitoterapia. 2007;78:426-429.

[96] Galati E.M, Monforte M.T, Kirjavainen S, Forestieri A.M, and Trovato A. Il Farmaco, 1994;49:709.

[97] Crespo M.E, Galvez J, Cruz T, Ocete M.A, and Zarzuelo A. Antiinflammatory activity of diosmin and hesperidin in rat colitis induced by TNBS. Planta Medica. 1999;65:651-653.

[98] Hitzenberger G. Therapeutic effectiveness of flavonoids shown on the example of DaflonC4 500 mg. Wein. Med. Wochenschr. 1997;174:409.

[99] Rezai-Zadeh K, Douglas Shytle R, Bai Y, Tian J, Hou H, Mori T, Zeng J., Obregon D., Town T., and Tan, J. Flavonoid-mediated presenilin-1 phosphorylation reduces Alzheimer's disease beta-amyloid production. Journal of Cellular and Molecular Medicine. 2009;13:574-88.

[100] Lacombe C, Lelievre J.C, Bucherer C, and Grimaldi A. Activity of Daflon 500 mg on the hemorheological disorders in diabetes. International Angiology. 1989;8:45-48.

[101] Valensi P.E, Behar A, De-Champvallins M.M, Attalah M, Boulakia F.C, and Attali J.R. Effects of a purified micronized flavonoid fraction on capillary filtration in diabetic patients. Diabet Med. 1996;13:882-888.

[102] Manuel Y, Keenoy B, Vertommen J, and De Leeuw I. The effect of flavonoid treatment on the glycation and antioxidant status in type 1 diabetic patients. Diabetes Nutrition and Metabolism. 1999;12:256-263.

[103] Tanaka T. Makita H., Kawabata K., Mori H., Kakumoto M and Satoh K. Carcinogenesis. 1997;18: 957.

[104] Tirkey N, Pilkhwal S, Kuhad A, and Chopra K. Hesperidin, a citrus bioflavonoid, decreases the oxidative stress produced by carbon tetrarchloride in rat liver and kidney. BMC Pharmacology. 2005;5:2.

[105] Jung U.J, Lee M.K, Park Y.B, Kang M.A and Choi M.S. Effect of citrus flavonoids on lipid metabolism and glucose-regulating enzyme mRNA levels in type-2 diabetic mice. International Journal of Biochemistry and Cell Biology. 2006;38:1134-1145.

[106] Kaur G, Tirkey N, Chopra K. Beneficial effect of hesperidin on lipopolysaccharide-induced hepatotoxicity. Toxicology. 2006;226: 152-160.

[107] Pari L. and Srinivasan S. Antihyperglycemic effect of diosmin on hepatic key enzymes of carbohydrate metabolism in streptozotocin-nicotinamide-induced diabetic rats, Biomedicine and Pharmacotherapy. 2010;64(7):477-481.

[108] Silambarasan T and Raja B. Diosmin, a bioflavonoid reverses alterations in blood pressure, nitric oxide, lipid peroxides and antioxidant status in DOCA-salt induced hypertensive rats. European Journal of Pharmacology. 2012;679(1): 81-89.

[109] Kraft K. Artichoke leaf extract—recent findings reflecting effects on lipid metabolism, liver and gastrointestinal tracts. Phytomedicine. 1997;4(4), 369-378.

[110] Ross J.A and Kasum C.M. Dietary flavonoids: bioavailability, metabolic effects, and safety. Annual Review of Nutrition. 2002;22:19-34.

[111] Choi J.S, Choi Y.J, Park S.H, Kang J.S, and Kang Y.H. Flavones mitigate tumor necrosis factor-alpha-induced adhesion molecule upregulation in cultured human endothelial cells: role of nuclear factor-kappa B. Journal of Nutrition. 2004;134:1013–9.

[112] Loizzo M.R, Said A, Tundis R, Rashed K, Statti G.A, Hufner.A., and Menichini.F. Inhibition of angiotensin converting enzyme (ACE) by flavonoids isolated from Ailanthus excelsa (Roxb) (Simaroubaceae). Phytotherapy Research. 2007;21:32–6.

[113] Ma X, Li Y.F, Gao Q, Ye Z.G, Lu X.J, Wang H.P, Jiang, H.D., Bruce, I.C. and Xia, Q. Inhibition of superoxide anionmediated impairment of endothelium by treatment with luteolin and apigenin in rat mesenteric artery. Life Sciences. 2008;83:110–7.

[114] Xu K., Liu B., Ma Y., Du J., Li G., Gao H., Zhang Y. and Ning Z. Physicochemical Properties and Antioxidant Activities of Luteolin-Phospholipid Complex. Molecules. 2009;14:3486-93.

[115] Horvathova K., Chalupa I., Sebova L., Tothova D., Vachalkova A. Protective effect of quercetin and luteolin in human melanoma HMB-2 cells. Mutation Research. 2005;565:105-12.

[116] Odontuya G., Hoult J.R., and Houghton P.J. Structure-activity relationship for antiinflammatory effect of luteolin and its derived glycosides. Phytotherapy Research. 2005;19: 782-6.

[117] Cheng I.F. and Breen K. On the ability of four flavonoids, baicilein, luteolin, naringenin, and quercetin, to suppress the Fenton reaction of the iron-ATP complex. Biometals. 2000;13:77-83.

[118] Hu C, and Kitts D.D. Luteolin and luteolin-7-O-glucoside from dandelion flower suppress iNOS and COX-2 in RAW264.7 cells. Molecular and Cellular Biochemistry. 2004;265:107-113.

[119] Wruck C.J., Claussen M., Fuhrmann G., Romer L., Schulz A., Pufe T., Waetzig V., Peipp M., Herdegen T., Gotz M.E. Luteolin protects rat PCl2 and C6 cells against MPP+ induced toxicity via an ERK dependent Keapl-Nrf2-ARE pathway. Journal of Neural Transmission. 2007;72:57-67.

[120] Choi B.M, Lim D.W, Lee J.A, Gao S.S, Kwon D.Y, and Kim B.R. Luteolin suppresses Cisplatin-induced apoptosis in auditory cells: possible mediation through induction of heme oxygenase-1 expression. Journal of Medicinal Food. 2008;11:230-6.

[121] Qiusheng Z., Yuntao Z., Rongliang Z., Dean G., Changling L. Effects of verbascoside and luteolin on oxidative damage in brain of heroin treated mice. Pharmazie. 2005;60:539-43.

[122] Manju V., Balasubramaniyan V., Nalini N. Rat colonic lipid peroxidation and antioxidant status: the effects of dietary luteolin on 1,2-dimethylhydrazine challenge. Cellular and Molecular Biology Letters. 2005;10: 535-51.

[123] Zarzuelo A., Jiménez I., Gámez M.J., Utrilla P., Fernadez I., Torres M.I., and Osuna I. Effects of luteolin 5-O-b-rutinoside in streptozotocin-induced diabetic rats. Life Sciences. 1996;58, 2311–2316.

[124] Kim J. S., Kwon C. S., and Son K. H. Inhibition of alpha-glucosidase and amylase by luteolin, a flavonoid. Bioscience, Biotechnology and Biochemistry. 2000;64(11): 2458-61.

[125] Ding L, Jin D, and Chen X. Luteolin enhances insulin sensitivity via activation of PPARγ transcriptional activity in adipocytes. Journal of Nutrition and Biochemistry; 2010;21(10): 941-7.

[126] Bohm F, Tinkler J.H, and Truscott T.G. Carotenoids protect against cell membrane damage by the nitrogen dioxide radical. Natural Medicine. 1995;1:98-99.

[127] Porrini M and Riso P. Lymphocyte lycopene concentration and DNA protection from oxidative damage is increased in women after a short period of tomato consumption. Journal of Nutrition. 2000;130:189-192.

[128] Arab L. and Steck S. Lycopene and cardiovascular disease. American Journal of Clinical Nutrition. 2000;71: 1691S-5S.

[129] Kuhad A., Sethi R. and Chopra K. Lycopene attenuates diabetes-associated cognitive decline in rats. Life Sciences. 2008;83:128–134.

[130] Agarwal S, and Rao A.V. Tomato Lycopene and Its Role in Human Health and Chronic Diseases. Canadian Medical Association Journal. 2000;163(6) : 739.

[131] Basuny A.M, Mostafat D.M. and Azouz A. Supplementation of polyunsaturated oils with lycopene as natural antioxidant and antipolymerization during heating process. Minia Journal of Agricultural Research and Development. 2006;26: 449-469.

[132] Basuny A.M, Gaafar A.M. and Arafat S.M. Tomato lycopene is a natural antioxidant and can alleviate hypercholesterolemia. African Journal of Biotechnology. 2009;23: 6627-6633.

[133] Hisao G, Fong T.H, Tzu N.H, Lin K.H, Chou D.S, and Sheu J.R. A potent antioxidant, lycopene, affords neuroprotection against microglia activation and focal cerebral ischemia in rats. In Vivo. 2004;18: 351- 356.

[134] Gunasekera R.S, Sewgobind K., Desai S., Dunn L, Black H.S., McKeehan W.L, and Patil B. Lycopene and lutein inhibit proliferation in rat prostate carcinoma cells. Nutrition and Cancer. 2007;58:171–177.

[135] Akbaraly N.T, Faure H., Gourlet V., Favier A. and Berr, C. Plasma carotenoid levels and cognitive performance in an elderly population: Results of the EVA Study. Journals of Gerontology, Series A, 2007;62: 308–316.

[136] Riso P., Visioli F., Grande S., Guarnieri S., Gardana C., Simonetti P., Porrini M. Effect of a tomato-based drink on markers of inflammation, immunomodulation, and oxidative stress. Journal of Agriculture and Food Chemistry. 2006;54, 2563–2566.

[137] Krinsky N.I. Carotenoids as antioxidants. Nutrition. 2001;17: 815-817.

[138] Mortensen A., Skibsted L.H., Truscott T.G. The interaction of dietary carotenoids with radical species. Archives of Biochemistry and Biophysics. 2001;385, 13–19.

[139] oung A.J. and Lowe G.M. Antioxidant and prooxidant properties of carotenoids. Archives of Biochemistry and Biophysics. 2001;385, 20–27.

[140] El-Agamey A., Lowe, G.M., McGarvey D.J., Mortensen A., Phillip D.M, Truscott T.G., Young A.J. Carotenoid radical chemistry and antioxidant or pro-oxidant properties. Archives of Biochemistry and Biophysics. 2004;430:37–48.

[141] Krinsky N.I and Johnson E.J. Carotenoid actions and their relation to health and disease. Molecular Aspects of Medicine. 2005;26: 459–516.

[142] Polidori M.C., Mecocci P., Stahl W., Parente B., Cecchetti R., Cherubini A., Cao P., Sies H., Senin U. Plasma levels of lipophilic antioxidants in very old patients with Type 2 diabetes. Diabetes/Metabolism Research and Reviews. 2000;16:15–19.

[143] Coyne T, Ibiebele T.I, Baade P.D, Dobson A, McClintock C, Dunn S, Leonard D, Shaw J. Diabetes mellitus and serum carotenoids: Findings of a population-based study in Queensland, Australia. American Journal of Clinical Nutrition. 2005;82: 685–693.

[144] Ford E.S, Will J.C, Bowman B.A, and Narayan K.M. Diabetes mellitus and serum carotenoids findings from the Third National Health and Nutrition Examination Survey. American Journal of Epidemiology. 1999;149:168-176.

[145] Kuhad A., and Chopra K. Lycopene ameliorates thermal hyperagesia and cold allodynia in STZ-induced diabetic rat. Indian Journal of Experimental Biology. 2008;46:108-111.

[146] Krul C, Luiten-Schuite A, Tenfelde A, van Ommen B, Verhagen H, and Havenaar R. dAntimutagenic activity of green tea and black tea extracts studied in a dynamic in vitro gastrointestinal model. Mutation Research. 2001;474:71–85.

[147] Schmidt M, Schmitz H.J, Baumgart A, Guedon D, Netsch M.I, Kreuter M.H, Schmidlin C.B, and Schrenk, D. Toxicity of green tea extracts and their constituents in rat hepatocytes in primary culture. Food Chemistry and Toxicology. 2005;43:307– 14.

[148] Sutherland B.A., Rosanna M.A., Rahman, Appleton I. Mechanisms of action of green tea catechins, with a focus on ischemia-induced neurodegeneration Journal of Nutritional Biochemistry. 2006;17:291– 306.

[149] Ruch R.J, Cheng S.J, and Klaunig J.E. Prevention of cytotoxicity and inhibition of intercellular communication by antioxidant catechins isolated from Chinese green tea. Carcinogenesis. 1989;10:1003–8.

[150] Guo Q, Zhao B, Li M, Shen S, and Xin W. Studies on protective mechanisms of four components of green tea polyphenols against lipid peroxidation in synaptosomes. Biochim Biophys Acta; 1996;1304:210– 22.

[151] Sawai Y and Sakata K. NMR analytical approach to clarify the antioxidative molecular mechanism of catechins using 1,1- diphenyl-2-picrylhydrazyl. Journal of Agriculture and Food Chemistry. 1998;46:111 –4.

[152] Kashima M. Effects of catechins on superoxide and hydroxyl radical. Chemical and Pharmaceutical Bulletin (Tokyo). 1999;47:279– 83.

[153] Nanjo F, Mori M, Goto K, and Hara Y. Radical scavenging activity of tea catechins and their related compounds. Bioscience Biotechnology Biochemistry.1999;63:1621–3.

[154] Zhao B, Guo Q, and Xin W. Free radical scavenging by green tea polyphenols. Methods in Enzymology. 2001;335:217–31.

[155] Sang S, Tian S, Wang H, Stark R.E, Rosen R.T, Yang C.S, and Ho C.T. Chemical studies of the antioxidant mechanism of tea catechins: radical reaction products of epicatechin with peroxyl radicals. Bioorganic and Medicinal Chemistry. 2003;11:3371– 8.

[156] Grinberg L.N, Newmark H, Kitrossky N, Rahamim E, Chevion M, and Rachmilewitz E.A. Protective effects of tea polyphenols against oxidative damage to red blood cells. Biochemistry and Pharmacology. 1997;54:973– 8.

[157] Seeram N.P and Nair M.G. Inhibition of lipid peroxidation and structure–activity-related studies of the dietary constituents anthocyanins, anthocyanidins, and catechins. Journal of Agriculture and Food Chemistry. 2002;50:5308– 12.

[158] Anderson R.F, Fisher L.J, Hara Y, Harris T, Mak W.B, Melton L.D, and Packer J.E. Green tea catechins partially protect DNA from hydroxyl radical induced strand breaks and base damage through fast chemical repair of DNA radicals. Carcinogenesis; 2001;22:1189– 93.

[159] Skrzydlewska E, Ostrowska J, Farbiszewski R, and Michalak K. Protective effect of green tea against lipid peroxidation in the rat liver, blood serum and the brain. Phytomedicine. 2002;9:232– 8.

[160] Anderson R.A and Polansky M.M. Tea enhance insulin activity. Journal of Agriculture and Food Chemistry. 2002;50: 7182-7186.

[161] Sabu M.C, Smitha K, and Kuttan R. Anti-diabetic activity of green tea polyphenols and their role in reducing oxidative stress in experimental diabetes. Journal of Ethnopharmacology. 2002;83:109-116.

[162] Tsuneki H, Ishizuka M, Terasawa M, Wu J.B, Sasaoka T, and Kimura I. Effect of green tea on blood glucose levels and serum proteomic patterns in diabetic (db/db) mice and on glucose metabolism in healthy humans. BMC Pharmacology. 2004;4:18-27.

[163] Fukino Y, Shimbo M, Aoki N, Okubo T, and Iso H. Randomized controlled trial for an effect of green tea consumption on insulin resistance and inflammation markers. Journal of Nutritional Science and Vitaminology (Tokyo); 2005;51:335-342.

[164] Rizvi S.I, Abu Zaid M, Anis R, and Mishra N. Protective role of tea catechins against oxidation-induced damage of type 2 diabetic erythrocytes. Clinical and Experimental Pharmacology and Physiology. 2005;32:70–75.

[165] Rizvi S.I, and Abu Zaid M. Impairment of sodium pump and Na/H exchanger in erythrocytes from NIDDM patients. Effect of tea catechins. Clinica Chimica Acta. 2005;354: 59–67

[166] Qin B., Panickar K.S., and Anderson R.A. Cinnamon: Potential role in the prevention of insulin resistance, metabolic syndrome, and type 2 diabetes. Journal of Diabetes Science and Technology. 2010;4: 685–693.

[167] Sirichai A., Weerachat S., Aramsri M., Sathaporn N., and Sirintorn Y. Cinnamic Acid and Its Derivatives Inhibit Fructose-Mediated Protein Glycation. International Journal of Molecular Sciences. 2012;13:1778-1789.

[168] Lee E.J., Kim S.R., Kim J., and Kim Y.C. Hepatoprotective phenylpropanoids from Scrophularia buergeriana roots against CCl4-induced toxicity: Action mechanism and structure-activity relationship. Planta Medica. 2002;68: 407–411.

[169] Natella F., Nardini M., Di, Felice M., and Scaccini C. Benzoic and cinnamic acid derivatives as antioxidants: Structure-activity relation. Journal of Agriculture and Food Chemistry.1999;47:1453–1459.

[170] Liu I.M., Hsu F.L, Chen C.F, and Cheng J.T. Antihyperglycemic action of isoferulic acid in streptozotocin-induced diabetic rats. British Journal of Pharmacology. 2000;129: 631–636.

[171] Shahidi F. and Naczk M. Cereals, legumes and nuts. In " Phenolics in Food and Nutra ceuticals, CRC press, Boca Raton, 2004;17-166.

[172] Nenadis N., Lazaridou O. and Tsimidou M. Use of reference compounds in antioxidant activity. Pancreas. 2007;15(3): 246-50.

[173] Kanchana G., Shyni W.J, Rajadurai M. and Periasamy R. Evaluation of Antihyperglycemic Effect of Sinapic Acid in Normal and Streptozotocin-Induced Diabetes in Albino Rats. Global Journal of Pharmacology. 2011;5(1): 33-39.

[174] Masoko P., Mmushi T. J., Mogashoa M. M., Mokgotho M. P., Mampuru L. J., and Howard R.L. "In vitro evaluation of the antifungal activity of Sclerocarya birrea extracts against pathogenic yeasts," African Journal of Biotechnology. 2008;7: 3521–3526.

[175] Njume C., Afolayan A. J., Green E., and Ndip R. N. "Volatile compounds in the stem bark of Sclerocarya birrea (Anacardiaceae) possess antimicrobial activity against drug-resistant strains of Helicobacter pylori. International Journal of Antimicrobial Agents. 2011;38(4): 319-324

[176] Dieye A.M, Sarr A, Diop S.N, Ndiaye M, Sy G.Y, Diarra M, Rajraji G.I, Ndiaye S.A and Faye B. Medicinal plants and the treatment of diabetes in Senegal: survey with patients. Fundamental and Clinical Pharmacology. 2008;22: 211–216.

[177] Dimo T., Rakotonirina S.V., Tan P.V., Azay J, Dongo E, Kamtchouing P, and Cros G. Effect of Sclerocarya birrea (Anacardiaceae) stem bark methylene chloride/methanol extract on streptozotocin-diabetic rats. Journal of Ethnopharmacology. 2007;110: 434–438.

[178] Kirtikar, K. R. and Basu, B. D. Indian Medicinal Plants, Bishen Singh Mahendra Pal Singh, Dehradun,, 1998;2(7):22462247.

[179] DeFeudis F.V, Papadopoulos V and Drieu K. Gingko biloba extracts and cancer: a research area in its infancy. Fundamentals of Clinical Pharmacology. 2003;17: 405- 17.

[180] Takeoka G.R and Dao L.T. Antioxidant constituent of almond [Prunus dulcis (Mill.) D.A. Webb.] hulls. Journal of Agriculture and Food Chemistry. 2003;51: 496-501.

[181] Van Rensburg W.J, Ferreira D, Malan E and Steenkamp J.A. Tyrosinase catalysed biphenyl construction from flavan-3-ol substrates. Phytochemistry. 2000;53: 285-92.

[182] Kumar R.S, Rajkapoor B, Perumal P, Dhanasekaran T, Josea M.A. and Jothimanivannan C. Antitumor Activity of Prosopis glandulosa Torr. on Ehrlich Ascites Carcinoma (EAC) Tumor Bearing Mice. Iranian Journal of Pharmaceutical Research. 2011;10: 505-510.

[183] Siddhuraju P. Antioxidant activity of polyphenolic compounds extracted from defatted raw and dry heated Tamarindus indica seed coat. LWT Food Science and Technology. 2007;40:982-990.

[184] Maiti R, Das U.K and Ghosh D (). Attenuation of Hyperglycemia and Hyperlipidemia in Streptozotocin- Induced Diabetic Rats by Aqueous Extract of Seed of Tamarindus indica. Biological and Pharmaceutical Bulletin. 2005;28:1172-1176.

[185] Martinello F, Soaresm S.M and Franco J.J. Hypolipidemic and antioxidant activities from Tamarindus indica L. pulp fruit in hypercholestromic hamsters. Food and Chemical Toxicology. 2006;44:810-818.

[186] Sudjaroen Y, Haubner R, Wu°rtele G, Hull W.E, Erben G, Spiegelhalder B, Changbumrung S, Bartsch H and Owen R.W (). Isolation and structure elucidation of phenolic antioxidants fromTamarind (Tamarindus indica L.) seeds and pericarp. Food and Chemical Toxicology. 2005;43:1673-1682.

[187] Mahmoudzades-Sagheb H, Heidari Z, Shahraki M and Moudi B. A stereological study of effects of aqueous extract of Tamarindus indica seeds on pancreatic islets in Streptozotocin-induced diabetic rats. Pakistan Journal of Pharmaceutical Sciences. 2010;23:427-434.

[188] Lebovitz, H.E. Postprandial hyperglycemic state: importance and consequences. Diabetes Research and Clinical Practice. 1998;40: S27–S28.

[189] DeFronzo R.A. Pharmacologic Therapy for Type 2 Diabetes Mellitus. Annals of Internal Medicine. 1999;131:281-303.

[190] Bailey C.J. Potential new treatments for type 2 diabetes. Trends in Pharmacological Sciences. 2000;1(7):259-65

15

Oxidative Stress and Diabetic Complications: The Role of Antioxidant Vitamins and Flavonoids

Omolola R. Ayepola, Nicole L. Brooks and Oluwafemi O. Oguntibeju

1. Introduction

Diabetes mellitus is a group of disorders of multiple aetiologies resulting from a defect in insulin secretion, insulin action, or both. Insulin deficiency in turn leads to chronic hyperglycemia (very high blood glucose levels) with disturbances in carbohydrate, fat and protein metabolism [1]. The two major types of diabetes mellitus (DM) are insulin dependent (IDDM) - type 1 and non -insulin dependent (NIDDM) -type 2. Type 1 DM is characterized by a specific destruction of the pancreatic β cells commonly associated with immune-mediated damage [2]. Individuals with type 2 DM display a gradual change in glucose homeostasis due to insulin resistance and/or decreased insulin secretion [3].

Sustained hyperglycemia leads to the progressive development of long-term microvascular and macrovascular complications which causes morbidity and mortality among those affected [4, 5]. Although glycemic control has long been the mainstay for preventing the progression of diabetic complications, there is far less evidence that these interventions reverse diabetic complications [6]. Also, limitations in intensive glycemic treatment such as difficulty in achieving and/or maintaining tight glycemic control [7], incidence of hypoglycemia and increased mortality [8, 9] suggest an urgent need for alternative and/or complementary therapies to this disorder.

Hyperglycemia-induced oxidative stress is now recognized as the driving force for the development of diabetic complications [10]. Oxidative stress in diabetes results in stimulation of the polyol pathway, formation of advanced glycation end products (AGE), activation of protein kinase C (PKC) and subsequent formation of reactive oxygen radicals [11, 12]. Hyperglycemia, not only generates more reactive oxygen species (ROS), but also attenuates antioxidative mechanisms by scavenging enzymes and substances [13].

2. The complications of diabetes mellitus (DM)

The injurious effects of hyperglycemia are separated into microvascular (involving small vessels such as capillaries) and macrovascular complications (involving large vessels, such as arteries and veins). Microvascular complications include diabetic nephropathy, neuropathy and retinopathy while macrovascular complications include coronary artery disease, peripheral arterial disease and stroke [5].

Diabetic nephropathy is a major cause of end-stage renal disease worldwide. It is a progressive decline in the glomerular filtration rate, characterized by glomerular hyperfiltration, glomerular and tubular epithelial hypertrophy, increased urinary albumin excretion, increased basement membrane thickness and mesangial expansion with the accumulation of extracellular matrix proteins (ECM) [14]. Alteration of the permeability characteristics of the glomerular capillary wall manifests clinically as abnormal albuminuria [15]. Microalbuminuria progresses to end-stage renal disease through a number of stages including normoalbuminuria, microalbuminuria and macroalbuminuria [16].

Diabetic retinopathy results from the damage of the small vasculature of the retina, multi cellular and the light sensitive tissue at the back of the eye. It is a major cause of visual impairment worldwide [17, 18]. The retina capillaries are lined with endothelial cells responsible for maintaining the blood retinal barrier, and are surrounded by smooth muscle cells, pericytes, which provide tone to the vessels [18]. The vascular lesions that are identified at the early stage of diabetic retinopathy include pericytes disappearance from capillaries resulting in pericyte ghosts, obliteration of capillaries and small arterioles, gradual thickening of vascular basement membrane, increased permeability of endothelial cells, and formation of microaneurysms (i.e. weakening of vessel walls that results in the projection of a balloonlike sac), vessel leakage, exudate, and hemorrhage [19, 20].

Neuropathies are characterized by a progressive loss of nerve fiber function. A widely accepted definition of diabetic neuropathy is "the presence of symptoms and/or signs of peripheral nerve dysfunction in people with mellitus after exclusion of other causes" [21]. In the peripheral nervous system, diabetes causes a progressive deterioration of sensory nerves and damage to motor nerves [22]. Diabetic neuropathy is ultimately the leading cause of lower extremity amputation [23]. Peripheral neuropathy is thought to develop because of cellular damage to endothelial cells, affecting nerve blood flow and also damage to the neurons affecting conductivity of impulses [23]. Signs and symptoms of diabetic neuropathy include decrease or no sweating, numbness, or tingling, and some sort of burning sensation, weakness and loss of reflexes [24].

Both type I and type II diabetes are powerful and independent risk factors for coronary artery disease (CAD), stroke, and peripheral arterial disease [25, 26, 27]. Diabetics have a 2- to 4-fold higher risk for cardiovascular events [28] and nearly 80% of diabetes-associated deaths are caused by cardiovascular disease (CVD) [29]. Atherosclerosis, (excessive accumulation of lipids, cholesterol, inflammatory cells, and connective tissue in the vessel wall) accounts for more than 80% of the CVD-associated death and disability [30, 31]. Formation of atherosclerotic plaques can result in occlusion of vessel lumen and a rapid cessation in blood flow to target tissue [32]. Hyperglycemia, increased free fatty acids, and insulin resistance induce a large number of alterations at the cellular level that contribute to vascular dysfunction and accelerate the atherosclerotic process. These include increased oxidative stress, decreased bioavailability of NO, disturbances of intracellular signal transduction and increased production of several prothrombotic factors [32, 33].

3. Role of oxidative stress in diabetic complications

Reactive oxygen species (ROS) and reactive nitrogen species (RNS) are the terms collectively describing free radicals and other non-radical reactive derivatives also called oxidants. Biological free radicals are highly unstable molecules which are products of normal cellular metabolism. They have electrons available to react with various organic substrates such as lipids, proteins and deoxyribonucleic acid (DNA). Free radicals are well recognized for playing a dual role as both deleterious and beneficial species, since they can be either harmful or beneficial to living systems [34]. At low or moderate levels free radicals (ROS and RNS) exerts beneficial effects such as defence against infectious agents, induction of a mitogenic response and the maturation process of cellular structures [35-37]. ROS include superoxide anion ($O_2^{\cdot-}$), hydroxyl ($^{\cdot}OH$), hydrogen peroxide (H_2O_2) and hypochlorous acid (HOCl) while RNS include nitric oxide ($^{\cdot}NO$), nitrogen dioxide ($NO_2^{\cdot-}$) and peroxynitrite ($OONO^-$) [38, 39]. High concentrations of free radicals on the other hand result in deleterious processes that can damage cell structures due to oxidative stress [40, 41].

Free radicals produced under physiological conditions are maintained at steady state levels by endogenous or exogenous antioxidants (externally supplied through foods or supplements) which act as free radical scavengers. However, oxidative stress occurs when the production of free radicals overwhelms the detoxification capacity of cellular antioxidant system causing biological damage [42-44]. The endogenous antioxidants (Table 1) comprise of the enzymatic antioxidants such as superoxide dismutase (SOD), glutathione peroxidase (GPx), glutathione reductase (GR), catalase (CAT), and non-enzymatic antioxidants including glutathione (GSH), α lipoic acid, vitamins C and E [39, 45, 46]. On the other hand, the exogenous antioxidants include micronutrients and other exogenously administered compounds such as vitamin E, vitamin C, trace metals (selenium, manganese, zinc), carotenoids and flavonoids [39, 44, 47].

Antioxidants	Cellular location	Role	Reference
Enzymatic Antioxidants			
(A) Catalase	Peroxisomes	Decomposition of H_2O_2 to water and oxygen	[48]
(B) Glutathione peroxidase	Cytoplasm, mitochondria, and nucleus	Detoxifies H_2O_2 and lipid peroxides with simultaneous oxidation of GSH and generation of GSSG	[49]
(C) Glutathione reductase	Cytoplasm, mitochondria, and nucleus	Recycles Glutathione disulfide back to glutathione using the cofactor NADPH	[50]
(D) Superoxide dismutase	Cytoplasm, nucleus lysosomes, mitochondria	Conversion of superoxide radical to H_2O_2	[51]
Non enzymatic antioxidants			
(A) GSH	Cytoplasm, mitochondria and nucleus	Acts as a cofactor for antioxidant enzymes (GPx, GST), regenerates other antioxidants such as Vitamins C and E to their active forms	[52]
(B) Vitamin-E	Membrane	Directly scavenge singlet oxygen, peroxyl and superoxide radicals , protects against peroxidation of membrane lipids	[34]
(C) Vitamin-C	Cytosol	Acts synergistically with vitamin E to terminate radical inducedlipid peroxidation	[34, 53]
(D) α-Lipoic acid	Cell membrane and cytoplasm	Increases glutathione and vitamin C levels	[54]

Table 1. Role of antioxidants in the protection against free radical damage

Numerous experimental evidences have highlighted a direct link between oxidative stress and diabetes through the measurement of oxidative stress biomarkers in both diabetic patient and rodents. As shown in Table 2, a hyperglycemic state can lead to an increase in the levels of oxidative DNA damage markers such as 8-hydroxy-2′-deoxyguanosine (8-OHdG) and 8-oxo-7, 8-dihydro-2'-deoxyguanosine (8-oxodG); lipid-peroxidation products measured as thiobarbituric acid-reactive substances (TBARS); protein oxidation products such as nitrotyrosine and carbonyl levels and also lower the activity of antioxidant enzymes. Cell culture studies using pancreatic beta cells, aortic smooth muscle cells and endothelial cells have also provided evidence for an increase in ROS production in diabetes [55, 56].

Due to their ability to directly oxidize and damage DNA, proteins, and lipids, free radicals are believed to play a key role in the onset and progression of late-diabetic complications [57]. In the absence of an appropriate condensation by antioxidant defense network, increased oxidative stress leads to activation of stress-sensitive intracellular signaling pathways and the formation of gene products that cause cellular damage and contribute to late diabetic complications [58-61].

	Antioxidants and macromolecules	Evidence of oxidative stress	Target tissue/organ	References
Animals	Enzymatic antioxidants	↓ SOD,CAT,GR, GPX	Liver, Pancreas, Liver, kidney	[62-64]
	Non-enzymatic antioxidant	↓ Vit E and C	Liver, kidney	[64]
		↓ GSH /GSSG,GSH	Kidney, hippocampus. Retina, Heart	[65] [66] [67] [68]
	Lipids	↑ TBARS, lipid peroxides, MDA	Kidney	[69-70]
	DNA	↑ 8-OHdG, 8-OHG	Plasma, Liver, Kidney	[71-72]
	Protein	↑ Nitrotyrosine	kidney Retina	[73] [67]
	Reactive oxygen species	↑ ROS	Hippocampus	[66]
Humans	Enzymatic antioxidants	↑ SOD,CAT, GPX	Erythrocyte	[74]
	Non enzymatic antioxidants	↓ GSH	Erythrocyte	[75]
	Lipid	↑ F2-Isoprostanes ↑ MDA	Urine Erythrocyte	[76] [77]
	DNA	↑ 8-OHdG	Urine	[78-79]
	Protein	↑ Nitrotyrosine Protein carbonyl	Plasma	[80, 81]

Table 2. Experimental evidence supporting the involvement of oxidative stress

4. Pathways of free radical generation in diabetes mellitus and its associated complications

In diabetes, ROS is thought to be generated through increased polyol pathway [82], increased formation of advanced-glycation end products (AGEs) [83] and protein kinase C (PKC) activation [84].

4.1. Aldose reductase pathway and ROS generation

Aldose reductase is the rate limiting enzyme of the polyol pathway. The nicotinamide adenine dinucleotide phosphate (NAD(P)H)-requiring aldose reductase, catalyses the reduction of glucose to sorbitol followed by the oxidation of sorbitol to fructose by NAD+ dependent sorbitol dehydrogenase. At normal blood glucose concentration (5.5 mM), aldose reductase catalyzed reaction represents less than 3% of total glucose utilization [85]. However, hyperglycemia results in saturation of hexokinase and more than 30% of glucose is directed into the polyol pathway [86]. In a diabetic state, polyol pathway increases in tissues that do not require insulin for cellular glucose uptake, such as retina, kidney, peripheral nerves and blood vessels [87].

The overall reaction of the polyol pathway leads to a shortage of intracellular NAD(P)H and a surplus of NADH, i.e, a reductive imbalance. Increased NADH generation during conversion of sorbitol to fructose provides substrate for NADH oxidase to generate ROS [88]. NADH serves as a source of electrons in complex 1 of the electron transport chain resulting in increased mitochondrial generation of superoxide radical. In diabetic cells, oxidative phosphorylation in mitochondria is enhanced due to increase flux of electron donors into the electron transport chain. This drives the inner mitochondrial membrane potential upward causing blockage of electron transfer inside complex III [89]. Electrons back up to coenzyme Q results and electrons are transferred one at a time to molecular oxygen, generating superoxide. DNA damage by superoxide and peroxynitrite results in the activation of poly (ADP-ribose) polymerase (PARP), a DNA repair enzyme. PARP reduces the activity of glyceraldehyde-3- phosphate dehydrogenase (GAPDH) (an enzyme of the glycolytic pathway which catalyses the conversion of glyceraldehydes -3 phosphate to 1, 3 biphosphoglycerate) by ADP- ribosylation [90, 91]. A consequence of GAPDH inhibition by PARP is an increase in triose phosphate pool, upstream of GAPDH and increase flux of intermediates into the damaging pathways of diabetic complications.

The polyol pathway also results in reduction in the bioavailability of NAD(P)H. The reduced bioavailability of NAD(P)H negatively affects the antioxidant defence system by depleting glutathione (GSH) a very important antioxidant. This is because the activity of GSH reductase, an antioxidant enzyme that generates GSH from its oxidized form (GSSH) depends on NAD(P)H. Depletion of NAD(P)H also decreases the synthesis of nitric oxide (NO), a vaculo-protective agent. NAD(P)H serves as a cofactor for nitric oxide synthase (NOS) which synthesizes NO from L-arginine. If endothelial nitric oxide synthase (eNOS) lack its substrate, L-arginine or one of its co-factor, it may produce superoxide radical ($\cdot O_2^{\cdot-}$) instead of NO and this is referred to as "uncoupled state of nitric oxide"[92]. Nitric oxide performs several physiological roles such as inhibition of platelet activation, vascular relaxation [93] and acts as an anti-inflammatory agent by reducing platelet aggregation and adhesion [94]. These properties inhibit atherogenesis and protect the blood vessel. Reduced bioavailability of NO level will therefore increase inflammation, enhance thrombosis and disrupt the integrity of endothelial cells. Reduction in NO has been documented in diabetes subjects with nephropathy [95]. Superoxide anion directly quenches NO by forming highly reactive peroxynitrite ($ONOO^-$) which initiates lipid peroxidation, oxidizes sulfhydryl group in protein and nitrates amino acids such as tyrosine, thereby affecting many signal transduction pathways. The polyol pathway serves as a main source of ROS generation in the retina [96]. In addition, sorbitol accumulation has been implicated in osmotic swelling of the eye lens and cataractogenesis [97].

4.2. Advanced glycation end product (AGEs) formation and ROS generation in diabetic complications

Glucose can react spontaneously with free amino groups of protein to form Schiff bases. These Schiff bases through complex reactions such as amadori rearrangement, dehydration and condensation forms cross-linked heterogeneous fluorescent derivatives called advanced glycation end products (AGEs). Advanced glycation end products constitute a heterogeneous group of molecules formed by non-enzymatic reactions of reducing sugars, ascorbate and other carbohydrates with amino acids, lipids and nucleic acids [98, 99]. Glycation end product's adducts such as pyraline, pentosidine and N- Carboxy- methyl lysine (CML) are found to be elevated in diabetic tissues [100 - 102].

Once formed, AGEs can cause tissue damage by two main pathways which are: (1) formation of cross links that alter protein structure and function and, (2) interaction of AGE with AGE-cell surface receptors on the surfaces of various cells such as endothelial cells, macrophages, neurons, and smooth-muscle cells resulting in activation of cell signaling and gene expression that induces oxidative stress and inflammation [98, 99; 102-105]. Oxidative stress can accelerate AGE formation while AGE formation can also amplify the production of more ROS resulting in a vicious cycle of AGE formation and oxidative stress.

AGE's mediate some of their effect via interaction with some receptors that have been shown to bind to these chemical moieties. Among these receptors, Receptor for Advanced Glycation End products (RAGE) is the most extensively studied [106]. Evidence from numerous studies suggest that AGE's are involved in a vicious cycle of inflammation, generation of ROS and increased production of AGE's. Ligand RAGE interaction results in activation of pathways such as p21ras, erk1/2 (p44/p42), MAP kinases, p38 and SAPK/JNK MAP kinases [107-109]. A consequence of the activation of these pathways is the nuclear translocation of transcription factor, Nuclear Factor Kappa B (NF-KB). Translocation of NF-KB to the nucleus increases the transcription of a number of proteins such as, vascular endothelial growth factor (VEGF), monocyte chemoattractant protein-1 (MCP-1), vascular cell adhesion molecule-1 (VCAM-1) and intracellular adhesion molecule-1 (ICAM-1) and pro-inflammatory cytokines such as interleukin (IL)-1β, IL-6, 1L-18 and tumour necrosis factor (TNF)-α which are centrally involved in the endothelial recruitment of neutrophil and subsequent development or progression of atherosclerotic plaque [109-112].

The gene regions of NF-KB are located at the promoter region of RAGE. Moreover, binding of NF-KB to the promoter region of RAGE results in up-regulation of RAGE itsel. Interaction of AGE with RAGE generates more oxidative stress and this further potentiates the formation of AGE's [109, 113]. Generation of ROS by ligand stimulated RAGE activation is mediated at least in part via activation of NADPH oxidase [114]. Other mechanisms by which AGE's may be linked to increased generation of ROS is by reducing the activities of enzymatic antioxidant such as SOD and CAT, lowering of glutathione stores, and activation of PKC [107, 115, 116].

Increased renal AGE in diabetic animals and patients have been linked to structural abnormality observed in diabetic nephropathy such as mesangial expansion, glomerular basement membrane thickening and tubulointerstitial fibrosis [117]. Advanced Glycation End Product's level is increased with decreased renal function in type 1 diabetic patients [118]. Evidence from clinical studies indicates a correlation between progression of diabetic retinopathy and the level of AGE in serum and retinal blood vessels of diabetic patients [100, 119]. In diabetes, increased AGE's are observed within retinal capillary cells and causes pericyte loss in diabetic retinopathy [120]. AGE's induce toxic effects on retinal pericytes by causing oxidative stress and subsequent apoptosis [121].

High levels of serum AGE's have been documented in patients with type 2 diabetes mellitus and coronary heart disease [122]. Glycation increases susceptibility of low density lipoprotein (LDL) to oxidative modification which is considered a critical step in its atherogenicity [123]. Glycation end products can also enhance atherosclerosis by trapping LDL in the subendothelium and decrease the recognition of AGE-modified LDL by LDL receptor [124]. Modification of LDL and its increased localization in vessels increases foam cell production and accelerates atherosclerosis development [125]. Oxidative stress induces AGE's formation on collagen leading to cross-linking which is considered to play a role in diabetic cardiomyopathy [126]. The intermolecular collagen cross-linking caused by AGE increases vascular stiffness and interferes with arterial blood flow [127, 128] and this partly explains the diastolic dysfunction and systolic hypertension seen in diabetic subjects.

4.3. Protein kinase C (PKC) activation and ROS generation in diabetic complications

PKC activation is related to vasoconstriction, proliferation and overgrowth of smooth muscle cells as well as accelerated synthesis of extracellular matrix proteins, and thus plays significant roles in the onset and progression of vascular cell dysfunction in diabetes mellitus [129-131]. Two major pathways have been implicated in the activation of PKC in hyperglycemia. Persistent and excessive activation of several PKC isoforms result primarily from enhanced *de novo* synthesis of diacylglycerol (DAG) from glucose via increase in triose phosphate availability [90, 105, 132, 133]. There is also evidence that the interaction between AGE's and their cell-surface receptors can result in enhanced activity of PKC isoforms [134, 135].

PKC likely regulates diabetic complications on multiple levels such as activation of eNOS, NAD(P)H oxidase, phospholipase A_2 (PLA_2), endothelin-1 (ET-1), Vascular endothelial growth factor (VEGF), Transforming growth factor-β (TGF-β), and by activating NF-KB. Diacylglycerol activated PKC alters the gene expression of key proteins leading to decrease blood flow, capillary occlusion, inflammation, free radicals generation and damage to cellular macromolecule [130-132, 136, 137].

High glucose levels can stimulate ROS production via a PKC-dependent activation of NAD(P)H oxidase in cultured aortic endothelial cells, smooth muscle cells, and renal mesangial cells [84]. Nicotinamide adenine dinucleotide phosphate oxidase, which is primarily found in phagocytic cells, is the main source of ROS in non-phagocytic cells such as mesangial cells, endothelial cells [138], fibroblasts [139], podocytes [140] and smooth muscle cells [141]. The expression of NAD(P)H oxidase components is up-regulated in vascular tissues from animal models of diabetes and in patients with diabetes and coronary artery disease [142-144]. Experimental evidence indicates that NAD(P)H oxidase-dependent production of ROS may cause DNA damage in diabetic renal tissues leading to the development of nephropathy [145]. Increased activity of the NAD(P)H oxidase has also been reported in the retina of diabetic rats suggesting its involvement in the development of diabetic retinopathy [146].

5. Antioxidant as therapeutic agents in the management of diabetes mellitus

Despite efforts to control blood glucose, tissue and organ damage are cumulative over many years in most diabetic patients. Varying degrees of hyperglycemia are virtually unavoidable in subjects with diabetes mellitus and glycemic memory has been used to describe the development of diabetes-related complications in diabetic patients even after normoglycemia has been restored and initial glycemic environment is remembered in the target organs [105,147]. It is noteworthy that ROS has been implicated as a major cause of the metabolic memory after glucose normalization due to the chains of reactions leading to cell damage and loss of cellular function. Due to the implication of hyperglycemia-induced oxidative stress in diabetes, these patients should in theory benefit from antioxidant supplementation. The beneficial effect of antioxidants has been reported in animal models of diabetes and in diabetic patients [50, 148]

6. Vitamins

Vitamin E is a fat-soluble vitamin. It has been shown that plasma α-tocopherol concentrations are lower in diabetics compared to controls [58] and appear to be even lower in diabetics with complications such as microangiopathy than in diabetics without complications [81]. Administration of Vitamin E has proven to be beneficial in preventing cellular damage by inhibition of lipid peroxidation, protein oxidation, protein glycations and platelet aggregation [149-151] Vitamin E supplementation for two weeks (600 mg/day) lowered urinary F2-isoprostanes (a marker of lipid oxidation) in type 2 diabetics [152]. It was shown in a study that a decrease in plasma F2-isoprostanes was seen in type 2 diabetic patients after six weeks supplementation with Vitamin E [153].

Oxidative stress in the kidney of diabetics is usually associated with tissue damage that interferes with proper organ function, causing an increase in urinary protein excretion and blood urea nitrogen (BUN) [154]. Vitamin E supplementation (1000 IU/kg diet) to diabetic rats for 4 weeks significantly reduced urinary protein excretion and BUN suggesting a beneficial effect on kidney function [154]. Inhibitory effect of Vitamin E on glycation of hemoglobin in type I and type 2 diabetic rats has been documented [151, 155]. The ability of vitamin E to inhibit AGE's might be due to its antioxidant effect on the autoxidative pathways of AGE formation [156]. Vitamin E administration has also reduced oxidation of low density lipoprotein (LDL) and development of atherosclerosis [157].

Numerous studies have shown that vitamin E normalized parameters of oxidative stress and inhibited vascular abnormalities caused by hyperglycemia-induced production of DAG and PKC activation in the retina, glomerulus and macrophages [158-160]. Supplementation with vitamin E reduced basement membrane thickening in diabetic rat retina and reduced vascular endothelial growth factor (VEGF) and aldose reductase activity, the abnormalities associated with diabetic retinopathy [161]. Dietary supplementation of vitamin E (2000 IU/kg) to diabetic rats for 8 weeks had cardioprotective effects which was simultaneously associated with an ability of vitamin E to blunt diabetes-induced amplification of myocardial 8-*iso* PGF2 and oxidized GSSG formation [162]. Clinical trials with vitamin E provided evidence that vitamin E may improve cardiovascular function [163, 164]. However, most large studies with vitamin E have not yielded positive benefits for decreasing the development or progression of diabetic microvascular and cardiovascular pathologies or mortality [165, 166].

Vitamin C is an antioxidant vitamin which plays an important role in protecting free radical-induced damage and a decrease in basal vitamin C levels has been documented in type 2 DM. Treatment of diabetic rats with vitamin C significantly decreased renal malondialdehyde, albuminuria, proteinuria, glomerular and tubulointerstitial sclerosis, suggesting the role of vitamin C in suppressing the progression of renal injury in diabetic rats [167]. Vitamin C also improved diabetes-induced endothelial dysfunction in a rat model by enhancing NO bioavailability [168].

The beneficial effects of vitamin C supplementation in humans are controversial. A study reported that vitamin C may improve glycemic control, lowering both fasting blood glucose and glycated haemoglobin (HbA1c) [169]. Chronic oral administration of vitamin C to patients with type 2 diabetes causes a decline in plasma free radicals that is associated with improved whole body glucose disposal [170,171] and improved endothelial function [172]. Recently, another study reported a reduction in the malondialdehyde (MDA) level, a major product of oxidative damage in both fasting and postprandial states of type 2 diabetic patients after vitamin C (1000 mg day^{-1}) supplementation for 6 weeks although no effect was observed on lipid profiles [173]. Some studies have indicated that the intra-arterial infusion of vitamin c restores endothelium-dependent vasodilation in patients with type 1 or type 2 diabetes [174, 175] suggesting that hyperglycemia-induced oxidative stress mediates endothelial dysfunction in diabetic patients.

However, in contrast to these promising results, other studies showed no beneficial effect with vitamin C treatment. Chen and colleagues [176] concluded that a high oral dose of vitamin C therapy was ineffective at improving endothelial dysfunction and insulin resistance in type 2 DM. It is important to note that complete replenishment of vitamin C levels was not achieved in the subjects. This is crucial since high concentrations of vitamin C (>80 μM) has been documented as a requirement for the preservation of NO-dependent endothelial function as vitamin C only competes with NO for superoxide anion at these high concentrations [177-178]. Also, in another study, no beneficial effects of oral vitamin C supplementation (1.5 g daily for 3 weeks) was observed on blood pressure, oxidative stress, and endothelial function in type 2 diabetes [179].

7. Flavonoids

Flavonoids (bioflavonoids) are a diverse group of polyphenols (phenyl benzopyrans) which function as phytochemicals [180]. Flavonoids are well-known for their multi-directional biological activities including anti-diabetic efficacy. Experimental evidence has shown that flavonoids exhibits anti-inflammatory [181], anticarcinogenic [182], antiviral [183] and antiallergic properties. These effects are generally associated with free radical scavenging activity of flavonoids. The antioxidant effects of flavonoids are enhanced by the number and position of hydroxyl groups in the molecule. The catechol structure, presence of unsaturation and 4-oxo function in the C-ring also contributes to their radical scavenging activity [184, 185]. Flavonoids may be capable of binding the transition metal ions, which play a role in glycoxidation, thus preventing metal-catalysed formation of hydroxyl radicals or related species from H_2O_2 [186].

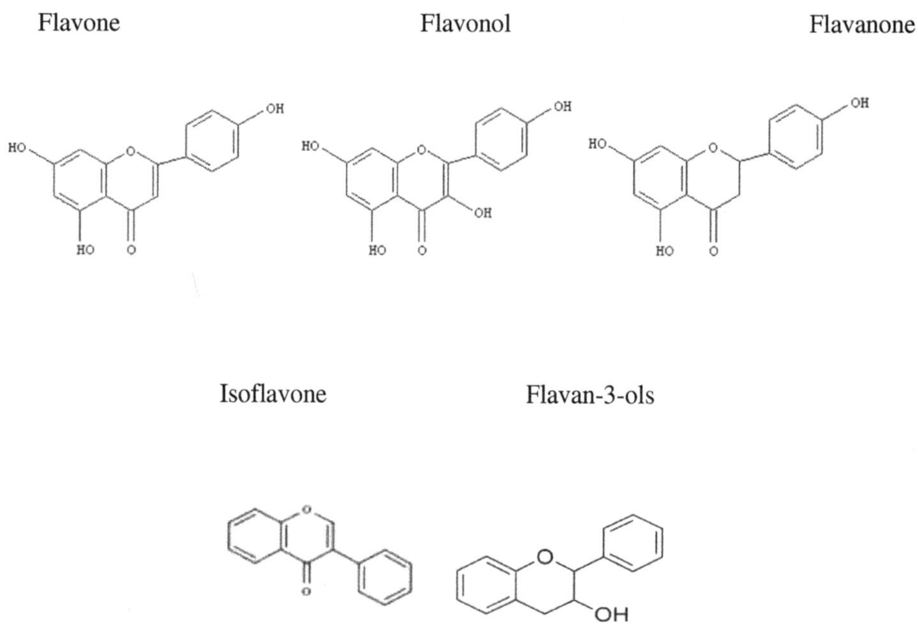

Figure 1. Classes of flavonoids [187]

The potential beneficial effects of flavonoids in the prevention of diabetes mellitus and its associated complications have been investigated both *in vitro* and *in vivo* studies (Table 3). The inhibitory effect of flavonoids on glycation has been demonstrated and it is suggested that this effect is partly due to their antioxidant properties [188]. Epigallocatechin (EGC) has a beneficial effect in a rat model of diabetic nephropathy via suppressing hyperglycemia, proteinuria and lipid peroxidation. EGC also reduced renal accumulation of AGE's and their related oxidative stress [189]. Another study demonstrated the *in vitro* inhibitory effect of different flavonoids on pentosidine formation in collagen in the presence of glucose (250 mmol/L). The decreasing inhibitiory activity was observed from myricetin, quercetin, rutin, catechin and kaempferol in a structure and concentration dependent manner [190]. Kim and colleagues [191] also investigated the effect of quercetin, isoquercitrin, hyperin and cacticin on formation of AGE's *in vitro*. At a concentration of 50 mM, the percentages of inhibition were 1.0, 89.6, 92.0 and 40.5, respectively. The inhibitory effect of hyperin on AGE formation was 6.5 times higher than that of aminoguanidine, a known AGE inhibitor which showed 14.1% inhibition at a concentration of 50 μM.

Flavonoids, in addition to their antioxidant effect, possess inhibitory activity on aldose reductase pathway and can serve as a potential multifunctional agent in the prevention of diabetic retinopathy. Goodarzi *et al.* [192] showed that oral administration of quercetin and the flavanone, naringin to streptozotocin-induced diabetic rats significantly reduced aldose reductase activity in the lenses compared to control. Oral administration of two isoflavone compounds, tectorigenin and irigenin also inhibited sorbitol accumulation in the lenses of streptozotocin induced diabetic rats [193].

Activation of PKC contributes to the loss of capillary pericytes and thickening of vascular basement membrane (BM) in diabetic retinopathy [194]. Also PKC mediated alterations in vascular permeability, blood flow, formation and response to angiogenic growth factors contribute to retinal leakage, ischemia, and neovascularisation [195]. Therefore, PKC inhibitors can be targeted for the treatment of diabetic retinopathy. Hesperetin (Hsp), a flavanone found in citrus fruits and a potent antioxidant has retina vasculo-protective properties due to its strong anti-angiogenic effect via inhibiting VEGF and PKC-β pathways [196]. Modulation of endogenous biomarkers and inhibition of diabetes induced neuropathic pain was observed in diabetic rats after naringin (4′,5,7-trihydroxy flavonone 7-rhamnoglucoside) administration [197]. In the same study, a dose dependent decrease in the levels of oxidative-nitrosative stress, inflammatory mediators as well as apoptosis was documented in neural cells. The antioxidant properties of naringin may be a factor in the inhibition of neurodegeneration.

The soy isoflavone genistein (3 and 6mg/kg), administered by a subcutaneous injection to diabetic mice relieved peripheral painful neuropathy by reverting the proinflammatory cytokine and ROS overproduction. It also restored the inducible nitric oxide synthase (iNOS) and eNOS content and increased NO production in thoracic aorta although treatment had no effect on hyperglycemia [198]. The flavonoid luteolin (200 mg/kg), when administered to rats orally, protected against the progression of diabetes-induced cardiac dysfunction by attenuation of myocardial oxidative stress probably through its antioxidant properties [199].

In a double blind placebo-controlled study, the effects of daflon 500 (made up of flavonoids diosmin (90%) and hesperidin (10%)) was investigated in a group of 28 type 1 diabetic patients. Treatment with these flavonoids resulted in a decrease in HbA_{1C} which is associated with an increase in the level and activities of thiol-containing antioxidants such as glutathione peroxidase [200]. The *in vitro* protective effect of myricetin on protein oxidation and membrane lipid peroxidation of erythrocytes from diabetic patients was reported in a study by Pandey and co-workers [201].

The treatment of diabetic rats with rutin decreased fasting plasma glucose, glycosylated haemoglobin, thiobarbituric acid reactive substances and lipid hydroperoxides while levels of non-enzymatic antioxidants were increased [202]. In another study, rutin supplementation (500 mg tablets) to diabetic patients for 60 days decreased the levels of fasting blood glucose, blood pressure and improved lipid profiles in the diabetic subjects [203]. Rutin reduced blood glucose, ameliorated oxidative stress and inhibited the accumulation of extracellular matrix

(ECM) component and glomerular basement membrane thickening in the renal cortex of diabetic rats suggesting its renoprotective effect in experimental diabetic nephropathy [204]. The inhibitory effect of rutin on AGE formation in STZ-induced rats has also been shown [205].

Diosmin (DS) (diosmetin 7-*O*-rutinoside) is a natural flavone glycoside which can be obtained by dehydrogenation of the corresponding flavanone glycoside, hesperidin that is abundant in the pericarp of various citrus fruits [206]. Diosmin treatment of streptozotocin-nicotinamide induced diabetic rats, ameliorated oxidative stress in plasma and tissues as evidenced by improved glycemic and antioxidant status along with decreased lipid peroxidation [207]. Experimental evidence showed the potential of rutin, a flavonol to delay glomerulosclerosis of diabetic nephropathy (DN) due to its ability to inhibit cell hypertrophy and the accumulation of ECM mediated by TGF-β1/Smads and ROS signals in mesangial cells cultured by high glucose [208] Quercetin enhances endothelium-derived NO bioavailability, reduced blood glucose levels and oxidative stress in diabetic rats suggesting its beneficial effect in vascular function [209].

Classes of Flavonoid and Food sources	Selected examples	Target organ, tissue or cells	Mechanism of action	Reference
Flavonols (Brussel sprouts, apples, onion, curly kale, leek, beans, cherries, Citrus fruits, Cranberries)	Morin	Liver	Decreased MDA levels, Increased activity of SOD and GSH concentration.	[210]
		Hepatocytes	Decreased ROS production, DNA damage and apoptosis. Modulation of antioxidant enzymes; GSH, CAT, SOD and GPX.	[211]
	Rutin	Kidney, serum, urine	Lowered blood glucose and improved renal function. Increased total antioxidant capability activities of SOD, CAT and GPX. Lowered ECM accumulation and AGE formation. Decreased renal expression of TGF-β.	[204]
	Quercetin	Pancreas, serum, erythrocyte.	Lowered MDA and NO level, increased antioxidant enzyme activity and preservation of islet cells integrity.	[212]
		Kidney , serum, urine	Lowered blood glucose and improved renal function. Reduced renal lipid peroxides and increased activity of anti-oxidative enzymes; SOD and CAT and non-enzymatic antioxidant GSH.	[213]

Classes of Flavonoid and Food sources	Selected examples	Target organ, tissue or cells	Mechanism of action	Reference
Flavanones (Citus peel, Orange juice, grape fruit juice, lemon juice)	Hesperidin & Naringin	Liver, serum	Boost antioxidant system by increasing activities of SOD, GR, GPx, CAT and levels of non-enzymatic antioxidants; GSH, VIT-C and VIT-E. Decreased lipid peroxidation product, MDA and proinflammatory markers, TNF-α, IL-6.	[214]
	Hesperidin	Retina, plasma	Decreased aldose reductase activity and levels of AGE's, VEGF, ICAM-1, TNF-α, IL-1β and MDA while increasing SOD activity.	[215]
	Naringenin	Pancreas, heamoglobin, serum, plasma	Lowered fasting blood glucose, decreased hyperglycemia, glycated haemoglobin, MDA and markers of hepatic damage. Increased levels of insulin and enzymatic and non-enzymatic antioxidants.	[216]
		Kidney, liver serum, urine,	Improved glycemic control and elevated insulin level, reduced plasma levels of kidney dysfunction markers. Lowered renal activity and expression of NF-KB and pro-inflammatory cytokine and chemokine, suppression of PKC activity.	[217]
Flavanolols (Milk thistle, red onion, Siberian larch tree)	Silymarin	Kidney	Increased expression and activity of SOD, GPX, CAT. Decreased high blood glucose	[218]
Flavones (Parsley, pepper celery, broccoli capsicum)	Luteolin	Kidney	Decreased activity of SOD, MDA content and expression of Heme Oxygenase-1 (HO-1) protein.	[219]
		Aortic ring	Aortic Vasorelaxation, decrease in ROS production, increased activity of SOD, NOS and level of NO.	[220]
	Diosmin	Liver and kidney	Decreased TBARS and hydroperoxides. Increased activity of enzymatic antioxidants ;SOD, CAT, GPx, GST and GR and non-enzymatic antioxidants; GSH, Vitamin C and Vitamin E.	[207]

Classes of Flavonoid and Food sources	Selected examples	Target organ, tissue or cells	Mechanism of action	Reference
Flavones	Chrysin and luteolin	Serum and aorta	Aortic relaxation, decreased blood pressure, decreased lipidemia and serum AGE's. Increased NO generation	[221]
	Apigenin	Serum and liver	Increased insulin levels and decreased hyperglycemia. Normalized LPO and endogeneous antioxidants, CAT, SOD, GSH in the liver.	[222]
Flavan-3-ols (Red wine and red grapes, green and black tea)	Catechin	Thoracic aorta	Decreased hyperglycemia NADPH oxidase activity and ROS production. Increased insulin level, lowered blood pressure and improved aortic relaxation.	[223]
	Epicatechin	Pancreatic Islets, plasma, haemoglobin	Increased anti-inflammatory cytokines, IL-10, IL-12. Improved glucose tolerance and insulin levels and lowered HbA1C.	[224]
Isoflavones (Soy foods and legumes)	Genistein	Kidney	Decreased MDA level and expression of PKC and pro-inflammatory proteins such as NF-KB, MCP-1 and Cox-2. Activation of antioxidant enzymes and defense against oxidative damage via increase expression of Nrf2, a transactivator of antioxidant genes.	[225]
	Daidzein	Aorta	Maintenance of endothelium dependent relaxation and attenuation of oxidative stress via decrease MDA levels and increase SOD activity	[226]

Abbreviations: Find all citations in this journal (defECM: Extracellular matrix, MDA: Malondialdehyde, NO: Nitric oxide, NOS: Nitric oxide synthase, NADPH; nicotinamide adenine dinucleotide phosphate, LPO: Lipid peroxidation, Nrf2: NF-E2-related factor-2, Cox-2: Cyclooxygenase-2, TAOC: Total antioxidative capability

Table 3. Beneficial effects of some flavonoids in diabetes mellitus

The inherent antioxidative properties of some common antidiabetic drugs such as aminoguanidine, statins, thiazolidinediones, glibenclamide and repaglinide also provides an additional support to the involvement of oxidative stress in diabetes and therefore suggest that the use of antioxidants as therapeutic agents in diabetes is a promising approach [227-231].

8. Conclusion and future perspective

Increased ROS production has been suggested as a common pathway linking diverse pathogenic mechanisms of diabetic vascular complications. There are numerous evidences from animal studies on the beneficial effect of antioxidant vitamins supplementation in diabetes mellitus, but results from clinical studies are inconclusive. The antioxidant activity of some anti-diabetic drugs has also been shown to contribute significantly to their therapeutic effect. Biflavonoids as antioxidants are promising and attractive natural substances to enrich the current therapy options against diabetes. The overall positive results from animal studies suggest that the role of antioxidants cannot be underestimated in the quest to find effective therapies for diabetic complications. A multi-therapeutic approach to the treatment of diabetic complications might increase the chance of successful therapeutic intervention. In addition to maintaining glycemic control, blockage of pathways involved in the formation of free radicals with antioxidants is a promising approach to the treatment of hyperglycemia-mediated complications in humans. The bioactivity of flavonoids *in vivo* can be greatly influenced by metabolism and bioavailability and this information is limited in many studies. Limited clinical studies have been carried out to support the beneficial effects of flavonoids in the prevention of diabetic complications. In order to achieve the goal of using flavonoids in the management of diabetes mellitus, further investigation on the long and short-term effect of the ingestion of flavonoids in humans is warranted.

Author details

Omolola R. Ayepola[1], Nicole L. Brooks[2] and Oluwafemi O. Oguntibeju[1*]

*Address all correspondence to: oguntibejuo@cput.ac.za, bejufemi@yahoo.co.uk.

1 Nutrition and Chronic Disease Research Unit, Oxidative Stress Research Centre, Department of Biomedical Sciences, Faculty of Health and Wellness Sciences, Cape Peninsula University of Technology, Bellville, South Africa

2 Department of Wellness Sciences, Faculty of Health and Wellness Sciences, Cape Peninsula University of Technology, Cape Town, South Africa

References

[1] Bastaki, A. 2005. Diabetes mellitus and its treatment. *Int J Diab and Metab* 13(3): 111.

[2] Zhao, Y. 2011. Autoimmunity and Therapeutic Challenges of Type 1 Diabetes. *Transl Med*,1: 104e

[3] Ruhe, R.C. & McDonald, R.B. 2001. Use of antioxidant nutrients in the prevention and treatment of type 2 diabetes. *J Am Coll Nutr, 20* (sup5): 363S-369S.

[4] Resnick, H.E. & Howard, B.V. 2002. Diabetes and cardiovascular disease. *Annu Rev Med,* 53(1): 245-267.

[5] Fowler, M.J. 2008. Microvascular and macrovascular complications of diabetes. *Clin Diabetes,* 26(2): 77-82.

[6] Cook, M.N., Girman, C.J., Stein, P.P., Alexander, C.M. & Holman, R.R. 2005. Glycemic control continues to deteriorate after sulfonylureas are added to metformin among patients with type 2 diabetes. *Diabetes Care,* 28(5): 995-1000.

[7] Kowluru, R.A., Abbas, S.N. & Odenbach, S. 2004. Reversal of hyperglycemia and diabetic nephropathy: effect of reinstitution of good metabolic control on oxidative stress in the kidney of diabetic rats. *J Diabetes Complication,* 18(5): 282-288.

[8] Mayor, S. 2008. Intensive glucose lowering arm of diabetes trial is stopped after excess deaths. *Br Med J,* 336(7641): 407.

[9] Ismail-Beigi, F., Craven, T., Banerji, M.A., Basile, J., Calles, J., Cohen, R.M., Cuddihy, R., Cushman, W.C., Genuth, S. & Grimm Jr, R.H. 2010. Effect of intensive treatment of hyperglycaemia on microvascular outcomes in type 2 diabetes: an analysis of the ACCORD randomised trial. *The Lancet,* 376(9739): 419-430.

[10] Kawahito, S., Kitahata, H. & Oshita, S. 2009. Problems associated with glucose toxicity: Role of hyperglycemia-induced oxidative stress. *World J Gastroenterol:* 15(33): 4137.

[11] Ceriello, A. 2003. New insights on oxidative stress and diabetic complications may lead to a "causal" antioxidant therapy. *Diabetes Care,* 26(5): 1589-1596.

[12] Giacco, F. & Brownlee, M. 2010. Oxidative stress and diabetic complications. *Circ Res,* 107(9): 1058-1070.

[13] Zhang, C., Liu, J., Pan, H., Yang, X. & Bian, K. 2011. Mitochondrial dysfunction induced by excessive ROS/RNS-metabolic cardiovascular disease and traditional Chinese medicines intervention. *China J Chinese Mat med,* 36(17): 2423.

[14] Jain, M. 2012. Histopathological changes in diabetic kidney disease. *Clin Queries: Nephrol,* 1(2): 127-133.

[15] Lewis, E.J. & Xu, X. 2008. Abnormal Glomerular Permeability Characteristics in Diabetic Nephropathy Implications for the therapeutic use of low–molecular weight heparin. *Diabetes Care,* 31(Supplement 2): S202-S207.

[16] O'Connor, A.S. & Schelling, J.R. 2005. Diabetes and the kidney. *Am J Kidney Dis,* 46(4): 766-773.

[17] Marshall, S.M.m& Flyvbjerg, A. 2006. Prevention and early detection of vascular complications of diabetes. *Br Med J,* 333(7566): 475.

[18] Santos, J.M., Mohammad, G., Zhong, Q. & Kowluru, R.A. 2011. Diabetic retinopathy, superoxide damage and antioxidants. *Curr Pharm Biotechnol* 1;12(3):352-61

[19] Engerman, R.L. 1989. Pathogenesis of diabetic retinopathy. *Diabetes,* 38 (10): 1203-1206.

[20] Hammes, H. 2005. Pericytes and the pathogenesis of diabetic retinopathy. *Horm Metab Res,* 37(S 1): 39-43.

[21] American Diabetes Association: Standards of medical care in diabetes 2007 [Position Statement]. *Diabetes Care* 30:S4–S41, 2007

[22] Pazdro, R. & Burgess, J.R. 2010. The role of vitamin E and oxidative stress in diabetes complications. *Mech Ageing Dev,* 131(4): 276-286.

[23] Obrosova, I.G. 2009. Diabetes and the peripheral nerve. *Biochim Biophys Acta,* 1792(10): 931-940.

[24] Soumya, D. 2011. Late Stage Complications of Diabetes and Insulin Resistance. *J Diabetes Metabol,* 2:167

[25] Schwartz, C.J., Valente, A.J., Sprague, E.A., Kelley, J.L., Cayatte, A.J. & Rozek, M.M. 1992. Pathogenesis of the atherosclerotic lesion: implications for diabetes mellitus. *Diabetes Care,* 15(9): 1156-1167.

[26] American Diabetes association. Consensus Statement, 1993. Role of cardiovascular risk factors in prevention and treatment of macrovascular disease in diabetes. *Diabetes Care.* 16:72-78.

[27] Orchard, T.J., Costacou, T., Kretowski, A. & Nesto, R.W. 2006. Type 1 diabetes and coronary artery disease. *Diabetes Care,* 29(11): 2528-2538.

[28] Ding, H. & Triggle, C.R. 2005. Endothelial cell dysfunction and the vascular complications associated with type 2 diabetes: assessing the health of the endothelium. *Vasc Health Risk Manag,* 1(1): 55.

[29] Winer, N. & Sowers, J.R. 2004. Epidemiology of diabetes. *J Clin Pharmacol,* 44(4): 397-405.

[30] Epstein, F.H. & Ross, R. 1999. Atherosclerosis-an inflammatory disease. *New Engl J Med,* 340(2): 115-126.

[31] Libby, P., Ridker, P.M. & Hansson, G.K. 2011. Progress and challenges in translating the biology of atherosclerosis. *Nature,* 473(7347): 317-325.

[32] Funk, S.D., Yurdagul, A. & Orr, A.W. 2012. Hyperglycemia and endothelial dysfunction in atherosclerosis: lessons from type 1 diabetes. *Int J Vasc Med,* 2012:1-19.

[33] Creager, M.A., Lüscher, T.F., Cosentino, F. & Beckman, J.A. 2003. Diabetes and vascular disease pathophysiology, clinical consequences, and medical therapy: part I. *Circulation,* 108(12): 1527-1532.

[34] Valko, M., Leibfritz, D., Moncol, J., Cronin, M.T., Mazur, M. & Telser, J. 2007. Free radicals and antioxidants in normal physiological functions and human disease. *Int J Biochem Cell Biol,* 39(1): 44-84.

[35] Dröge, W. 2002. Free radicals in the physiological control of cell function. *Physiol Rev,* 82(1): 47-95.

[36] Pacher, P., Beckman, J.S. & Liaudet, L. 2007. Nitric oxide and peroxynitrite in health and disease. *Physiol Rev,* 87(1): 315-424.

[37] Sachdev, S. & Davies, K.J. 2008. Production, detection, and adaptive responses to free radicals in exercise. *Free Radic Biol Med,* 44(2): 215-223.

[38] Sies, H. 1997. Oxidative stress: Oxidants and antioxidants. *Exp Physiol., 82,* 291–295.

[39] Halliwell, B. & Gutteridge, J. M. C., 2007. *Free Radic Biol Med.* 4th. Edn, Clarendon Press, Oxford

[40] Bahorun, T., Soobrattee, M., Luximon-Ramma, V. & Aruoma, O. 2006. Free radicals and antioxidants in cardiovascular health and disease. *Internet J Med Update,* 1(2): 25-41.

[41] Halliwell, B. 2007. Biochemistry of oxidative stress. *Biochem Soc Trans,* 35(Pt 5): 1147-1150.

[42] Abdollahi, M., Ranjbar, A., Shadnia, S., Nikfar, S. & Rezaie, A. 2004. Pesticides and oxidative stress: a review. *Medical science monitor: Int Med J Exp and Clin Res,* 10(6): RA141-7.

[43] Ridnour, L.A., Thomas, D.D., Mancardi, D., Espey, M.G., Miranda, K.M., Paolocci, N., Feelisch, M., Fukuto, J. & Wink, D.A. 2004. The chemistry of nitrosative stress induced by nitric oxide and reactive nitrogen oxide species. Putting perspective on stressful biological situations. *Biol Chem,* 385(1): 1-10.

[44] Halliwell, B. 2011. Free radicals and antioxidants. *Trends Pharmacol Sci,* 32(3): 125-130.

[45] Fukai, T. & Ushio-Fukai, M. 2011. Superoxide dismutases: role in redox signaling, vascular function, and diseases. *Antioxid Redox Signal,* 15(6): 1583-1606.

[46] Lubos, E., Loscalzo, J. & Handy, D.E. 2011. Glutathione peroxidase-1 in health and disease: from molecular mechanisms to therapeutic opportunities. *Antioxid Redox Signal,* 15(7): 1957-1997.

[47] Pham-Huy, L.A., He, H. & Pham-Huy, C. 2008. Free radicals, antioxidants in disease and health. *Int J Biomed Sc:* 4(2): 89.

[48] Winterbourn, C.C. 1993. Superoxide as an intracellular radical sink. *Free Radic Biol Med,* 14(1): 85-90.

[49] Jurkovič, S., Osredkar, J. & Marc, J. 2008. Molecular impact of glutathione peroxidases in antioxidant processes. *Biochem Med,* 18(2): 162-174.

[50] Maritim, A., Sanders, R. & Watkins, 3.J. 2003. Diabetes, oxidative stress, and antioxidants: a review. *J Biochem and Mol Tox,* 17(1): 24-38.

[51] Zelko, I.N., Mariani, T.J. & Folz, R.J. 2002. Superoxide dismutase multigene family: a comparison of the CuZn-SOD (SOD1), Mn-SOD (SOD2), and EC-SOD (SOD3) gene structures, evolution, and expression. *Free Radic Biol Med,* 33(3): 337-349.

[52] Livingstone, C. & Davis, J. 2007. Review: Targeting therapeutics against glutathione depletion in diabetes and its complications. *Br J Diabetes Vasc Dis,* 7(6): 258-265.

[53] May, J.M., Qu, Z. & Morrow, J.D. 1996. Interaction of Ascorbate and-Tocopherol in Resealed Human Erythrocyte Ghosts. Transmembrane electron transfer and protection from lipid peroxidation. *J Biol Chem,* 271(18): 10577-10582.

[54] Smith, A., Shenvi, S., Widlansky, M., Suh, J. & Hagen, T. 2004. Lipoic acid as a potential therapy for chronic diseases associated with oxidative stress. *Curr Med Chem,* 11(9): 1135-1146.

[55] Inoguchi, T., Li, P., Umeda, F., Yu, H.Y., Kakimoto, M., Imamura, M., Aoki, T., Etoh, T., Hashimoto, T. & Naruse, M. 2000. High glucose level and free fatty acid stimulate reactive oxygen species production through protein kinase C--dependent activation of NAD (P) H oxidase in cultured vascular cells. *Diabetes,* 49(11): 1939-1945.

[56] Lee JL, Suh KS, Choi MC, Chon S, Oh S, Woo JT, Kim SW,Kim JW, Kim YS (2010). Kaempferol protects HIT-15 pancreatic beta-cells from 2-deoxy-D-ribose-induced oxidative damage. *Phytother Res* 24:419-423

[57] Rösen, P., Nawroth, P., King, G., Möller, W., Tritschler, H. & Packer, L. 2001. The role of oxidative stress in the onset and progression of diabetes and its complications: asummary of a Congress Series sponsored byUNESCO-MCBN, the American Diabetes Association and the German Diabetes Society. *Diabetes Metabol Res Rev,* 17(3): 189-212.

[58] Nourooz-Zadeh, J., Rahimi, A., Tajaddini-Sarmadi, J., Tritschler, H., Rosen, P., Halliwell, B. & Betteridge, D. 1997. Relationships between plasma measures of oxidative stress and metabolic control in NIDDM. *Diabetologia,* 40(6): 647-653.

[59] Brownlee, M. 2001. Biochemistry and molecular cell biology of diabetic complications. *Nature,* 414(6865): 813-820.

[60] Evans, J.L., Goldfine, I.D., Maddux, B.A. & Grodsky, G.M. 2002. Oxidative stress and stress-activated signaling pathways: a unifying hypothesis of type 2 diabetes. *Endocr Rev,* 23(5): 599-622.

[61] Shih, C., Wu, Y. & Lin, W. 2002. Antihyperglycaemic And Anti-Oxidant Properties Of Anoectochilus Formosanus in Diabetic Rats. *Clin Exp Pharmacol Physiol,* 29(8): 684-688.

[62] Manna, P., Das, J., Ghosh, J. & Sil, P.C. 2010. Contribution of type 1 diabetes to rat liver dysfunction and cellular damage via activation of NOS, PARP, IκBα/NF-κB,

MAPKs, and mitochondria-dependent pathways: Prophylactic role of arjunolic acid. *Free Radic Biol Med,* 48(11): 1465-1484.

[63] Hamden, K., Boujbiha, M.A., Masmoudi, H., Ayadi, F.M., Jamoussi, K. & Elfeki, A. 2009. Combined vitamins (C and E) and insulin improve oxidative stress and pancreatic and hepatic injury in alloxan diabetic rats. *Biomed Pharmacother,* 63(2): 95-99.

[64] Prabakaran D, Ashokkumar N. Protective effect of esculetin on hyperglycemia-mediated oxidative damage in the hepatic and renal tissues of experimental diabetic rats. *Biochimie.* 2013 95(2):366-73.

[65] Erejuwa, O.O., Sulaiman, S.A., Wahab, M.S.A., Salam, S.K.N., Salleh, M.S.M. & Gurtu, S. 2011. Comparison of antioxidant effects of honey, glibenclamide, metformin, and their combinations in the kidneys of streptozotocin-induced diabetic rats. *Int J Mol Sci,* 12(1): 829-843.

[66] Aragno, M., Mastrocola, R., Medana, C., Restivo, F., Catalano, M.G., Pons, N., Danni, O. & Boccuzzi, G. 2005. Up-regulation of advanced glycated products receptors in the brain of diabetic rats is prevented by antioxidant treatment. *Endocrinology,* 146(12): 5561-5567.

[67] Kowluru, R.A. & Kanwar, M. 2007. Effects of curcumin on retinal oxidative stress and inflammation in diabetes. *Nutr and metabol,* 4: 8

[68] Babu, P.V.A., Sabitha, K.E. & Shyamaladevi, C.S. 2006. Therapeutic effect of green tea extract on oxidative stress in aorta and heart of streptozotocin diabetic rats. *Chem Biol Interac,* 162(2): 114-120.

[69] Ramesh, B., Viswanathan, P. & Pugalendi, K.V. 2007. Protective effect of Umbelliferone on membranous fatty acid composition in streptozotocin-induced diabetic rats. *Eur J Pharmacol,* 566(1): 231-239.

[70] Haidara, M.A., Mikhailidis, D.P., Rateb, M.A., Ahmed, Z.A., Yassin, H.Z., Ibrahim, I.M. & Rashed, L.A. 2009. Evaluation of the effect of oxidative stress and vitamin E supplementation on renal function in rats with streptozotocin-induced Type 1 diabetes. *J Diabetes and Its Complications,* 23(2): 130-136.

[71] Rajavel, V., Sattar, A., Zubaid, M., Abdulla, M.A., Kassim, N.M. & Abdullah, N.A. 2012. Chronic Administration of Oil Palm (Elaeis guineensis) Leaves Extract Attenuates Hyperglycaemic-Induced Oxidative Stress and Improves Renal Histopathology and Function in Experimental Diabetes. *Evid Base Compl Alternative Med,* doi: 10.1155/2012/195367

[72] Park, K.S., Kim, J.H., Kim, M.S., Kim, J.M., Kim, S.K., Choi, J.Y., Chung, M.H., Han, B., Kim, S.Y. & Lee, H.K. 2001. Effects of insulin and antioxidant on plasma 8-hydroxyguanine and tissue 8-hydroxydeoxyguanosine in streptozotocin-induced diabetic rats. *Diabetes,* 50(12): 2837-2841.

[73] Figarola, J., Scott, S., Loera, S., Tessler, C., Chu, P., Weiss, L. & Hardy, J. 2003. LR-90 a new advanced glycation endproduct inhibitor prevents progression of diabetic nephropathy in streptozotocin-diabetic rats. *Diabetologia,* 46(8): 1140-1152.

[74] Likidlilid A, Patchanans N, Peerapatdit T, Sriratanasathavorn C, 2010. Lipid Peroxidation and Antioxidant Enzyme Activities in Erythrocytes of Type 2 Diabetic Patients. *J Med Assoc Thai,* 93 (6): 682-93

[75] Sekhar, R.V., McKay, S.V., Patel, S.G., Guthikonda, A.P., Reddy, V.T., Balasubramanyam, A. & Jahoor, F. 2011. Glutathione synthesis is diminished in patients with uncontrolled diabetes and restored by dietary supplementation with cysteine and glycine. *Diabetes Care,* 34(1): 162-167.

[76] Flores L, Rodela S, Abian J, Clària J, Esmatjes E, 2004 F2 isoprostane is already increased at the onset of type 1 diabetes mellitus: effect of glycemic control. *Metabolism.* 2004;53(9):1118-1120.

[77] Selvaraj, N., Bobby, Z. & Sathiyapriya, V. 2006. Effect of lipid peroxides and antioxidants on glycation of hemoglobin: an in vitro study on human erythrocytes. *Clin Chim Acta,* 366(1): 190-195.

[78] Goodarzi, M.T., Navidi, A.A., Rezaei, M. & Babahmadi-Rezaei, H. 2010. Oxidative damage to DNA and lipids: correlation with protein glycation in patients with type 1 diabetes. J *Clin Lab Anal,* 24(2): 72-76.

[79] Hinokio, Y., Suzuki, S., Hirai, M., Suzuki, C., Suzuki, M. & Toyota, T. 2002. Urinary excretion of 8-oxo-7, 8-dihydro-2′-deoxyguanosine as a predictor of the development of diabetic nephropathy. *Diabetologia,* 45(6): 877-882.

[80] Ceriello, A., Mercuri, F., Quagliaro, L., Assaloni, R., Motz, E., Tonutti, L. & Taboga, C. 2001. Detection of nitrotyrosine in the diabetic plasma: evidence of oxidative stress. *Diabetologia,* 44(7): 834-838.

[81] Martín-Gallán, P., Carrascosa, A., Gussinyé, M. & Domínguez, C. 2003. Biomarkers of diabetes-associated oxidative stress and antioxidant status in young diabetic patients with or without subclinical complications. *Free Rad Biol Med,* 34(12): 1563-1574.

[82] Chung, S.S., Ho, E.C., Lam, K.S. & Chung, S.K. 2003. Contribution of polyol pathway to diabetes-induced oxidative stress. *Journal of the American Society of Nephrology,* 14(suppl 3): S233-S236.

[83] Baynes, J.W. & Thorpe, S.R. 1999. Role of oxidative stress in diabetic complications: a new perspective on an old paradigm. *Diabetes,* 48(1): 1-9.

[84] Inoguchi, T., Sonta, T., Tsubouchi, H., Etoh, T., Kakimoto, M., Sonoda, N., Sato, N., Sekiguchi, N., Kobayashi, K. & Sumimoto, H. 2003. Protein kinase C–dependent increase in reactive oxygen species (ROS) production in vascular tissues of diabetes: role of vascular NAD (P) H oxidase. *Clin J Am Soc Nephrol,* 14(suppl 3): S227-S232.

[85] Morrison, A.D., Clements Jr, R.S., Travis, S.B., Oski, F. & Winegrad, A.I. 1970. Glucose utilization by the polyol pathway in human erythrocytes. *Biochem Biophys Res Comm,* 40(1): 199-205.

[86] González, R.G., Barnett, P., Aguayo, J., Cheng, H. & Chylack, L. 1984. Direct measurement of polyol pathway activity in the ocular lens. *Diabetes,* 33(2): 196-199.

[87] Stephen S.M. Chung, Eric C.M. HO, Karen S.L. Lam, and Sookja K. Chung, 2003. Contribution of Polyol Pathway to Diabetes-Induced Oxidative Stress. *J Am Soc Nephrol* 14: S233–S236

[88] Morre, D.M., Lenaz, G. & Morre, D.J. 2000. Surface oxidase and oxidative stress propagation in aging. *J Exp Biol,* 203(10): 1513-1521.

[89] Yang, X. & Trumpower, B.L. 1988. Protonmotive Q cycle pathway of electron transfer and energy transduction in the three-subunit ubiquinol-cytochrome c oxidoreductase complex of Paracoccus denitrificans. *J Biol Chem,* 263(24): 11962-11970.

[90] Du, X., Matsumura, T., Edelstein, D., Rossetti, L., Zsengellér, Z., Szabó, C. & Brownlee, M. 2003. Inhibition of GAPDH activity by poly (ADP-ribose) polymerase activates three major pathways of hyperglycemic damage in endothelial cells. *J Clin Investig,* 112(7): 1049-1057.

[91] Soriano, F.G., Virág, L., Jagtap, P., Szabó, É., Mabley, J.G., Liaudet, L., Marton, A., Hoyt, D.G., Murthy, K.G. & Salzman, A.L. 2001. Diabetic endothelial dysfunction: the role of poly (ADP-ribose) polymerase activation. *Nature Med,* 7(1): 108-113.

[92] Vásquez-Vivar, J., Kalyanaraman, B., Martásek, P., Hogg, N., Masters, B.S.S., Karoui, H., Tordo, P. & Pritchard, K.A. 1998. Superoxide generation by endothelial nitric oxide synthase: the influence of cofactors. *Proc Natl Acad Sci,* 95(16): 9220-9225.

[93] Mehta, J.L., Rasouli, N., Sinha, A.K. & Molavi, B. 2006. Oxidative stress in diabetes: a mechanistic overview of its effects on atherogenesis and myocardial dysfunction. *Int J Biochem Cell Biol,* 38(5): 794-803.

[94] Sharma, J., Al-Omran, A. & Parvathy, S. 2007. Role of nitric oxide in inflammatory diseases. *Inflammopharmacology,* 15(6): 252-259.

[95] Tessari, P., Cecchet, D., Cosma, A., Vettore, M., Coracina, A., Millioni, R., Iori, E., Puricelli, L., Avogaro, A. & Vedovato, M. 2010. Nitric oxide synthesis is reduced in subjects with type 2 diabetes and nephropathy. *Diabetes,* 59(9): 2152-2159.

[96] Mara, L. & Oates, P.J. 2008. Diabetic Retinopathy. In *The Polyol Pathway and Diabetic Retinopathy.* : Springer: 159-186. Contemporary Diabetes 2008:159-186

[97] Patel, D., Prasad, S., Kumar, R. & Hemalatha, S. 2011. Cataract: A major secondary complication of diabetes, its epidemiology and an overview on major medicinal plants screened for anticataract activity. *Asian Pac J Tropical Dis,* 1(4): 323-329.

[98] Vlassara, H. & Palace, M. 2002. Diabetes and advanced glycation endproducts. *J Intern Medicine,* 251(2): 87-101.

[99] Peppa, M., Uribarri, J. & Vlassara, H. 2004. The role of advanced glycation end products in the development of atherosclerosis. *Curr Diabetes Rep,* 4(1): 31-36.

[100] Stitt, A.W. 2001. Advanced glycation: an important pathological event in diabetic and age related ocular disease. *Br J Ophthalmol,* 85(6): 746-753.

[101] Wautier, J. & Guillausseau, P. 2001. Advanced glycation end products, their receptors and diabetic angiopathy. *Diabetes Metabol,* 27(5; PART 1): 535-544.

[102] Ahmed, N., 2005. Advanced glycation end products-role in pathology of diabetic complications. *Diabetes Res Clin Pract* 67, 3-21.

[103] Nishikawa, T., Edelstein, D., Du, X.L., Yamagishi, S., Matsumura, T., Kaneda, Y., Yorek, M.A., Beebe, D., Oates, P.J. & Hammes, H. 2000. Normalizing mitochondrial superoxide production blocks three pathways of hyperglycaemic damage. *Nature,* 404(6779): 787-790.

[104] Sourris, K.C. & Forbes, J.M. 2009. Interactions between advanced glycation end-products (AGE) and their receptors in the development and progression of diabetic nephropathy-are these receptors valid therapeutic targets. *Curr Drug Targets,* 10(1): 42-50.

[105] Giacco, F. & Brownlee, M. 2010. Oxidative stress and diabetic complications. *Circ Res,* 107(9): 1058-1070.

[106] Ramasamy, R., Vannucci, S.J., Du Yan, S.S., Herold, K., Yan, S.F. & Schmidt, A.M. 2005. Advanced glycation end products and RAGE: a common thread in aging, diabetes, neurodegeneration, and inflammation. *Glycobiology,* 15(7): 16R-28R.

[107] Yan, S.D., Schmidt, A.M., Anderson, G.M., Zhang, J., Brett, J., Zou, Y.S., Pinsky, D. & Stern, D. 1994. Enhanced cellular oxidant stress by the interaction of advanced glycation end products with their receptors/binding proteins. *J Biol Chem,* 269(13): 9889-9897.

[108] Lander, H.M., Tauras, J.M., Ogiste, J.S., Hori, O., Moss, R.A. & Schmidt, A.M. 1997. Activation of the receptor for advanced glycation end products triggers a p21 ras-dependent mitogen-activated protein kinase pathway regulated by oxidant stress. *J Biol Chem,* 272(28): 17810-17814.

[109] Goldin, A., Beckman, J.A., Schmidt, A.M. & Creager, M.A. 2006. Advanced glycation end products sparking the development of diabetic vascular injury. *Circulation,* 114(6): 597-605.

[110] Cybulski MI, Gimbrone MA., 1991. Endothelial expression of a mononuclear leukocyte adhesion molecule during atherogenesis. *Science.* 251:788-791

[111] Rubanyi, G.M. 1993. The role of endothelium in cardiovascular homeostasis and diseases. *J Cardiovasc Pharmacol,* 22: S15-S18.

[112] Schiekofer, S., Andrassy, M., Chen, J., Rudofsky, G., Schneider, J., Wendt, T., Stefan, N., Humpert, P., Fritsche, A. & Stumvoll, M. 2003. Acute hyperglycemia causes intracellular formation of CML and activation of ras, p42/44 MAPK, and nuclear factor κB in PBMCs. *Diabetes,* 52(3): 621-633.

[113] Barbosa, J.H., Oliveira, S.L. & Seara, L.T. 2008. The role of advanced glycation end-products (AGEs) in the development of vascular diabetic complications. *Arq Bras Endocrinol Metabol,* 52(6): 940-950.

[114] Wautier, M., Chappey, O., Corda, S., Stern, D.M., Schmidt, A.M. & Wautier, J. 2001. Activation of NADPH oxidase by AGE links oxidant stress to altered gene expression via RAGE. *Am J Physiol Endocrinol Metabol,* 280(5): E685-E694.

[115] Obrosova, I.G. 2002. How does glucose generate oxidative stress in peripheral nerve? *Int Rev Neurobiol,* 50: 3-35.

[116] Jiang, J., Wang, Z. & Li, D. 2004. Effects of AGEs on oxidation stress and antioxidation abilities in cultured astrocytes. *Biomed Environ Sc,* 17(1): 79-86.

[117] Yamagishi, S. & Matsui, T. 2010. Advanced glycation end products, oxidative stress and diabetic nephropathy. *Oxid Med and Cell Longev,* 3(2): 101-108.

[118] Miura, J., Yamagishi, S., Uchigata, Y., Takeuchi, M., Yamamoto, H., Makita, Z. & Iwamoto, Y. 2003. Serum levels of non-carboxymethyllysine advanced glycation end-products are correlated to severity of microvascular complications in patients with Type 1 diabetes. *J Diabetes Complications,* 17(1): 16-21.

[119] Ono, Y., Aoki, S., Ohnishi, K., Yasuda, T., Kawano, K. & Tsukada, Y. 1998. Increased serum levels of advanced glycation end-products and diabetic complications. *Diabetes Res Clin Prac,* 41(2): 131-137.

[120] Stitt, A.W. 2003. The role of advanced glycation in the pathogenesis of diabetic retinopathy. *Exp Mol Pathol,* 75(1): 95-108.

[121] Chen, B., Jiang, D. & Tang, L. 2006. Advanced glycation end-products induce apoptosis involving the signaling pathways of oxidative stress in bovine retinal pericytes. *Life Sci,* 79(11): 1040-1048.

[122] Kilhovd, B.K., Berg, T.J., Birkeland, K.I., Thorsby, P. & Hanssen, K.F. 1999. Serum levels of advanced glycation end products are increased in patients with type 2 diabetes and coronary heart disease. *Diabetes Care,* 22(9): 1543-1548.

[123] Bowie, A., Owens, D., Collins, P., Johnson, A. & Tomkin, G.H. 1993. Glycosylated low density lipoprotein is more sensitive to oxidation: implications for the diabetic patient? *Atherosclerosis,* 102(1): 63-67.

[124] Bucala, R., Makita, Z., Vega, G., Grundy, S., Koschinsky, T., Cerami, A. & Vlassara, H. 1994. Modification of low density lipoprotein by advanced glycation end products

contributes to the dyslipidemia of diabetes and renal insufficiency. *Proc Natl Acad Sci,* 91(20): 9441-9445.

[125] Sobenin, I., Tertov, V., Koschinsky, T., Bünting, C., Slavina, E., Dedovc, I. & Orekhov, A. 1993. Modified low density lipoprotein from diabetic patients causes cholesterol accumulation in human intimal aortic cells. *Atherosclerosis,* 100(1): 41-54.

[126] Goh, S. & Cooper, M.E. 2008. The role of advanced glycation end products in progression and complications of diabetes. *J Clin Endocrinol Metabol,* 93(4): 1143-1152.

[127] Eble, A.S., Thorpe, S.R. & Baynes, J.W. 1983. Nonenzymatic glucosylation and glucose-dependent cross-linking of protein. *J Biol Chem,* 258(15): 9406-9412.

[128] Cooper, M.E., Bonnet, F., Oldfield, M. & Jandeleit-Dahm, K. 2001. Mechanisms of diabetic vasculopathy: an overview. *Am J Hypertens,* 14(5): 475-486.

[129] Koya, D. & King, G.L. 1998. Protein kinase C activation and the development of diabetic complications. *Diabetes,* 47(6): 859-866.

[130] Meier, M. & King, G.L. 2000. Protein kinase C activation and its pharmacological inhibition in vascular disease. *Vasc Med,* 5(3): 173-185.

[131] Way, K., Katai, N. & King, G. 2001. Protein kinase C and the development of diabetic vascular complications. *Diabet Med,* 18(12): 945-959.

[132] Inoguchi, T., Battan, R., Handler, E., Sportsman, J.R., Heath, W. & King, G.L. 1992. Preferential elevation of protein kinase C isoform beta II and diacylglycerol levels in the aorta and heart of diabetic rats: differential reversibility to glycemic control by islet cell transplantation. *Proc Natl Acad Sci,* 89(22): 11059-11063.

[133] Shiba, T., Inoguchi, T., Sportsman, J.R., Heath, W.F., Bursell, S. & King, G.L. 1993. Correlation of diacylglycerol level and protein kinase C activity in rat retina to retinal circulation. *Am J Physiol Endocrinol Metabol,* 265(5): E783-E793.

[134] Derubertis, F.R. & Craven, P.A. 1994. Activation of protein kinase C in glomerular cells in diabetes: mechanisms and potential links to the pathogenesis of diabetic glomerulopathy. *Diabetes,* 43(1): 1-8.

[135] Thallas-Bonke, V., Thorpe, S.R., Coughlan, M.T., Fukami, K., Yap, F.Y., Sourris, K.C., Penfold, S.A., Bach, L.A., Cooper, M.E. & Forbes, J.M. 2008. Inhibition of NADPH oxidase prevents advanced glycation end product–mediated damage in diabetic nephropathy through a protein kinase C-α–dependent pathway. *Diabetes,* 57(2): 460-469.

[136] Klann, E., Roberson, E.D., Knapp, L.T. et al., 1998. A role for superoxide in protein kinase C activation and induction of long-term potentiation. *J Biol Chem.* 273: 4516–4522.

[137] Noh, H. & King, G. 2007. The role of protein kinase C activation in diabetic nephropathy. *Kidney Int,* 72(: S49-S53.

[138] Jones, S., O'donnell, V., Wood, J., Broughton, J., Hughes, E. & Jones, O. 1996. Expression of phagocyte NADPH oxidase components in human endothelial cells. *Am J Physiol Heart Circ Physiol,* 271(4): H1626-H1634.

[139] Pagano, P.J., Clark, J.K., Cifuentes-Pagano, M.E., Clark, S.M., Callis, G.M. & Quinn, M.T. 1997. Localization of a constitutively active, phagocyte-like NADPH oxidase in rabbit aortic adventitia: enhancement by angiotensin II. *Proc Natl Acad Sci,* 94(26): 14483-14488.

[140] Greiber, S., Münzel, T., Kästner, S., Müller, B., Schollmeyer, P. & Pavenstädt, H. 1998. NAD (P) H oxidase activity in cultured human podocytes: effects of adenosine triphosphate. *Kidney Int,* 53(3): 654-663.

[141] Patterson C, Ruef J, Madamanchi NR, Barry-Lane P, Hu Z, Horaist C, Ballinger CA, Brasier AR, Bode C, Runge MS, 1999: Stimulation of a vascular smooth muscle cell NAD(P)H oxidase by thrombin: evidence that p47phox may participate in forming this oxidase in vitro and in vivo. *J Biol Chem.* 274:19814–19822.

[142] Hink, U., Li, H., Mollnau, H., Oelze, M., Matheis, E., Hartmann, M., Skatchkov, M., Thaiss, F., Stahl, R.A. & Warnholtz, A. 2001. Mechanisms underlying endothelial dysfunction in diabetes mellitus. *Circ Res,* 88(2): e14-e22.

[143] Guzik, T.J., Mussa, S., Gastaldi, D., Sadowski, J., Ratnatunga, C., Pillai, R. & Channon, K.M. 2002. Mechanisms of increased vascular superoxide production in human diabetes mellitus Role of NAD (P) H oxidase and endothelial nitric oxide synthase. *Circulation,* 105(14): 1656-1662.

[144] Kim, Y.K., Lee, M., Son, S.M., Kim, I.J., Lee, W.S., Rhim, B.Y., Hong, K.W. & Kim, C.D. 2002. Vascular NADH oxidase is involved in impaired endothelium-dependent vasodilation in OLETF rats, a model of type 2 diabetes. *Diabetes,* 51(2): 522-527.

[145] Etoh, T., Kakimoto, M., Sonoda, N., Kobayashi, K., Kuroda, J., Sumimoto, H. & Nawata, H. 2003. Increased expression of NAD (P) H oxidase subunits, NOX4 and p22phox, in the kidney of streptozotocin-induced diabetic rats and its reversibity by interventive insulin treatment. *Diabetologia,* 46(10): 1428-1437.

[146] Ellis, E., Grant, M.B., Murray, F.T., Wachowski, M.B., Guberski, D.L., Kubilis, P.S. & Lutty, G.A. 1998. Increased NADH oxidase activity in the retina of the BBZ/Wor diabetic rat. *Free Radic Biol Med,* 24(1): 111-120.

[147] Ceriello, A., Ihnat, M.A. & Thorpe, J.E. 2009. The "metabolic memory": is more than just tight glucose control necessary to prevent diabetic complications? *J Clin Endocrinol Metabol,* 94(2): 410-415.

[148] Liu S, Lee I.M., Song Y, Van Denburgh M, Cook N.R., Manson J.E., Buring J.E., 2006. Vitamin E and risk of type 2 diabetes in the women's health study randomized controlled trial. *Diabetes,* 55:2856–62.

[149] Rhee, S., Jeong, Y. & Choi, J. 2005. Effects of vitamin E on phospholipase A2 activity and oxidative damage to the liver in streptozotocin-induced diabetic rats. *Ann Nutr Metabol,* 49(6): 392-396.

[150] Devaraj, S., Leonard, S., Traber, M.G., Jialal, I., 2008. Gamma-tocopherol supplementation alone and in combination with alpha-tocopherol alters biomarkers of oxidative stress and inflammation in subjects with metabolic syndrome. *Free Radic Biol Med.* 44:1203–1208

[151] Minamiyama, Y., Takemura, S., Bito, Y., Shinkawa, H., Tsukioka, T., Nakahira, A., Suehiro, S. & Okada, S. 2008. Supplementation of α-tocopherol improves cardiovascular risk factors via the insulin signalling pathway and reduction of mitochondrial reactive oxygen species in type II diabetic rats. *Free Radic Res,* 42(3): 261-271.

[152] Davi, G., Ciabattoni, G., Consoli, A., Mezzetti, A., Falco, A., Santarone, S., Pennese, E., Vitacolonna, E., Bucciarelli, T., Costantini, F., Capani, F., Patrono, C., 1999. In vivo formation of 8-iso-prostaglandin f2alpha and platelet activation in diabetes mellitus: effects of improved metabolic control and vitamin E supplementation. *Circulation.* 99, 224–229

[153] Wu, J.H., Ward, N.C., Indrawan, A.P., Almeida, C., Hodgson, J.M., Proudfoot, J.M., Puddey, I.B. & Croft, K.D. 2007. Effects of α-tocopherol and mixed tocopherol supplementation on markers of oxidative stress and inflammation in type 2 diabetes. *Clin Chem,* 53(3): 511-519.

[154] Montero, A., Munger, K.A., Khan, R.Z., Valdivielso, J.M., Morrow, J.D., Guasch, A., Ziyadeh, F.N. & Badr, K.F. 2000. F2-isoprostanes mediate high glucose-induced TGF-&bgr; synthesis and glomerular proteinuria in experimental type I diabetes. *Kidney Int,* 58(5): 1963-1972.

[155] Je, H., Shin, C., Park, H., Huh, I. & Sohn, U. 2001. The comparison of vitamin C and vitamin E on the protein oxidation of diabetic rats. *J Auton Pharmacol,* 21(5): 231-236.

[156] Schleicher, E.D., Wagner, E. & Nerlich, A.G. 1997. Increased accumulation of the glycoxidation product N (epsilon)-(carboxymethyl) lysine in human tissues in diabetes and aging. *J Clin Investig,* 99(3): 457.

[157] Jialal, I., Devaraj, S. & Venugopal, S. 2002. Oxidative stress, inflammation, and diabetic vasculopathies: the role of alpha tocopherol therapy. *Free Rad Res,* 36(12): 1331-1336.

[158] Sakamoto, W., Fujie, K., Handa, H., Ogihara, T. & Mino, M. 1989. In vivo inhibition of superoxide production and protein kinase C activity in macrophages from vitamin E-treated rats. *Int J Vitam Nutr Res,* 60(4): 338-342.

[159] Kunisaki, M., Bursell, S., Clermont, A.C., Ishii, H., Ballas, L.M., Jirousek, M.R., Umeda, F., Nawata, H. & King, G.L. 1995. Vitamin E prevents diabetes-induced abnormal

retinal blood flow via the diacylglycerol-protein kinase C pathway. *Am J Physiol Endocrinol Metabol,* 269(2): E239-E246.

[160] Koya, D., Lee, I., Ishii, H., Kanoh, H. & King, G.L. 1997. Prevention of glomerular dysfunction in diabetic rats by treatment with d-alpha-tocopherol. *Clin J Am Soc Nephrol,* 8(3): 426-435.

[161] Yülek, F., Or, M., Özoğul, C., Isik, A.C., Ari, N., Stefek, M., Bauer, V. & Karasu, C. 2007. Effects of stobadine and vitamin E in diabetes-induced retinal abnormalities: involvement of oxidative stress. *Arch Med Sc,* 38(5): 503-511.

[162] Hamblin M, Smith HM, Hill MF., 2007. Dietary supplementation with vitamin E ameliorates cardiac failure in type I diabetic cardiomyopathy by suppressing myocardial generation of 8-iso-prostaglandin F2-alpha and oxidized glutathione. *J Card Fail,* 13(10): 884-892.

[163] Boaz, M., Smetana, S., Weinstein, T., Matas, Z., Gafter, U., Iaina, A., Knecht, A., Weissgarten, Y., Brunner, D. & Fainaru, M. 2000. Secondary prevention with antioxidants of cardiovascular disease in endstage renal disease (SPACE): randomised placebo-controlled trial. *The Lancet,* 356(9237): 1213-1218.

[164] Skyrme-Jones, R.A.P., O'Brien, R.C., Berry, K.L. & Meredith, I.T. 2000. Vitamin E supplementation improves endothelial function in type I diabetes mellitus: a randomized, placebo-controlled study. *J Am Coll Cardiol,* 36(1): 94-102.

[165] Heart Outcomes Prevention Evaluation (HOPE) Study Investigators, 2000. Effects of ramipril on cardiovascular and microvascular outcomes in people with diabetes mellitus: results of the HOPE study and MICRO-HOPE substudy. *Lancet.* 355: 253-259.

[166] Lonn E, Yusuf S, Hoogwerf B, Pogue J, Yi Q, Zinman B, Bosch J, Dagenais G, Mann JFE, Gerstein HC, 2002. Effects of vitamin E on cardiovascular and microvascular outcomes in high-risk patients with diabetes: Results of the HOPE study and MICRO-HOPE substudy. *Diabetes Care.* 25:1919-1927.

[167] Lee, E.Y., Lee, M.Y., Hong, S.W., Chung, C.H. & Hong, S.Y. 2007. Blockade of oxidative stress by vitamin C ameliorates albuminuria and renal sclerosis in experimental diabetic rats. *Yonsei Med J,* 48(5): 847-855.

[168] Sridulyakul, P., Wongeak-in, N. & Patumraj, S. 2010. Increased nitric oxide level in diabetic rats from vitamin C supplementation: an in vivo detection using diaminofluorescein. *Asian Biomed,* 2(5): 371-379.

[169] Eriksson, J. & Kohvakka, A. 1995. Magnesium and ascorbic acid supplementation in diabetes mellitus. *Ann Nutr Metabol,* 39(4): 217-223.

[170] Paolisso, G., Balbi, V., Volpe, C., Varricchio, G., Gambardella, A., Saccomanno, F., Ammendola, S., Varricchio, M. & D'Onofrio, F. 1995. Metabolic benefits deriving from chronic vitamin C supplementation in aged non-insulin dependent diabetics. *J Am Coll Nutr,* 14(4): 387-392.

[171] Mullan, B.A., Young, I.S., Fee, H. & McCance, D.R. 2002. Ascorbic acid reduces blood pressure and arterial stiffness in type 2 diabetes. *Hypertension,* 40(6): 804-809.

[172] Regensteiner, J.G., Popylisen, S., Bauer, T.A., Lindenfeld, J., Gill, E., Smith, S., Oliver-Pickett, C.K., Reusch, J.E. & Weil, J.V. 2003. Oral L-arginine and vitamins E and C improve endothelial function in women with type 2 diabetes. *Vasc Med,* 8(3): 169-175.

[173] Mazloom, Z., Hejazi, N., Dabbaghmanesh, M.H., Tabatabaei, H.R., Ahmadi, A. & Ansar, H. 2011. Effect of vitamin C supplementation on postprandial oxidative stress and lipid profile in type 2 diabetic patients. *Pakistan J Biol Sci: PJBS,* 14(19): 900-904.

[174] Ting, H.H., Timimi, F.K., Boles, K.S., Creager, S.J., Ganz, P. & Creager, M.A. 1996. Vitamin C improves endothelium-dependent vasodilation in patients with non-insulin-dependent diabetes mellitus. *J Clin Investig,* 97(1): 22.

[175] Timimi, F.K., Ting, H.H., Haley, E.A., Roddy, M., Ganz, P. & Creager, M.A. 1998. Vitamin C improves endothelium-dependent vasodilation in patients with insulin-dependent diabetes mellitus. *J Am Coll Cardiol,* 31(3): 552-557.

[176] Chen, H., Karne, R.J., Hall, G., Campia, U., Panza, J.A., Cannon, R.O., Wang, Y., Katz, A., Levine, M. & Quon, M.J. 2006. High-dose oral vitamin C partially replenishes vitamin C levels in patients with type 2 diabetes and low vitamin C levels but does not improve endothelial dysfunction or insulin resistance. *Am J Physiol Heart Circ Physiol,* 290(1): H137-H145.

[177] Jackson, T.S., Xu, A., Vita, J.A. & Keaney, J.F. 1998. Ascorbate prevents the interaction of superoxide and nitric oxide only at very high physiological concentrations. *Circ Res,* 83(9): 916-922.

[178] Sherman, D.L., Keaney, J.F., Biegelsen, E.S., Duffy, S.J., Coffman, J.D. & Vita, J.A. 2000. Pharmacological concentrations of ascorbic acid are required for the beneficial effect on endothelial vasomotor function in hypertension. *Hypertension,* 35(4): 936-941.

[179] Darko, D., Dornhorst, A., Kelly, F., Ritter, J. & Chowienczyk, P. 2002. Lack of effect of oral vitamin C on blood pressure, oxidative stress and endothelial function in Type II diabetes. *Clin Sci,* 103(4): 339-344.

[180] Corradini, E., Foglia, P., Giansanti, P., Gubbiotti, R., Samperi, R. & Lagana, A. 2011. Flavonoids: chemical properties and analytical methodologies of identification and quantitation in foods and plants. *Nat Prod Res,* 25(5): 469-495.

[181] Middleton, E., Kandaswami, C. & Theoharides, T.C. 2000. The effects of plant flavonoids on mammalian cells: implications for inflammation, heart disease, and cancer. *Pharmacol Rev,* 52(4): 673-751.

[182] Batra P and Sharma AK, 2013 Anti-cancer potential of flavonoids: recent trends and future perspectives 3 *Biotechnology* DOI 10.1007/s13205-013-0117-5

[183] Selway, J.W. 1986. Antiviral activity of flavones and flavans. *Progr Clin Biol Res,* 213: 521-536.

[184] Rice-Evans, C.A., Miller, N.J. & Paganga, G. 1996. Structure-antioxidant activity relationships of flavonoids and phenolic acids. *Free Radic Biol Med,* 20(7): 933-956.

[185] Heim, K. E.; Tagliaferro, A. R.; Bobilya D. J. Flavonoid antioxidants: chemistry, metabolism and sructure-activity relationships. *J Nutr Biochem.* 2002, 13, 572-584

[186] Groot, H.d. & Rauen, U. 1998. Tissue injury by reactive oxygen species and the protective effects of flavonoids. *Fund Clin Pharmacol,* 12(3): 249-255.

[187] Narayana K.R., Reddy M.S., Chaluvadi M.R., Krishna D.R., 2001. Bioflavonoids classification, pharmacological, biochemical effects and therapeutic potential. *Indian J Physiol Pharmacol;* 33: 2-16.

[188] Wu, C. & Yen, G. 2005. Inhibitory effect of naturally occurring flavonoids on the formation of advanced glycation endproducts. *J Agr Food Chem,* 53(8): 3167-3173.

[189] Yamabe N, Yokozawa T, Oya T and Kim M, 2006. Therapeutic potential of (-) epigallocatechin 3-Ogallate on renal damage in diabetic nephropathy model rats. *J Pharmacol Exp Therapeut,* 319: 228-236.

[190] Urios, P., Grigorova-Borsos, A. & Sternberg, M. 2007. Flavonoids inhibit the formation of the cross-linking AGE pentosidine in collagen incubated with glucose, according to their structure. *Eur J Nutr,* 46(3): 139-146.

[191] Kim, H.Y., Lee, J.M., Yokozawa, T., Sakata, K. & Lee, S. 2011. Protective activity of flavonoid and flavonoid glycosides against glucose-mediated protein damage. *Food Chem,* 126(3): 892-895.

[192] Goodarzi, M., Zal, F., Malakooti, M. & Sadeghian, M.S.S. 2006. Inhibitory activity of flavonoids on the lens aldose reductase of healthy and diabetic rats. *Acta Medica Iranica,* 44(1).

[193] Jung, S.H., Lee, Y.S., Lee, S., Lim, S.S., Kim, Y.S. & Shin, K.H. 2002. Isoflavonoids from the rhizomes of Belamcanda chinensis and their effects on aldose reductase and sorbitol accumulation in streptozotocin induced diabetic rat tissues. *Arch Pharm Res,* 25(3): 306-312.

[194] Kim, J., Kim, J.H., Jun, H., Yu, Y.S. & Kim, K. 2010. Inhibition of protein kinase C δ attenuates blood-retinal barrier breakdown in diabetic retinopathy. *Am J Clin Pathol,* 176(3): 1517-1524.

[195] Frank, R.N., 2004. Diabetic retinopathy. *New Engl J Med.* 350: 48–58

[196] Kumar, B., Gupta, S.K., Srinivasan, B., Nag, T.C., Srivastava, S. & Saxena, R. 2012. Hesperetin ameliorates hyperglycemia induced retinal vasculopathy via anti-angiogenic effects in experimental diabetic rats. *Vasc Pharmacol,* 57(5): 201-207.

[197] Kandhare, A.D., Raygude, K.S., Ghosh, P., Ghule, A.E. & Bodhankar, S.L. 2012. Neuroprotective effect of naringin by modulation of endogenous biomarkers in streptozotocin induced painful diabetic neuropathy. *Fitoterapia,* 83(4): 650-659.

[198] Valsecchi, A.E., Franchi, S., Panerai, A.E., Rossi, A., Sacerdote, P. & Colleoni, M. 2011. The soy isoflavone genistein reverses oxidative and inflammatory state, neuropathic pain, neurotrophic and vasculature deficits in diabetes mouse model. Eur J Clin Pharmacol, 650(2): 694-702.

[199] Wang, G., Li, W., Lu, X., Bao, P. & Zhao, X. 2012. Luteolin ameliorates cardiac failure in type I diabetic cardiomyopathy. *J Diabetes Complications,* 26(4): 259-265.

[200] Manuel y Keenoy, B., Vertommen, J. & De Leeuw, I. 1999. The effect of flavonoid treatment on the glycation and antioxidant status in Type 1 diabetic patients. *Diabetes, Nutr Metabol,* 12(4): 256-263.

[201] Pandey, K.B., Mishra, N. & Rizvi, S.I. 2009. Myricetin may provide protection against oxidative stress in type 2 diabetic erythrocytes. *Int J Biosci,* 64(9): 626.

[202] Kamalakkannan, N. & Prince, P.S.M. 2006. Antihyperglycaemic and Antioxidant Effect of Rutin, a Polyphenolic Flavonoid, in Streptozotocin-Induced Diabetic Wistar Rats. *Basic Clin Pharmacol Toxicol,* 98(1): 97-103.

[203] Sattanathan, K., Dhanapal, C., Umarani, R. & Manavalan, R. 2011. Beneficial health effects of rutin supplementation in patients with diabetes mellitus. *JAPS,* 1(08): 227-231.

[204] Hao, H., Shao, Z., Tang, D., Lu, Q., Chen, X., Yin, X., Wu, J. & Chen, H. 2012. Preventive effects of rutin on the development of experimental diabetic nephropathy in rats. *Life Sci.*

[205] Cervantes-Laurean, D.D. Schramm, E.L. Jacobson, I. Halaweish, G.G. Bruckner, G.A., 2006. Boissonneault. Inhibition of advanced glycation end product formation on collagen by rutin and its metabolites. *J Nutr Biochem.* 17: 531–540

[206] Campanero, M.A., Escolar, M., Perez, G., Garcia-Quetglas, E., Sadaba, B. & Azanza, J.R. 2010. Simultaneous determination of diosmin and diosmetin in human plasma by ion trap liquid chromatography–atmospheric pressure chemical ionization tandem mass spectrometry: Application to a clinical pharmacokinetic study. *J Pharmaceut Biomed Anal,* 51(4): 875-881.

[207] Srinivasan S, Pari L, 2012. Ameliorative effect of diosmin, a citrus flavonoid against streptozotocin-nicotinamide generated oxidative stress induced diabetic rats. *Chem Biol Interact.* 195: 43–51

[208] Tang, D., Wei, Y., Gao, Y., Yin, X., Yang, D., Mou, J. & Jiang, X. 2011. Protective effects of rutin on rat glomerular mesangial cells cultured in high glucose conditions. *Phytother Res,* 25(11): 1640-1647.

[209] Machha, A., Achike, F.I., Mustafa, A.M. & Mustafa, M.R. 2007. Quercetin, a flavonoid antioxidant, modulates endothelium-derived nitric oxide bioavailability in diabetic rat aortas. *Nitric Oxide,* 16(4): 442-447.

[210] Alkhamees, O.A. 2013. Morin a Flavonoid Exerts Antioxidant Potential in Streptozotocin-induced Hepatotoxicity. *Br J Pharmacol Toxicol* 4(1): 10-17, 2013

[211] Kapoor, R. & Kakkar, P. 2012. Protective role of morin, a flavonoid, against high glucose induced oxidative stress mediated apoptosis in primary Rat hepatocytes. *PloS one,* 7(8): e41663.

[212] Coskun, O., Kanter, M., Korkmaz, A. & Oter, S. 2005. Quercetin, a flavonoid antioxidant, prevents and protects streptozotocin-induced oxidative stress and β-cell damage in rat pancreas. *Pharmacol Res,* 51(2): 117-123.

[213] Anjaneyulu, M. & Chopra, K. 2004. Quercetin, an anti-oxidant bioflavonoid, attenuates diabetic nephropathy in rats. *Clin Exp Pharmacol Physiol,* 31(4): 244-248.

[214] Mahmoud AM, Ashour MB, Abdel-Moneim A, Ahmed OM, 2012. Hesperidin and naringin attenuate hyperglycemia-mediated oxidative stress and proinflammatory cytokine production in high fat fed/streptozotocin-induced type 2 diabetic rats. *J Diabetes Complications.* 26: 483-490.

[215] Shi, X., Liao, S., Mi, H., Guo, C., Qi, D., Li, F., Zhang, C. & Yang, Z. 2012. Hesperidin Prevents Retinal and Plasma Abnormalities in Streptozotocin-Induced Diabetic Rats. *Molecules,* 17(11): 12868-12881.

[216] Annadurai, T., Muralidharan, A.R., Joseph, T., Hsu, M., Thomas, P. & Geraldine, P. 2012. Antihyperglycemic and antioxidant effects of a flavanone, naringenin, in streptozotocin–nicotinamide-induced experimental diabetic rats. *J Physiol Biochem,* 68(3): 307-318.

[217] Tsai, S., Huang, C., Mong, M., Kam, W., Huang, H. & Yin, M. 2011. Anti-inflammatory and antifibrotic effects of naringenin in diabetic mice. *J Agr Food Chem,* 60(1): 514-521.

[218] Soto, C., Pérez, J., García, V., Uría, E., Vadillo, M. & Raya, L. 2010. Effect of silymarin on kidneys of rats suffering from alloxan-induced diabetes mellitus. *Phytomedicine,* 17(14): 1090-1094.

[219] Wang, G.G., Lu, X.H., Li, W., Zhao, X. & Zhang, C. 2011. Protective effects of luteolin on diabetic nephropathy in STZ-induced diabetic rats. *Evid Base Compl Alternative Med,* article ID 323171, 7 pages.

[220] Qian, L., Wang, H., Chen, Y., Chen, F., Ma, Y., Bruce, I.C. & Xia, Q. 2010. Luteolin reduces high glucose-mediated impairment of endothelium-dependent relaxation in rat aorta by reducing oxidative stress. *Pharmacol Res,* 61(4): 281-287.

[221] El-Bassossy, H.M., Abo-Warda, S.M. & Fahmy, A. 2013. Chrysin and Luteolin Attenuate Diabetes-Induced Impairment in Endothelial-Dependent Relaxation: Effect on Lipid Profile, AGEs and NO Generation. *Phytother Res*. doi: 10.1002/ptr.4917.

[222] Panda, S. & Kar, A. 2007. Apigenin (4 ', 5, 7-trihydroxyflavone) regulates hyperglycaemia, thyroid dysfunction and lipid peroxidation in alloxan-induced diabetic mice. *J Pharm Pharmacol*, 59(11): 1543-1548.

[223] Ihm, S., Lee, J., Kim, S., Seung, K., Schini-Kerth, V.B., Chang, K. & Oak, M. 2009. Catechin prevents endothelial dysfunction in the prediabetic stage of OLETF rats by reducing vascular NADPH oxidase activity and expression. *Atherosclerosis*, 206(1): 47-53.

[224] Fu, Z., Yuskavage, J. & Liu, D. 2013. Dietary Flavonol Epicatechin Prevents the Onset of Type 1 Diabetes in Nonobese Diabetic Mice. *J Agr Food Chem*, 61(18): 4303-4309.

[225] Kim, M.J. & Lim, Y. 2013. Protective Effect of Short-Term Genistein Supplementation on the Early Stage in Diabetes-Induced Renal Damage. *Mediat Inflamm*, 2013: 1-14

[226] Roghani, M., Vaez Mahdavi, M., Jalali-Nadoushan, M., Baluchnejadmojarad, T., Naderi, G., Roghani-Dehkordi, F., Taghi Joghataei, M. & Kord, M. 2013. Chronic Administration of Daidzein, a Soybean Isoflavone, Improves Endothelial Dysfunction and Attenuates Oxidative Stress in Streptozotocin-induced Diabetic Rats. *Phytother Res*, 27(1): 112-117.

[227] Fukui, T., Noma, T., Mizushige, K., Aki, Y., Kimura, S. & Abe, Y. 2000. Dietary troglitazone decreases oxidative stress in early stage type II diabetic rats. *Life Sci*, 66(21): 2043-2049.

[228] Dobsak P, Courderot-Masuyer C, Siegelova J, Svacinova H, Jancik J, Vergely-Vanriessen C, Rochette, 2001. Antioxidant properties of aminoguanidine: a paramagnetic resonance test. *Scripta Med* (BRNO) 74: 45–50.

[229] Elmalí, E., Altan, N. & Bukan, N. 2004. Effect of the sulphonylurea glibenclamide on liver and kidney antioxidant enzymes in streptozocin-induced diabetic rats. *Drugs in R & D*, 5(4): 203-208

[230] Haendeler, J., Hoffmann, J., Zeiher, A.M. & Dimmeler, S. 2004. Antioxidant effects of statins via s-nitrosylation and activation of thioredoxin in endothelial cells a novel vasculoprotective function of statins. *Circulation*, 110(7): 856-861.

[231] Gumieniczek, A., Hopkała, H., Roliński, J. & Bojarska-Junak, A. 2005. Antioxidative and anti-inflammatory effects of repaglinide in plasma of diabetic animals. *Pharmacol Res*, 52(2): 162-166.

Permissions

All chapters in this book were first published by InTech Open; hereby published with permission under the Creative Commons Attribution License or equivalent. Every chapter published in this book has been scrutinized by our experts. Their significance has been extensively debated. The topics covered herein carry significant findings which will fuel the growth of the discipline. They may even be implemented as practical applications or may be referred to as a beginning point for another development.

The contributors of this book come from diverse backgrounds, making this book a truly international effort. This book will bring forth new frontiers with its revolutionizing research information and detailed analysis of the nascent developments around the world.

We would like to thank all the contributing authors for lending their expertise to make the book truly unique. They have played a crucial role in the development of this book. Without their invaluable contributions this book wouldn't have been possible. They have made vital efforts to compile up to date information on the varied aspects of this subject to make this book a valuable addition to the collection of many professionals and students.

This book was conceptualized with the vision of imparting up-to-date information and advanced data in this field. To ensure the same, a matchless editorial board was set up. Every individual on the board went through rigorous rounds of assessment to prove their worth. After which they invested a large part of their time researching and compiling the most relevant data for our readers.

The editorial board has been involved in producing this book since its inception. They have spent rigorous hours researching and exploring the diverse topics which have resulted in the successful publishing of this book. They have passed on their knowledge of decades through this book. To expedite this challenging task, the publisher supported the team at every step. A small team of assistant editors was also appointed to further simplify the editing procedure and attain best results for the readers.

Apart from the editorial board, the designing team has also invested a significant amount of their time in understanding the subject and creating the most relevant covers. They scrutinized every image to scout for the most suitable representation of the subject and create an appropriate cover for the book.

The publishing team has been an ardent support to the editorial, designing and production team. Their endless efforts to recruit the best for this project, has resulted in the accomplishment of this book. They are a veteran in the field of academics and their pool of knowledge is as vast as their experience in printing. Their expertise and guidance has proved useful at every step. Their uncompromising quality standards have made this book an exceptional effort. Their encouragement from time to time has been an inspiration for everyone.

The publisher and the editorial board hope that this book will prove to be a valuable piece of knowledge for researchers, students, practitioners and scholars across the globe.

List of Contributors

Erland Johansson
EJSelenium Consultant Ltd, Uppsala, Sweden

Tuomas Westermarck, P. Kaipainen and M. Kaski
Rinnekoti Research Center, Helsinki, Finland

Paul Ek
Laboratory of Analytical Chemistry, Åbo Academy, Finland

Faik Atroshi
Department of Pharmacology and Toxicology, University of Helsinki, Finland

Arno Latvus
Hankintatukku Oy, Museokatu, Helsinki, Finland

Sangeeta Shukla, Neelu Sinha and Amita Jaswal
School of Studies in Zoology, Jiwaji University, Gwalior, India

Margarita G. Skalnaya
Center for Biotic Medicine, Moscow, Russia

M. Iivanainen
Rinnekoti Research Centre, FIN Espoo, Finland
Department of Child Neurology, University of Helsinki, Finland

Shirly Ekvall and Valli Ekvall
University Affiliated Cincinnati Center for Developmental Disabilities, Children's Hospital Medical Center, Cincinnati, Ohio, USA
University of Cincinnati, Cincinnati, Ohio, USA

Eileen Harper
Providence Everett Medical Center, Seattle, Washington, USA

Wei Pan
University of Cincinnati, Cincinnati, Ohio, USA

Guntars Selga, M. Sauka, L. Aboltina, A. Davidova and D. Kheder
Department of Oral and Maxillofacial Surgery, Faculty of Dentistry, Rīga Stradiņš University, Rīga, Latvia

T. Määttä
Kainuu Social and Health Care Joint Authority, Finland

T. Tervo-Määttä
Department of Teacher Education, University of Oulu, Finland

A. Taanila
Institute of Health Sciences, University of Oulu, Finland
Unit of General Practice, University Hospital of Oulu, Finland

Elżbieta Płonka-Półtorak
Antiepileptic Outpatient Clinic, Provincial Hospital No. 2, Lwowska, Rzeszow, Poland

Sakaewan Ounjaijean
Research Institute for Health Sciences, Chiang Mai University, Chiang Mai, Thailand

Suthat Fucharoen
Thalassemia Research Center, Institute of Bioscience, Mahidol University, Nakorn Pathom, Thailand

Somdet Srichairatanakool
Department of Biochemistry, Faculty of Medicine, Chiang Mai University, Chiang Mai, Thailand

A Skesters and A Silova
Rīga Stradiņš University, Rīga, LV, Latvia

Nicole L. Brooks
Department of Wellness Sciences, Faculty of Health & Wellness Sciences, Cape Peninsula University of Technology, Bellville, South Africa

Ayodeji B. Oyenihi
Department of Biochemistry, School of Life Sciences, University of KwaZulu-Natal, Durban, South Africa

Oluwafemi O. Oguntibeju
Oxidative Stress Research Centre, Departments of Biomedical Sciences, Faculty of Health and Wellness Sciences, Cape Peninsula University of Technology, Bellville, South Africa

Guillaume Aboua
Department of Biomedical Sciences, Faculty of Health and Wellness Sciences, Cape Peninsula University of Technology, Bellville, South Africa

Omolola R. Ayepola
Nutrition and Chronic Disease Research Unit, Oxidative Stress Research Centre, Department of Biomedical Sciences, Faculty of Health and Wellness Sciences, Cape Peninsula University of Technology, Bellville, South Africa

Index

www.ingramcontent.com/pod-product-compliance
Lightning Source LLC
LaVergne TN
LVHW062233200926
848484LV00006B/1530